D1757687

3 0116 00539 9918

This book is due for return not later than the last date stamped below, unless recalled sooner.

Current Topics in Microbiology and Immunology

Volume 340

Current Topics in Microbiology and Immunology

Previously published volumes

Further volumes can be found at springer.com

Takashi Saito · Facundo D. Batista

Editors

Immunological Synapse

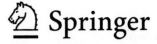 Springer

Editors
Takashi Saito, PhD
Lab. Cell Signaling
RIKEN Research Center for
Allergy & Immunology
1-7-22 Suehiro-cho, Tsuirumi-ku
Yokohama, Kanagawa
230-0045 Japan
saito@rcai.riken.jp

Facundo D. Batista, PhD
Cancer Research UK
London Research Institute
44 Lincoln's Inn Fields
London WC2A 3PX
United Kingdom
facundo.batista@cancer.org.uk

ISSN 0070-217X
ISBN: 978-3-642-03857-0   e-ISBN: 978-3-642-03858-7
DOI 10.1007/978-3-642-03858-7
Springer Heidelberg Dordrecht London New York

Library of Congress Control Number: 2009941066

Cover design: WMXDesign GmbH, Heidelberg, Germany

Printed on acid-free paper

Springer is part of Springer Science+Business Media (www.springer.com)

Preface

The proper physiological functioning of most eukaryotic cells requires their assembly into multi-cellular tissues that form organized organ systems. Cells of the immune system develop in bone marrow and lymphoid organs, but as the cells mature they leave these organs and circulate as single cells. Antigen receptors (TCRs) of T cells search for membrane MHC proteins that are bound to peptides derived from infectious pathogens or cellular transformations. The detection of such specific peptide–MHC antigens initiates T cell activation, adhesion, and immune-effectors functions. Studies of normal and transformed T cell lines and of T cells from transgenic mice led to comprehensive understanding of the molecular basis of antigen-receptor recognition and signaling. In spite of these remarkable genetic and biochemical advances, other key physiological mechanisms that participate in sensing and decoding the immune context to induce the appropriate cellular immune responses remain unresolved.

TCR recognition is tightly regulated to trigger sensitive but balanced T cell responses that result in the effective elimination of the pathogens while minimizing collateral damage to the host. The sensitivity of TCR recognition has to be properly tempered to prevent unintended activation by self-peptide–MHC complexes that cause autoimmune diseases. It is likely that once the TCR is engaged by a peptide–MHC and TCR signaling begins, additional regulatory mechanisms, involving other receptors, would increase the fidelity of the response. Such mechanisms that interpret TCR recognition within physiological settings may provide excellent targets for selective manipulation of immune responses, either enhancing or suppressing the immunity. However, the study of T cell activation under physiological conditions faces many technical challenges.

Cloned T cell lines and TCR transgenic mice can address the extremely low frequency of antigen-specific T cells within the circulating mature lymphocytes. Anti-receptor antibodies and soluble purified receptor–ligands are commonly used to selectively engage a particular receptor, even within a polyclonal lymphocyte population, without engaging any of the many other receptors on the immune cells. Such approaches were instrumental for identifying the molecular and functional role of adhesion receptors (LFA-1), co-stimulatory receptors (CD4, CD8, CD28), and inhibitory receptors (CTLA-4), to name just a few. However, these precise reductionist experiments were not designed to explain the remarkable sensitivity of the T cells and the complex-integrative mechanisms that decode TCR recognition and execute the necessary response. The study of T cell interactions with live APCs, where all activating and inhibitory receptors would be able to bind their physiological counter-receptors, may be more physiologically appropriate to address these issues.

Molecular imaging, using immunofluorescence microscopy, enabled the study of specific cellular interactions of immune cells. Biophysical considerations predicted that the receptors in T cell that bound their counter-receptors on the membrane of the APC would stabilize the cell contact. Moreover, the extent of receptor clustering at the contact is a quantitative and qualitative measure of receptor–ligand interactions. The first such studies used cloned NKT cells, CTL, and CD4 T cells and demonstrated that these T cells formed antigen-specific cell conjugates with their target cells or antigen-presenting cells (APCs). Immunofluorescence microscopy of these cellular conjugates demonstrated remarkable TCR-specific molecular rearrangements at the T–APC cell contact area, known today as the immune synapse. The TCR clustered at the synapse in an antigen-specific manner. Surprisingly, LFA1 and CD4 clustered only when the TCR was engaged, demonstrating that the interactions of LFA1 with ICAM and of CD4 with MHC depended on TCR signals. Thus, engagement of one receptor can affect the responses of other receptors, even without direct physical intermolecular interactions between them.

On the basis of similar consideration, molecular imaging was introduced to identify the intracellular proteins that are involved in signaling and cell adhesion. Immunofluorescence microscopic localization of cytoskeletal proteins identified talin as a key adhesion protein that associates with activated LFA1 and clusters at the synapse. Interestingly, minimal TCR signaling that is not sufficient to productively activate the T cells, or treatment with PMA, is sufficient to cause clustering of talin. Thus, imaging can detect different molecular responses to TCR activation and link them to different cellular outcomes.

In another cytoskeletal system, the microtubule network also responded to activation in the T–APC conjugates. The microtubule-organizing center (MTOC) and its associated Golgi apparatus reoriented within minutes in the T cell to face the synapse. Unlike the clustering of talin, MTOC reorientation is induced only in productively activated T cells. Intracellular imaging demonstrated that the role of this early MTOC/Golgi reorientation is to direct the secretion from activated T cells. In CTLs, cytotoxic proteins are directed toward the specific target cells to maximize their effective killing while limiting the damage to innocent bystander cells. In CD4 cells, selective cytokines are directed toward the activating B cells to maximize proliferation and differentiation of antigen-specific B cells that will produce relevant neutralizing antibodies.

Imaging of intracellular proteins detected many of the known proteins that participate in the biochemical pathways of T cell activation at the synapse. Molecular imaging can also be used as a screen to identify new proteins that regulate

T cell functioning. Such a screen identified PKCθ at the synapse, unlike any of the other PKC isoforms. Disruption of the PKCθ gene in mice demonstrated that PKCθ is essential for T cell proliferation and IL2 production.

The development and use of multilabel three-dimensional deconvolution microscopy was a turning point in the study of the immune synapse. The biggest surprising finding is that two intracellular proteins, talin and PKCθ, that cluster at the synapse in response to TCR signaling are spatially segregated at the contact, with PKCθ at the center surrounded by a ring of talin. This spatial segregation is mirrored also for receptors, with TCR clustering at the center surrounded by a ring of LFA1. Thus, multiple receptors that are uniformly distributed in the membrane of unbound T cells cluster upon cell conjugation, but rather than just clustering randomly they formed distinct SupraMolecular Activation Clusters (SMACs). These molecular structures are not seen when the TCR bound an antagonistic peptide, suggesting that restructuring of the synapse and SMAC formation are essential for T cell functioning. It is important to note that distinct molecular and structural changes take place on both the T cell and the APC side of the synapse.

From the time of these initial reports many laboratories extensively studied the structure and function of the synapse in different setups. The use of live cell imaging provided new insights on the kinetic nature of this immune cell junction. Quantitative imaging and mathematical modeling are continually challenging our views of the synapse. The use of new imaging techniques including TIRF and FRET, which will be discussed in this issue, provide even higher resolution and identify the detailed kinetics of TCR–microcluster formation. On the other extreme, multiphoton intravital imaging provides new insights on the dynamics of T cell interactions with dendritic cells in live mice. The intravital imaging provides the essential physiological data and context for the T–APC contacts but lacks the molecular resolution provided by other microscopic methods. New imaging techniques, that are developed continually, are likely to evolve our understanding of T cell function in health and disease.

Interestingly, it appears that human lymphotropic retroviruses like HIV and HTLV1 use the immune synapse to evade elimination. HIV and HTLV1 hijack the endogenous machinery of Golgi/MTOC reorientation and directed secretion to spread stealthily between interacting cells. Such localized viral transmission within confined cell contacts, which are referred to as virological synapses, may limit the access of soluble neutralizing antibodies to the transmitted viruses and may explain how they evade these antibodies. Moreover, these viruses can induce structural alterations of the synapse to reduce anti-viral immunity.

Although the importance of the immune synapse as a dynamic cell junction that regulates intercellular communication and viral transmission is universally recognized, many of the quantitative and qualitative details remain unsettled. The plasticity of this cell junction has to accommodate many very different binding partners and control the fate of interacting cells. It is likely that developmental changes in the state of the T cells or the APCs can impact the structure of the synapse. It is hoped that uncovering the ordered molecular rearrangement at the membrane will provide the long sought after clues for the remarkable functional sensitivity of T lymphocytes. These dynamic molecular interactions may eventually explain how engagement of the same TCR can generate different outcomes that resolve the immune challenges. The reviews in this issue present a broad slice of the many diverse topics that are currently intensely debated.

Baltimore   Abraham Kupfer

The Immunological Synapse Enters
Its Second Decade...

The aim of this current volume is to highlight the recent advances in investigations of the "Immunological Synapse", marking the 10-year anniversary of its initial visualization. From the decade since the discovery of the Immunological Synapse between T cells and B cells, the term has been extended to a variety of immune cells including T cells, B cells, and NK cells, and it has been established as a common feature of activation in immune cells and cellular communication for antigen recognition. Indeed, the Immunological Synapse structure displays the central characteristics of antigen recognition by immune cells including self/non-self discrimination, activation through assembly of signaling molecules, cell–cell communication to determine cell polarity for cell movement/attachment, cytokine secretion, and cytotoxicity.

During the past decade, concurrent advances in imaging technology have enabled the more intricate dissection of the Immunological Synapse at the molecular level, allowing the analysis of the spatiotemporal dynamics of assembly and dissociation of various receptors and signaling molecules associated with downstream pathways. These investigations have contributed to reshaping our understanding of the structure and function of the Immunological Synapse from the assumptions based on the original descriptions. This progress is elegantly illustrated by the widely held current view that antigen recognition and activation signals are induced primarily not from the central cluster as originally postulated, but rather from microscopic clusters of immunoreceptor located within the periphery of the synapse. For this volume we have invited a number of key researchers, who have made a significant contribution to the advances within the field, to offer their perspectives and current understanding of the molecular processes underlying the formation and function of the Immunological Synapse. The volume includes chapters discussing the organization, diversity, signaling, dynamics of Immunological Synapse and also cellular communication at the Immunological Synapse.

We fully anticipate that the next decade will be characterized by similar exciting and groundbreaking progress in terms of our understanding of immune cell activation and immune system regulation, particularly in vivo function and visualization of the Immunological Synapse and cellular activation. Employing state-of-the-art imaging technologies including TIRFM and MPM, we have already been able to gain some insights into the spatiotemporal dynamics of lymphocyte activation both in vitro at the molecular level and in vivo at the cellular level. Thus, these strategies have enabled a glimpse of new insights concerning the various factors regulating Immunological Synapse, such as the underlying cytoskeleton and the structure of secondary lymphoid tissues, which may play an important role in the regulation of immune cell activation in vivo.

Facundo Batista and Takashi Saito

Contents

Contributors

Andrés Alcover   Unité de Biologie Cellulaire des Lymphocytes, Département d'Immunologie, Institut Pasteur, CNRS, URA1961, 28, rue Docteur Roux. F-75724 Paris Cedex 15. France, andres.alcover@pasteur.fr

Stephen C. Bunnell   Department of Pathology, Tufts University Medical School, Jaharis Bldg., Rm. 512, 150 Harrison Ave., Boston, MA 02111, USA, Stephen.Bunnell@tufts.edu

Yolanda R. Carrasco   Department of Immunology and Oncology, National Centre of Biotechnology/CSIC, Darwin 3, UAM-Campus de Cantoblanco, Madrid E-28049, Spain, ycarrasco@cnb.csic.es

Rita Lucia Contento   Laboratory of Adaptive Immunity, I.R.C.C.S. Istituto Clinico Humanitas, Via Manzoni 113, 20089 Rozzano, Milan, Italy

Daniel M. Davis   Division of Cell and Molecular Biology, Sir Alexander Fleming Building, Imperial College London, South Kensington, London SW7 2AZ, UK, d.davis@imperial.ac.uk

Junsang Doh   School of Interdisciplinary Bioscience and Bioengineering and Department of Mechanical Engineering, Pohang University of Science and Technology, San31, Hyoja-dong, Nam-Gu, Pohang, Gyeongbuk, 790-784, Korea, jsdoh@postech.ac.kr

Bastian Dornbach   Helmholtz Centre for Infection Research, Inhoffenstr. 7, D-38124 Braunschweig, Germany

Loïc Dupré   INSERM, U563, Section Dynamique Moléculaire des Interactions Lymphocytaires, Toulouse, F-31300 France; Centre de Physiopathologie de Toulouse Purpan, Université Toulouse III Paul-Sabatier, Toulouse, F-31400 France

Michael L. Dustin   Helen L. and Martin S. Kimmel Center for Biology and Medicine in the Skirball Institute for Biomolecular Medicine and Department of Pathology, NYU School of Medicine. New York, NY 10016, USA, michael.dustin@med.nyu.edu

Philipp Eissmann   Division of Cell and Molecular Biology, Sir Alexander Fleming Building, Imperial College London, South Kensington, London SW7 2AZ, UK

Nicholas R.J. Gascoigne   Department of Immunology and Microbial Science, The Scripps Research Institute, 10550 North Torrey Pines Rd., La Jolla, CA 92037, USA, and Department of Immunology, University of Texas MD Anderson Cancer Center, 7455 Fannin, Houston, TX 77030, USA, Gascoigne@scripps.edu

Matthias Gunzer   Institute of Molecular and Clinical Immunology, Otto-von-Guericke University, Leipziger Str. 44, D-39120 Magdeburg, Germany, matthias.gunzer@med.ovgu.de

John A. Hoerter   Department of Immunology and Microbial Science, The Scripps Research Institute, 10550 North Torrey Pines Rd., La Jolla, CA 92037, USA, and Department of Immunology, University of Texas MD Anderson Cancer Center, 7455 Fannin, Houston, TX 77030, USA

Matthew F. Krummel   Department of Pathology and Biological Imaging Development Center, University of California San Francisco, 513 Parnassus Ave, San Francisco, CA 94143-0511, USA, Matthew.Krummel@ucsf.edu

Barbara Molon   Istituto Oncologico Veneto I.R.C.C.S., Via Gattamelata 64, 35128 Padua, Italy

Susan K. Pierce   Laboratory of Immunogenetics, National Institute of Allergy and Infectious Diseases, National Institutes of Health, Rockville, MD 20852, USA, spierce@niaid.nih.gov

Peter Reichardt   Institute of Molecular and Clinical Immunology, Otto-von-Guericke University, Leipziger Str. 44, D-39120 Magdeburg, Germany

Takashi Saito   Laboratory for Cell Signaling, RIKEN Research Center for Allergy and Immunology, 1-7-22 Suehiro-cho, Tsurumi-ku, Yokohama

230-0045, Japan and WPI Immunology Frontier Research Center, Suita, Osaka 565-0081, Japan, saito@rcai.riken.jp

Maria-Isabel Thoulouze Unité de Biologie Cellulaire des Lymphocytes, Département d'Immunologie, Institut Pasteur, CNRS, URA1961, 28, rue Docteur Roux. F-75724 Paris Cedex 15. France, marie-isabelle.thoulouze@pasteur.fr

Pavel Tolar Laboratory of Immunogenetics, National Institute of Allergy and Infectious Diseases, National Institutes of Health, Rockville, MD 20852, USA

Salvatore Valitutti INSERM, U563, Section Dynamique Moléculaire des Interactions Lymphocytaires, Toulouse, F-31300 France; Centre de Physiopathologie de Toulouse Purpan, Université Toulouse III Paul-Sabatier, Toulouse, F-31400 France, svalitu@inserm.fr

Antonella Viola Laboratory of Adaptive Immunity, Department of Translational Medicine, University of Milan, I.R.C.C.S. Istituto Clinico Humanitas, Via Manzoni 113, 20089 Rozzano, Milan, Italy, antonella.viola@humanitas.it

Pia P. Yachi Department of Immunology and Microbial Science, The Scripps Research Institute, 10550 North Torrey Pines Rd., La Jolla, CA 92037, USA, and Department of Immunology, University of Texas MD Anderson Cancer Center, 7455 Fannin, Houston, TX 77030, USA

Tadashi Yokosuka Laboratory for Cell Signaling, RIKEN Research Center for Allergy and Immunology, 1-7-22 Suehiro-cho, Tsurumi-ku, Yokohama 230-0045, Japan, yokosuka@rcai.riken.jp

Tomasz Zal Department of Immunology and Microbial Science, The Scripps Research Institute, 10550 North Torrey Pines Rd., La Jolla, CA 92037, USA, and Department of Immunology, University of Texas MD Anderson Cancer Center, 7455 Fannin, Houston, TX 77030, USA

Insights into Function of the Immunological Synapse from Studies with Supported Planar Bilayers

Michael L. Dustin

Contents

Abstract Innate and adaptive immunity is dependent upon reliable cell–cell communication mediated by direct interactions of cell surface receptors with ligands integrated into the surface of apposing cells or bound directly to the surface as in complement deposition or antibody mediated recognition through Fc receptors. Supported lipid bilayers formed on glass surfaces offer a useful model system in which to explore some basic features of molecular interactions in immunological relevant contacts, which include signal integration and effector functions through immunological synapses and kinapses. We have exploited that lateral mobility of molecules in the supported planar bilayers and fluorescence microscopy to develop

M.L. Dustin
Helen L. and Martin S. Kimmel Center for Biology and Medicine in the Skirball Institute for Biomolecular Medicine and Department of Pathology, NYU School of Medicine, New York, NY 10016, USA
e-mail: michael.dustin@med.nyu.edu

T. Saito and F.D. Batista (eds.), *Immunological Synapse*,   1
Current Topics in Microbiology and Immunology 340,
DOI 10.1007/978-3-642-03858-7_1, © Springer-Verlag Berlin Heidelberg 2010

a system for measurement of two-dimensional affinities and kinetic rates in the contact area, which is of immunological interest. Affinity measurements are based on a modified Scatchard analysis. Measurements of kinetic rates are based on fluorescence photo bleaching after recovery at the level of the entire contact area. This has been coupled to a reaction–diffusion equation that allows calculation of on- and off-rates. We have found that mixtures of ligands in supported planar bilayers can effectively activate T lymphocytes and simultaneously allow monitoring of the immunological synapse. Recent studies in planar bilayers have provided additional insights into organization principles of cell–cell interfaces. Perennial problems in understanding cell–cell communication are yielding quantitative measurements based on planar bilayers in areas of ligand-driven receptor clustering and the role of the actin cytoskeleton in immune cell activation. A major goal for the field is determining quantitative rules involved in signaling complex formation by innate and adaptive receptor systems.

Abbreviations

BCR	B-cell antigen receptor
LFA	Lymphocyte function associated
PKC	Protein kinase C
SMAC	Supramolecular activation cluster
TCR	T-cell antigen receptor
TIRF	Total internal reflection fluorescence

1 Introduction: Role of Receptor–Ligand Interaction in Immunity

Innate and adaptive immunity depend upon the ability of various immune effector cells to directly engage and communicate with other cell types via receptor–ligand interactions at membrane interfaces (Springer 1990). Innate immune mechanisms like the alternative and lectin mediated complement systems and adaptive immunity mediated by antibodies and T-cell receptors are dependent upon interactions of membrane-attached molecules. At the physical level these interactions are relatively poorly understood because they are more difficult to quantify than the interactions of soluble ligands with cell surface receptors that mediate cytokine dependent immune regulation. However, there are examples of cytokines that are presented in Trans by a receptor subunit on one cell to a distinct signaling subunit expressed by another cell and many chemokines may be biologically presented on the surface of other cells to stimulate leukocyte activation and motility (Lucas et al. 2007; Woolf et al. 2007). These relatively new examples can be combined with the large numbers of interactions between immunoglobulin super family members, C-type lectin family receptors and integrin family members that are abundant in regulation of innate and adaptive immunity. The emergency of precise physical methods like surface Plasmon resonance and differential scanning calorimetry has enabled measurement of adhesion molecule interactions in 3D, solution systems. These interactions tend to have a relatively low affinity and fast dissociation rates, consistent with mediating dynamic cell–cell interactions (Van Der Merwe and Davis 2003). A challenge of each of these receptor types is to measure interactions in the contact areas and to relate these measurements to function. While the physiological cell–cell interactions can be difficult to plumb by any of the current methods, the use of model systems is providing insight into these interactions.

The classical methods for studying this type of recognition in the immune system are to measure contact dependent functional end points without explicitly addressing the interaction process or to directly measure conjugate formation between cells. Adhesion or contact dependence is established by separating the cells suspected of interaction with a filter with pores too small for the cells to pass through (Lomnitzer and Rabson 1981). If the function persists then it is assumed that it is not contact dependent, whereas when the function is eliminated it is assumed that adhesion is required. The direct measurement of conjugate formation uses microscopy, flow cytometry or bulk cell quantification to determine the fraction of each cell type that is interacting at a given time point (Shaw et al. 1986). This often involved application of some force to separate non- or weakly adherent cells, such as vortexing in flow cytometry-based assay or some washing procedures. Adhesion to substrates can be directly visualized by interference reflection microscopy (Izzard and Lochner 1976), which allows quantification of the contact area and certain aspects of the membrane curvature at the edges of the contact, which can be related to adhesive energy (Kloboucek et al. 1999). All of these assays assess a process that is mediated by many interactions without providing any quantitative information. At the other extreme, rolling adhesion and probabilistic adhesion tests based on limiting contact area and time, but performing many trials, both operate at the level of single interactions, but provide limited insight into interactions in established contact areas that mediate most forms of immune cell communication (Pierres et al. 1996; Zhang et al. 2005). The model system based upon supported planar bilayers has provided most of the available quantitative data on molecular interactions underlying cell adhesion. This is an area in which my lab has been particularly active and I will review results based on this system obtained in my lab and others.

2 Degrees of Freedom in Immune Cell Activation

Studies in the late 1970s grappled with the issue of how immune cells like mast cells were activated. It was well established that globular proteins like albumin with multiple haptens (small molecules that are bound by antibodies) covalently attached to this nanoscale scaffold were potent stimuli for activation of macrophages and mast cells through Fc receptors when the effector cells were pre-incubated with a IgG or IgE antibodies, respectively, specific for the hapten. The haptens had only one degree or freedom relative to each other — that of rotation, and binding to cell surface receptors was well known to induce small receptor clusters in the same time frame as effector functions were activated (Metzger 1992) (Fig. 1a–b). Phospholipid anchored haptens in large vesicles were nonclustered and freely mobile, with two additional degrees of translational movement, yet they could trigger activation of effector cells that interacted directly with the large vesicles. This ability of monovalent ligands to trigger immune cell activation conflicted with the observation that soluble monovalent haptens, having six degrees of freedom were unable to activate cells and that only dimeric or oligomeric haptens were able to trigger immune cell functions by *cross-linking* the receptors (Metzger 1992; Schlessinger et al. 1976). Signaling activity in microaggregates generated by antibody cross-linker has been directly visualized (Stauffer and Meyer 1997). It had been argued by the proponents of the cross-linking model that the curvature of the vesicles would effectively cluster the immune cell antibody receptors by focusing them at a point defined by the point of minimal separation between the cell membrane and the spherical vesicle (Fig. 1c). In order to test this McConnell and colleagues incorporated the same phospholipid hapten into a supported planar monolayer deposited on a flat alkylated glass surface from Langmuir–Blodgett films (Hafeman et al. 1981). The antibody-hapten complexes were mobile in this monolayer as in the vesicle membranes and they still triggered activation of an oxidative burst and secretion of the lysosomal protein cathepsin B onto the surface. McConnell and colleagues visualized the accumulation of the fluorescently tagged antibodies in the contact area, but encountered problems with accelerated photo bleaching in contact areas with the activated immune cells so could not document the pattern of receptor engagement that led to activation (Fig. 1d–g). Transformed mast cells that bound to supported bilayers presenting laterally mobile IgE evolved small patches of IgE that were interpreted as microaggregates of ~100 receptors per <0.1 μm^2 spot (Weis et al. 1982). This increased density of receptors in a small area was proposed to arise due to topological constraints of small membrane projections such as microvilli. This mechanism of clustering has not been confirmed nor is it clear that complexes assembled by membrane curvature-driven aggregation would have sufficient integrity to initiate signaling (McKeithan 1995). Nonetheless, these experiments framed an enduring enigma of how apparently monovalent ligands in a fluid phospholipid bilayer can achieve receptor clusters and activation without an apparent mechanism for cross-linking.

3 Planar Bilayers and the Proof of MHC–Peptide Complexes

The ligands that mediate activation of T lymphocytes are MHC–peptide complexes that are highly asymmetric type I transmembrane proteins with large extracellular domains and relatively small cytoplasmic domains. The monolayers used in the

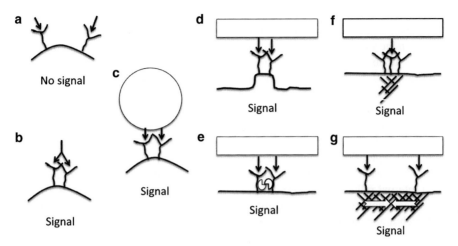

Fig. 1 Models for triggering immunoreceptors. It is unlikely that any "one fits all" model exists for immunoreceptors since they have strikingly different F-actin requirements. The *line on the bottom* represents the cell membrane that the *Y-shaped* figures are the cell surface receptor. The *arrows* represent ligands. The *sphere* is a liposome and the *rectangular shapes* represent fluid supported bilayers. (**a**) Monovalent engagement does not activate most immunoreceptors in general. A possible exception has been reported for certain antiTCR Fab (Gil et al. 2002). (**b**) Cross-linking with antibodies activates most immunoreceptors, at least transiently. (**c**) IgG on liposomes activates Fcε receptor. In order to active a TCR beads need to be larger than 3-µm diameter (Mescher 1992). (**d**) The early planar bilayer experiments with Fc receptors reacting to dimensionally constrained monovalent Ig Fc revealed that receptors could form clusters that were capable of signaling. This has been explained by assuming that membrane projections allow concentration of receptors and ligands to support adhesion, but it not clear this would satisfy kinetic proofreading criteria. (**e**) *Trans* and *cis* interactions might cooperate to promote microaggregate formation and signaling (Reich et al. 1997; Tolar et al. 2009). (**f**) F-actin dependent nucleation of a microaggregate by a single MHC–peptide complex. This is not proven, but implied by titration data. (**g**) F-actin and myosin IIA dependent force consistent with particle size requirements (Galbraith et al. 2002; Mescher 1992)

above study were deposited on the alkylated glass from an air-water interface, a method requiring organic solvents that are not compatible with membrane proteins. McConnell's lab and others overcame this problem by making the observation that supported bilayers can be formed simply by incubating aqueous solutions of unilamellar liposome with a clean glass coverslip or with small beads (Babbitt et al. 1985; Brian and McConnell 1984; Gay et al. 1986; Watts and McConnell 1986). Transmembrane proteins-like MHC class I and class II antigens are readily incorporated into unilamellar liposomes by detergent dialysis. After fusion of these proteoliposomes to glass surfaces the MHC molecules were laterally immobile. These experiments were performed not to study adhesion per se, but to determine if purified allogeneic or specific antigen bearing MHC molecules could functionally activate T cells since MHC molecules had been shown by genetic studies to control the responses of T cells to foreign antigens. Activation of T cells under these conditions required interaction with 1,000 MHC–peptide complexes (Watts and

McConnell 1986), which probably reflects the requirements for MHC–peptide complexes to activate T cells with little or no support for other adhesion ligands found on the surface of natural antigen presenting cells. It should be noted that fluid bilayer membranes are not biologically passive and that they will bind fibronectin from serum and support adhesion of immune cells without explicit incorporation of adhesion ligands (Bonte and Juliano 1986). In later studies we found that even higher levels of pure MHC–peptide complexes were required to mediate adhesion (Dustin et al. 1996b). This suggests that serum attachment factors did contribute to the earlier functional interactions. An interesting study demonstrated that T-cell antigen receptor (TCR) could actually facilitate the interaction of antigenic peptides with empty MHC molecules based on fluorescence resonance energy studies using total internal reflection fluorescence (TIRF) spectroscopy (Watts et al. 1986). It is no longer thought that TCR facilitates loading of peptides on MHC molecules, although it appeared to do so in these experiments. This study foreshadowed more recent studies that have combined TIRF microscopy with supported planar bilayers to probe the question of how freely diffusing monomeric MHC–peptide complexes activate T cells.

4 Determination of Two-Dimensional Affinity

The generation of monoclonal antibodies that block the function of allogeneic cytotoxic T lymphocytes, which is a type of immune cell important in transplant rejection, identified two adhesion pathways that play a prominent role in human and rodent immune responses. These molecules were initially defined as lymphocyte function associated-1 (LFA-1), LFA-2 and LFA-3 (Sanchez-Madrid et al. 1982). Analysis of blocking of adhesion by pair-wise combinations of these antibodies revealed that LFA-2 (CD2) and LFA-3 (CD58) were in the same pathway, whereas LFA-1 was in a separate pathway (Shaw et al. 1986). A screen for antibodies that were raised to B lymphoblasts (Epstein–Barr virus immortalized cells) from LFA-1 deficient patients and could block LFA-1 dependent aggregation of normal B lymphoblasts identified ICAM-1 as a surface molecule in the same pathway with LFA-1 (Rothlein et al. 1986). Supported planar bilayers were used to provide compelling evidence that CD58 and ICAM-1 were ligands for CD2 and LFA-1, respectively (Dustin et al. 1987a; Dustin et al. 1988; Dustin and Springer 1988; Marlin and Springer 1987). In parallel studies, we found that half of the CD58 on nucleated cells and all of the CD58 on erythrocytes were glycosylphosphatidylino-sitol (GPI) lipid-anchored, with the other half on nucleated cells having a trans-membrane domain and short cytoplasmic tail (Dustin et al. 1987b). As noted above, the McConnell lab had found that antibodies bound to lipid-linked haptens were laterally mobile in supported bilayers above the transition temperature. This sug-gested that a GPI-anchored molecule-like CD58 should also be laterally mobile. We purified the transmembrane form of CD58 from cells that had a biosynthetic defect in production of GPI anchors and compared this to CD58 from erythrocytes

(Hollander et al. 1988). We found that the mobile GPI-anchored CD58 was considerably more active in supported planar bilayers than the immobile transmembrane form (Chan et al. 1991). We speculated that the greater activity of the laterally mobile form of CD58 might be due to its ability to accumulate in the contact area by diffusion and trapping. We tested this by fluorescently labeling the CD58 while protecting the active site using the function-blocking antibody. This fluorescent CD58 was incorporated into a supported planar bilayer and we imaged the interface using a laser scanning microscope system to detect movement of the labeled CD58 after $CD2^+$ T cells were added. We were able to quantify the density binding of CD2 to CD58 in the T cell–bilayer interface (Dustin et al. 1996a). We were then able to perform a Scatchard analysis using this binding data, which was linear and suggested a 2D dissociation constant (K_d) of 21 molecules/μm^2. The 2D K_d measurement has subsequently been refined by modeling CD2 diffusion on cells (Dustin et al. 1997b; Zhu et al. 2006, 2007) and measuring the exclusion of freely diffusing molecules from the contact area (Bromley et al. 2001; Dustin et al. 2007a) (Fig. 2). The formation of contracts is dependent upon the 2D K_d more than on the kinetics of the interactions, making the 2D K_d an important parameter (Shao et al. 2005).

5　Kinetic Rates of Interactions in Contact Area

While contact formation is largely dependent upon the 2D affinity, signaling reactions are dependent upon the kinetic rates of the receptor–ligand interactions (McKeithan 1995). We noted early in our studies of the CD2–CD58 interaction in the planar bilayer system that when CD58 was photobleached by a focused laser beam that fluorescence recovered rapidly even when a large proportion of fluorescence in the contact area was destroyed (Dustin et al. 1996a). This observation suggests that the bleached CD58 is rapidly dissociating from and being replaced by bright CD58 molecules that diffuse in from outside the contact area. We later designed a system with a laser beam that could be defocused to bleach CD58 in the entire contact area (Dustin 1997). In this case, fluorescence can only recover due to dissociation of interactions followed by new binding with a recovery process governed by the single reaction rate constant $k_f(CD2 + CD58) + k_b$, where k_f and k_b are the forward and reverse rates, respectively. Cheng Zhu's lab determined the diffusion reaction equations needed to calculate k_f and k_b from the fluorescence photo bleaching after recovery time course (Tolentino et al. 2008; Wu et al. 2008). We refer to this method as contact fluorescence recovery after photobleaching (contact FRAP). Interestingly, the fitting of the recovery data revealed a k_b of 0.074/s, which is at least 100-fold slower than the solution k_b of 7.8/s (van der Merwe et al. 1994). The apparent k_f was 0.015 μm^2/s. It seems very unlikely that conditions in the contact area would result in a 100-fold stabilization of the CD2–CD58 bond, so the most likely explanation is that the dissociated CD58 tend to rebind the same CD2 many times prior to actually diffusing away

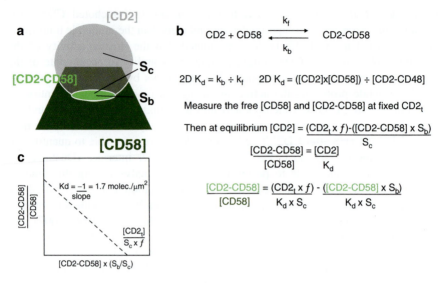

Fig. 2 Model for calculation of 2D dissociation constant. (**a**) The sphere represents a T cell expressing CD2 that interacts with a plane representing a supported bilayer reconstituted with different densities of purified FITC–CD58. The cell adheres and the system reaches equilibrium in 20–40 min at 24°C. The bilayer fluorescence and contact area fluorescence were measured. It is also important to use a distinct non-binding, but similar-sized protein (such as mouse CD48) labeled with a different dye, like Cy5, to determine the level of exclusion of free CD58 from the contact area, which is usually 20–40%. This is due to steric crowding in the contact area and is used to calculate the free [CD58] in the contact area. Measurements are made on 50–100 cells per data point. Each data point is a different starting CD58 density usually in the range of 10–1,000 molecules/μm^2. (**b**) Derivation of the Golan–Zhu plot (Zhu et al. 2007). The S_b is the area of the contact between cell and bilayer measured based on CD58 accumulation and CD48 exclusion. S_c is the area of the entire cell. f is the fractional mobility of CD2 on the surface of the T cell. This is essentially a modified Scatchard plot (Scatchard 1949) that allows the proportion of the total amount of CD2 (CD2$_t$) to vary based on its lateral mobility and mass-action driven partitioning into the contact area. (**c**) A schematic of a Golan–Zhu plot. Typically four to five densities of CD58 would be tested to provide equally distributed points along the line. The 2D K_d value is based on the best-controlled published data (Dustin et al. 2007a). This paper also describes a model for bridge formation by the CD58-Fc chimeric drug alefacept

and allowing for exchange only after a half-time of about 10 s. This duration of interaction suggests that CD2–CD58 interactions have a sufficient effective duration to contribute to TCR signaling processes and may also account for recent evidence for direct signaling through CD2–CD58 interactions (Kaizuka et al. 2009). Extensive measurements have not been made for the TCR–MHC–peptide interaction, but data from a single MHC–peptide density allowed an estimate of the 2D K_d for the 2B4 TCR interaction with I-E^k with moth cytochrome C peptide 88–103 of 10 molecules/μm^2, in the same range as the CD2–CD58 interaction (Grakoui et al. 1999). This convergence is significant since the 3D interaction of the TCR has a similar affinity, but a slower on and off rate in solution compared to CD2–CD58 (Grakoui et al. 1999; van der Merwe et al. 1994).

6 Tandem Low-Affinity Interactions Have Additional Limitations

The low affinity Fc receptors, CD16 and CD32, play an important role in binding to particles and cell surfaces coated with antibodies. Unlike the high affinity IgG FcR and the IgE FcR the, the low affinity receptors do not bind monovalent antibodies in solution. Surprisingly, they can also synergize with relatively low CD58–IgG1 Fc chimera in forming tandem low affinity bridges between cells (Dustin et al. 2007a). Such low affinity bridges may be important in the function of low affinity natural antibodies antibodies. These systems also face significant competition from high concentrations of circulating antibodies, such that a high degree of IgFc aggregation may be essential to activate these receptors (Dustin et al. 2007a).

7 Segregation of Adhesion Molecules by Size

Adhesion systems involved in immune cell activation normally operate in combinations rather than one at a time. Springer speculated that adhesion molecule size would be important for the organization of contact areas by forcing segregation of adhesion receptors like CD2–CD58, which span about 15 nm, and larger adhesion receptors like LFA-1–ICAM-1, which appeared capable of spanning greater than 30 nm (Springer 1990). It is been confirmed that contacts established by the CD2–CD58 adhesion mechanism generate uniform intermembrane spacing of 13 nm (Choudhuri et al. 2005; Milstein et al. 2008). The spacing generated by the integrin LFA-1 is a more complex issue. Integrins are large, non-covalent heterodimers with a globular domain connected to the membrane by two legs (Luo et al. 2007). LFA-1 activity is regulated by TCR signaling (Dustin and Springer 1989) and has three affinity states with K_d of 1 mM, 10 μM and 100 nM (Shimaoka et al. 2003). The complete crystal structure of the platelet fibrinogen receptor αIIbβ3 demonstrated that integrins have a "genu" or knee like structure that allows the legs to bend such that the binding site can exist anywhere from 5 to 25 nm from the membrane (Zhu et al. 2008). Electron microscopy studies demonstrate that higher affinity conformations correlate with more extended genus (Luo et al. 2007), it remains possible that affinity and bending/extension may be independent. This would allow variable intermembrane spacing, which is in fact observed in the contact areas between T cells and planar bilayers containing LFA-1 (Shaw and Dustin 1997). When CD58 and ICAM-1 are incorporated into the same planar bilayer-activated T cells, they form a contact in which the accumulation of CD58 and ICAM-1 appear to be completely segregated with interaction domains on a readily resolved micron scale (Dustin et al. 1998). More recently, we have performed experiments with engineered versions of CD48 that change the intermembrane spacing for different ligands binding to the same receptor, mouse CD2. CD2, CD58 and CD48 are all members of the immunoglobulin superfamily that are built from tandem arrays of small β-sandwich domains that are about 4 nm long. Van der Merwe and colleagues generated extended forms of CD48 by adding Ig domains from CD2 or CD22, with the natural binding sites of these spacer domains mutated (Wild et al. 1999). The extended forms of CD48 inhibit antigen recognition by T-cell hybridomas and primary T cells (Milstein et al. 2008; Wild et al. 1999). Addition of Ig-like domains might be expected to increase intermembrane spacing by up to 4 nm per domain, but van der Merwe and we observed that spacing was increased by 1 nm per domain (Choudhuri et al. 2005; Milstein et al. 2008). We observed that a 1 nm difference in size did not force segregation, but a 2 or 3-nm spacing difference led to complete segregation in a narrow range of ligand concentrations in which the two systems coexisted (Milstein et al. 2008). Outside this narrow range the more functionally abundant ligand occupied the entire contact area. Therefore, robust lateral segregation over a wide range of ligand densities, as observed for CD58 and ICAM-1 containing bilayers likely reflects both the physical process in the extracellular space, and active membrane/cytoskeletal processes that allow adhesion systems to establish competitive niches within the contact area.

8 Formation of the Immunological Synapse

The immunological synapse started as a model that cytotoxic T-cell function could be equated to that of a neural synapse stabilized by LFA-1 and with TCR acting as a ligand gated Ca^{2+} channel to trigger delivery of secretory vesicles to the target cells upon engagement with antigen (Norcross 1984). The TCR was soon shown to operate based on a tyrosine kinase cascade to activate phospholipase C-γ as a pathway to cytoplasmic Ca^{2+} elevation (Samelson et al. 1986) and this specific model was largely set aside. Imaging studies 10 years later revealed a specific organization of TCR in a central micron scale structure and LFA-1 as forming an annular disc surrounding the TCR cluster in the interface between antigen specific T cells and antigenic MHC–peptide complex bearing B cells (Monks et al. 1998). Kupfer described these patterns of terms of supramolecular activation clusters (SMACc) since they appeared to involve thousands of non-covalently associated molecules and were correlated with T-cell activation (Monks et al. 1998). Paul Allen, Andrey Shaw and I proposed that these SMACs together constituted an immunological synapse (Dustin et al. 1998; Dustin and Shaw 1999). We went on to use the supported planar bilayer containing GPI anchored ICAM-1 and a range of biological active, GPI anchored MHC–peptide complexes to reveal the pathway to formation of the immunological synapse. Surprisingly, this was based on centripetal transport of TCR engaged MHC–peptide complexes that were initially engaged in the periphery of the expanding contact area, in what appeared at a coarse grained view as pattern inversion (Grakoui et al. 1999). Unlike prior studies with antigen receptor triggering and bilayers, this system explicitly addressed the position of essential adhesion and specificity controlling elements to reveal a carefully orchestrated process. A surprising finding was that the TCR–MHC–peptide interactions in the central SMAC appeared to be stable over hours, which suggested an extreme version of the rebinding process that was revealed in the contact-FRAP studies above. We will address this later in this chapter. These dynamic images led to a number of models for the role of F-actin and the potential of the synapse to mediate processes like directed secretion and asymmetric cell division (Dustin and Chan 2000; Dustin and Cooper 2000).

Those interested in more technical information on planar bilayer formation and flexible methods for ligand deposition for immunological synapse reconstition are referred to a recently published protocol (Dustin et al. 2007b) and video describing some of these methods (http://www.jove.com/index/details.stp?ID=947).

9 Microclusters Drive Activation

The fundamental signaling machinery of the immunological synapse was not apparent in early coarse-grained views. Kupfer found that the protein kinase C-θ and the Src family kinase Lck were accumulated in or near the central SMAC (Monks et al. 1998), but subsequent studies revealed a rapid loss of TCR proximal signaling in this region and persistence of signaling elements in the periphery where LFA-1 appeared to dominate (Freiberg et al. 2002; Krummel et al. 2000; Lee et al. 2002). Models were developed to accommodate a flexible role of the central SMAC in signal termination when signaling was strong and signal enhancement when signaling is weak (Lee et al. 2003). A break-through in understanding signaling dynamics in the immunological synapse was made by returning to the basic technological platform introduced by McConnell in 1982 – TIRF microscopy on supported bilayers. In key observations first made by Varma, microclusters of TCR were observed to continually form in the periphery of the immunological synapse and stream inwards to the formed central SMAC (Varma et al. 2006). TIRF was essential to reduce background to a level where the small aggregates, with as few as ten receptors each, were visible (Varma et al. 2006). In an important test of the significance of these structures, we showed that antiMHC–peptide complex antibody immediately blocked the formation of the microclusters and signaling was fully extinguished as the last microclusters reach the central SMAC after about 2 min. Thus, the thousands of TCR accumulated in the cSMAC were insufficient to sustain Ca^{2+} signals (Varma et al. 2006). This basic finding was backed by studies that demonstrated the presence of active signaling molecules only in the microclusters and not in the central SMAC (Campi et al. 2005; Yokosuka et al. 2005, 2008). Earlier studies had demonstrated TCR signaling molecules associated with antiCD3 induced micro aggregates (Bunnell et al. 2002), but the advantage of the supported bilayers system over the immobile solid support is that the signaling and inactivation is a spatiotemporal process that allows deconvolution of the significant signaling and nonsignaling structures in the TCR "life-cycle." An interesting hybrid system has been developed by the Grove's lab based on using electron beam lithography to general nanoscale metallic lines on the substrate that partition of the bilayer into various geometric patterns. The compartments defined by the metallic lines allow the formation of microclusters, but prevent the transport of these clusters across the lines. A 1×1-μm grid allows the formation of many small microclusters that cannot be transported centrally to form a central SMAC and this manipulation actually measurably increased signaling (Mossman et al. 2005). The planar bilayer system can also be adapted to use natural MHC–peptide ligands or antiCD3 antibodies for studies on polyclonal T cells or cells with TCR of unknown specificity (Kaizuka et al. 2007). The mobility of molecules in the planar bilayers also allow for sorting within the plasma membrane interface. Saito and colleagues discovered that CD28–CD80 interactions are initially co-localized with TCR–MHC–peptide interactions in microclusters, but are sorted into a distinct compartment at the boundary between the central and peripheral SMACs (Yokosuka et al. 2008). This mode of rearrangement would not be possible with immobile ligands. While the smallest TCR microcluster that can be tracked have greater than ten TCR, a single MHC–peptide may be sufficient to trigger a microcluster based on titration data (Varma et al. 2006). However, direct observations are needed to test this possibility. These studies have advanced our understanding of TCR signaling processes in the synapse, but also have left us with the same fundamental question that faced McConnell in 1982 – how do freely diffusing monovalent ligands trigger formation of clusters. It is possible that the solution to this problem will be different for different receptor systems.

10 Modes of T-Cell Signal Integration

There are many lines of evidence that recognition of agonist MHC–peptide complexes in T cells delivers a stop signal, a prerequisite to form a synapse (Dustin et al. 1996b, 1997a, 1998; Grakoui et al. 1999; Mempel et al. 2004; Negulescu et al. 1996). However, it is also clear that T cells can integrate signals while migrating over the surface of antigen presenting cells (Gunzer et al. 2000; Mempel et al. 2004; Skokos et al. 2007). The Greek routes of synapse can translate as "joined together," which implies a high degree of monogamy. Position stability is a characteristic of neural synapses and has been part of the definition of immunological synapses (Dustin 2008; Dustin and Colman 2002; Dustin et al. 1998; Grakoui et al. 1999). Therefore, the ability of T cell to integrate TCR signals on the move, which is likely due to asymmetric adhesions that form microclusters at or near the leading edge, represents a different class of contacts. I have proposed the term "kinapse" to describe these mobile cell–cell interfaces – literally a "moving junction." The kinapse has not been extensively studied using bilayers systems, but some rules have been established. For example, PKCθ activity surprisingly favors kinapse formation while WASP activity favors synapse formation (Sims et al. 2007). The scaffold for the kinapse is likely to be talin and integrin dependent motility (Smith et al. 2005).

11   B Lymphocytes Acquire Antigen by Force

While T lymphocytes bind antigens only when they are presented on the surface of cells with MHC–peptide ligands, B lymphocytes bind intact antigens many of which are soluble. Batista considered the possibility that physiological acquisition of antigens by the B-cell antigen receptor (BCR) in vivo would involve binding of surface presented complexes through an immunological synapse and developed cellular and supported bilayer-based tools to study this process (Batista et al. 2001; Carrasco et al. 2004). In order to present a wide variety of purified proteins to B cells, Batista and colleagues developed methods to monobiotinylate proteins and then to capture these to the planar bilayer using biotinylated lipids and streptavidin, which can be fluorescently labeled for visualization. This has been a generally useful method for attaching many proteins to bilayers, particularly antibodies. The only caveate with this approach is that the exact valency of the system is not defined. Streptavidin likely binds to the bilayer through biotin binding sites and then can probably capture up to two monobiotinylated antibodies. B lymphocytes will form a similarly organized immunological synapse with microclusters converging on a central SMAC, but the biological imperative for the B lymphocyte is to pull the antigen off the surface such that the contraction and force dependent extraction are directly related to the B lymphocyte's subsequent ability to present antigens to T cells (Fleire et al. 2006). Interestingly, signaling by primary B cells in response to dimensionally constrained monovalent ligands on a planar bilayer requires CD19 (Depoil et al. 2008). Perhaps CD19 is a factor needed for aggregation of BCR by monovalent ligands. While the Batista lab works with mature primary B lymphocytes, the Pierce lab has focused on a complementary model based on a plasmacytoma cell line lacking BCR subunits (Tolar et al. 2005). They have reconstituted this cell line with fluorescent protein tagged BCR subunits and have used this to monitor changes in the intramolecular spacing of the cytoplasmic domains of the receptor complexes. The advantage of using the cell line is that all BCR subunits are fluorescently tagged and the disadvantage is that signaling requirements may differ due to the maturity of the cell line and potential differences related to transformation. The results were nonetheless interesting in that the authors were able to observe increased spacing of the cytoplasmic domains of the BCR by fluorescence resonance energy transfer (Tolar et al. 2005). These findings are consistent with recent work showing that key tyrosine phosphorylation sites are buried in the plasma membrane and dissociate upon activation (Xu et al. 2008). More recently, they have offered a novel solution to the old problem of receptor triggering by monovalent ligands, in this case short peptides with hexahistidine at the C-termini bound to Ni chelating lipids. This is a useful strategy for attaching any recombinant proteins that can be generated with a hexahistidine to decahistidine tag in a monovalent form. They have demonstrated that the extra Ig like domain that is spliced into the heavy chain of cell surface BCR undergoes a weak, lateral homophilic interaction that facilitates aggregation of engaged BCR (Tolar et al. 2009). This is conceptually similar to earlier models for TCR aggregation (Reich et al.

1997). A model based on a ligand-dependent release of an aggregation domain from an inhibitory interaction, which then can propagate to neighboring unligated receptors could account for the ability of one or a few ligands to nucleate larger receptor clusters. It remains unclear how F-actin would facilitate this process. One notion would be that the conformational change involved in exposure of this oligomerization domain requires a force generated by the actin cytoskeleton.

12   The F-Actin Machine Behind the Synapse

A striking contrast between Fc receptor systems studied by Metzger and McConnell and the TCR system that we have focused on is that immunological synapse formation, TCR signaling and microcluster formation are all F-actin dependent (Bunnell et al. 2002; Campi et al. 2005; Grakoui et al. 1999; Varma et al. 2006), whereas signaling through the Fcε receptor is enhanced when F-actin is depolymerized (Torigoe et al. 2004). In fact, the acquisition of F-actin independence by TCR microclusters is a property associated with inactivation of signaling in the central SMAC (Varma et al. 2006). How is F-actin involved in the immunological synapse? The TCR is directly linked to F-actin polymerizing machinery via Vav, which activates both Rac and CDC42 (Fischer et al. 1998). Integrins like LFA-1 may also contribute to this process. Rac activates the Wave2 complex, which activates both Arp2/3 and Formin mediated actin polymerization in lamellipodia (Gomez et al. 2007; Nolz et al. 2006). CDC42 activates WASp, which is another activator of the Arp2/3 complex involved in formation of filopodia and podosomes (Carman et al. 2007). TCR microclusters appear to form in lamellipodium like structures on planar bilayers containing ICAM-1 and MHC–peptide complexes (Kaizuka et al. 2007; Sims et al. 2007). Therefore the F-actin structures that are associated with microcluster formation and transport are dynamic, branched F-actin networked formed by Arp2/3. However when WAVE2 is knocked down, early TCR signaling proceeds normally suggesting that alternative pathways, perhaps WASp-based, are fully functional (Nolz et al. 2006). T cells express myosin IIA, but its function in synapse formation and signaling is controversial (Jacobelli et al. 2004; Wülfing and Davis 1998). A requirement for force generation in T-cell activation is consistent with a distinct size threshold for T-cell activation by MHC–peptide-coated particles (Mescher 1992). Sheetz found that bead size thresholds for focal adhesion formation are attributable to force dependence of this process (Galbraith et al. 2002). Myosin IIA knock down by siRNA and treatment with the myosin II specific inhibitor blebbistatin both block the translocation of TCR microclusters and impair signaling at a step between Src family kinase activation and phosphorylation of ZAP-70 and LAT (Ilani et al. 2009). TCR and integrin microclusters appear to form normally in the absence of myosin IIA. The immunological synapse is radially symmetric, like a spreading fibroblast with a radial lamellipodium (Sims et al. 2007). The symmetry of this system is promoted by WASp and suppressed by PKCθ to control the stability of the immunological synapse (Sims et al. 2007). The role of PKCθ in immunological synapse stability was surprising, but the result, originally obtained with naïve $CD4^+$ helper T lymphocytes (a type of immune cell that orchestrates many cells in the adaptive immune response), has been extended to cytotoxic T lymphocytes (Beal et al. 2008). The radially symmetric lamellipodium is characterized by a 3–5 μm wide annular region of centripetal F-actin flow, which dissipates in the central region occupied by the central SMAC (Kaizuka et al. 2007). TCR and LFA-1 microclusters are transported toward the center. The coupling to centripetally moving actin will exert forces on the integrin that are sufficient, in simulations, to induce conformational changes that increase integrin affinity (Zhu et al. 2008). Short-lived LFA-1 microclusters tend to dissociate in the F-actin depleted center and thus accumulate in the peripheral SMAC, perhaps because of the force dependence of maintaining high affinity LFA-1 (Zhu et al. 2008). TCR microclusters that achieve actin independence are transported to the central SMAC. Shorter-lived TCR microclusters may disappear at the boundary between the central and peripheral SMACs. The coupling between TCR microclusters and F-actin flow is not perfect and is based on speed; the TCR microclusters appear to be linked to the F-actin ~40% of the time. The generation of chrome barriers in planar bilayers using e-beam lithography has been extended to the fine analysis of microcluster movement (DeMond et al. 2008). It was found that microclusters navigate around barriers as long as the barrier was angled toward the center of the synapse. This confirmed the notion that there is a molecular "clutch" between the TCR and integrin clusters and the F-actin flow that allows the microclusters to display a mixture of diffusive and directed movement. This clutch appears to operate in both directions since immobile integrin clusters appear to be able to slow the centripetal F-actin flow with consequences for stability of signaling complexes (Nguyen et al. 2008). These observations point to important missing information in our understanding of lateral mobility of free and engaged ligands in the plasma membranes of different types of antigen-presenting cells. Synaptic patterns differ between B cells and dendritic cells as APC, with B-cells resembling structures formed with supported planar bilayers (Grakoui et al. 1999; Monks et al. 1998) and dendritic cells displaying more disrupted patterns (Brossard et al. 2005; Tseng et al. 2008). This suggests limited mobility or a high degree of compartmentalization, which is consistent with the demonstrated role of the actin cytoskeleton on antigen presenting function of dendritic cells (Al-Alwan et al. 2001a; Al-Alwan et al. 2001b). Understanding how both sides of the immunological synapse influence each other is an important area for future research in which planar bilayers will play an important role; for example, by reconstituting the dynamics of live antigen presenting cell molecules to T-cell surface receptors reconstituted in supported bilayers.

The physical processes that control the size of microclusters are not clear. It is interesting that TCR microclusters exclude CD45 from regions about 0.5 μm across by TIRFM (Varma et al. 2006). Similarly, the segregated patterns formed in mixed contacts with two receptor–ligand systems differing in intermembrane spacing differing by 2–3 nm and protein enriched domains formed when two planar bilayers form intermembrane junctions are all on the scale of 0.5–1 μm (Milstein et al. 2008; Parthasarathy and Groves 2006; Varma et al. 2006). This suggests that the length scale of membrane fluctuations may govern the size of microclusters. Modeling takes into account, membrane bending parameters that support this model (Weikl and Lipowsky 2004). A major gap in our current understanding is how dynamic F-actin contributes with membrane properties to TCR microcluster formation. One idea may come from studies of integrin microcluster formation, which is also F-actin dependent. High-speed imaging two-color TIRFM has demonstrated that α-actinin cross-linked F-actin serves as a scaffold for integrin cluster formation, rather than as a reaction to initial integrin engagement-based adhesion (Choi et al. 2008). For integrins, this process is initially myosin IIA independent, but nascent clusters rapidly undergo myosin IIA dependent maturation, which appears also to be the case for TCR clusters. The high sensitivity of TCR to a small number of ligands may require a preformed, actin-dependent scaffold.

13   What Is the Function of the Immunological Synapse?

The immunological synapse pattern has captured our imagination and led to a great deal of speculation, but deriving hard evidence for specific functions has been challenging. This is because manipulations that control the dynamic synaptic patterns often have direct biochemical effects on the cell that confound interpretation of results. Furthermore, since the SMACs are interdependent, it is difficult to manipulate them independently. In many cases the functional ideas about the synapse reflect working models with varying degrees of experimental support. Here are three functions for which there is experimental support:

1. *Stop signal*: The symmetry of the immunological synapse results in an arrest of T-cell mobility in 2D in vitro systems (Sims et al. 2007). The arrows in Fig. 3 represent the centripetal F-actin flow observed directly by speckle microscopy (Kaizuka et al. 2007). Since integrin adhesion molecules are linked to this F-actin flow the net traction is zero and the cell remains in place. If symmetry is broken the cell migrates (Sims et al. 2007). Synapse symmetry in vitro and T–DC interaction time in vivo are well correlated in genetic experiments (Sims et al. 2007). Stop signals increase dwell time with APC and may be important in signal integration during afferent and efferent phases of immune responses (Skokos et al. 2007), but this remains a working model since in vivo swarming, presumably mediated by local chemokine gradients, may be able to achieve the same advantages for signal integration.

2. *Directed secretion*: The cSMAC is an actin depleted zone at the center of the immunological synapse and thus appears to be an ideal location for directed secretion (Stinchcombe et al. 2006) (Fig. 3). This process can be observed directly using supported planar bilayers (Beal et al. 2008; Liu et al. 2009). The gain in efficiency of killing in going from a partial to complete pSMAC ring is about threefold (Beal et al. 2008). While the pSMAC does not appear to act as a tight gasket, it may dynamically contain large complexes through a continual inward transport of adhesion molecules that generate partial barriers (Kaizuka et al. 2007).

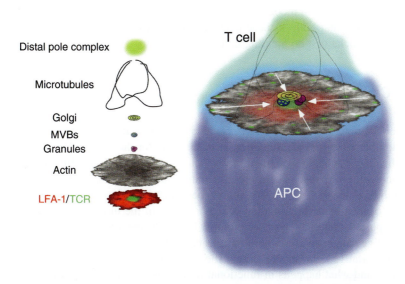

Fig. 3 Functional anatomy of the immunological synapse. A composite figure generated from independently acquired fluorescence micrographs of GFP-actin speckles (Kaizuka et al. 2007) and ICAM-1 and MHC-peptide complexes in supported bilayers (Grakoui et al. 1999). The legend is on the left. The arrows indicate the direction of F-actin speckle movement. *Green signals* in the periphery represent microclusters and these were added to represent peripheral formation of TCR and LFA-1 microclusters, which were too faint to detect in the original micrographs, but have subsequently been detected in many studies using TIRFM illumination or nanofabricated barriers to capture the microclusters (Campi et al. 2005; Mossman et al. 2005; Varma et al. 2006; Yokosuka et al. 2005). Structural elements with defined or strongly suspected functions include: (1) the symmetry F-actin/integrin ring to stop migration, (2) the F-actin depleted central domain for signal termination, multivesicular body formation and directed secretion, and (3) the polarized microtubule array and distal pole complex to establish the spindle axis for asymmetric cell division

3. *Asymmetric cell division*: This is a fundamental principle in biology for generation of differentiated cells from stem cells. The termination of the synapse by
   asymmetric cell division might give rise to unequal daughter cells fated for
   memory (stem cell-like) and effector cells (terminally differentiated) (Dustin
   and Chan 2000). T cells appear to undergo LFA-1-ICAM-1 dependent early
   asymmetric divisions that give rise to memory cell precursors early in response
   to infection in vivo (Chang et al. 2007). This idea has been challenged by others
   for studies suggest that memory cells arise from effector cells, rather than being
   set aside early in responses (Wherry and Ahmed 2004). However, there are
   many common elements in these models and it is agreed that early events in the
   time frame of the first synapse formed by a naïve T cell set the stage for
   generation of memory T cells. Furthermore, it has been confirmed that loss of
   ICAM-1 from antigen presenting cells prevents synapse formation at a standard
   antigen dose and impairs effector and memory responses (Scholer et al. 2008),
   which is compatible with either model. The major difference in the models is
   that the identifiable memory cell precursor divides, relatively few times in the

asymmetric division model and many times in the effector survival model. It is conceivable that both of these pathways are utilized with whichever can fill a memory niche first dominating in a given response.

14 Conclusions

Supported bilayer technology has provided important insights into immune cell function including the identification of the ligands for the TCR, CD2 and LFA-1, the chemistry and physics of adhesion and the formation and function of the immunological synapse. There are still many questions to be addressed and the planar bilayer technology will continue to be useful due to its ability to simulate key aspects of membrane presentation of ligands. One of the most valuable aspects of the supported planar bilayer technology has been the ability to collect highly quantitative data in an area where this has been challenging: the cell–cell interface. This quantitative data should bridge the gap between physics-based theories of adhesion and what happens in functional interfaces. Further discoveries regarding the function of the immunological synapse are likely on the horizon. Integration of planar bilayer technology with in vitro cell–cell and in vivo imaging will likely lead to valuable synergy. A problem with imaging the cell–cell interface is the random orientation and the relatively poor axial resolution and slow acquisition in 3D. One approach to this is to orient the cell–cell contact so that the synapse is in one focal plane. This has been very difficult, even with relatively flat adherent cells, but recent studies using laser tweezers to orient cell–cell conjugates have shown promise and generate data in cell–cell interfacts that appears to be of similar quality to the data obtained with the planar bilayer system (Oddos et al. 2008). Imaging of fluorescence from tagged molecules like TCR or ZAP-70 has been challenging in vivo. However, fluorescence intensity and FRET reporters have started to find applications in vivo (Breart et al. 2008). A new generation of two-photon microscopes with improved sensitivity, better objectives and the wider use of dispersion compensation to optimize excitation efficiency should provide greater potential to validate results in vivo and further inspire bilayer-based experiments to access underlying mechanisms.

Acknowledgments I thank the members of my lab who have contributed to many of the studies highlighted in this commentary. I thank Mike Sheetz for discussion of implications of bead size threshold for TCR stimulation.

References

Al-Alwan MM, Rowden G, Lee TD, West KA (2001a) Fascin is involved in the antigen presentation activity of mature dendritic cells. J Immunol 166:338–345
Al-Alwan MM, Rowden G, Lee TD, West KA (2001b) The dendritic cell cytoskeleton is critical for the formation of the immunological synapse. J Immunol 166:1452–1456

Babbitt BP, Allen PM, Matsueda G, Haber E, Unanue ER (1985) Binding of immunogenic peptides to Ia histocompatibility molecules. Nature 317:359–361

Batista FD, Iber D, Neuberger MS (2001) B cells acquire antigen from target cells after synapse formation. Nature 411:489–494

Beal AM, Anikeeva N, Varma R, Cameron TO, Norris PJ, Dustin ML, Sykulev Y (2008) Protein kinase C{theta} regulates stability of the peripheral adhesion ring junction and contributes to the sensitivity of target cell lysis by CTL. J Immunol 181:4815–4824

Bonte F, Juliano RL (1986) Interactions of liposomes with serum proteins. Chem Phys Lipids 40:359–372

Breart B, Lemaitre F, Celli S, Bousso P (2008) Two-photon imaging of intratumoral CD8+ T cell cytotoxic activity during adoptive T cell therapy in mice. J Clin Invest 118:1390–1397

Brian AA, McConnell HM (1984) Allogeneic stimulation of cytotoxic T cells by supported planar membranes. Proc Natl Acad Sci USA 81:6159–6163

Bromley SK, Iaboni A, Davis SJ, Whitty A, Green JM, Shaw AS, Weiss A, Dustin ML (2001) The immunological synapse and CD28-CD80 interactions. Nat Immunol 2:1159–1166

Brossard C, Feuillet V, Schmitt A, Randriamampita C, Romao M, Raposo G, Trautmann A (2005) Multifocal structure of the T cell – dendritic cell synapse. Eur J Immunol 35:1741–1753

Bunnell SC, Hong DI, Kardon JR, Yamazaki T, McGlade CJ, Barr VA, Samelson LE (2002) T cell receptor ligation induces the formation of dynamically regulated signaling assemblies. J Cell Biol 158:1263–1275

Campi G, Varma R, Dustin ML (2005) Actin and agonist MHC–peptide complex-dependent T cell receptor microclusters as scaffolds for signaling. J Exp Med 202:1031–1036

Carman CV, Sage PT, Sciuto TE, de la Fuente MA, Geha RS, Ochs HD, Dvorak HF, Dvorak AM, Springer TA (2007) Transcellular diapedesis is initiated by invasive podosomes. Immunity 26:784–797

Carrasco YR, Fleire SJ, Cameron T, Dustin ML, Batista FD (2004) LFA-1/ICAM-1 interaction lowers the threshold of B cell activation by facilitating B cell adhesion and synapse formation. Immunity 20:589–599

Chan PY, Lawrence MB, Dustin ML, Ferguson LM, Golan DE, Springer TA (1991) Influence of receptor lateral mobility on adhesion strengthening between membranes containing LFA-3 and CD2. J Cell Biol 115:245–255

Chang JT, Palanivel VR, Kinjyo I, Schambach F, Intlekofer AM, Banerjee A, Longworth SA, Vinup KE, Mrass P, Oliaro J, Killeen N, Orange JS, Russell SM, Weninger W, Reiner SL (2007) Asymmetric T lymphocyte division in the initiation of adaptive immune responses. Science 315:1687–1691

Choi CK, Vicente-Manzanares M, Zareno J, Whitmore LA, Mogilner A, Horwitz AR (2008) Actin and alpha-actinin orchestrate the assembly and maturation of nascent adhesions in a myosin II motor-independent manner. Nat Cell Biol 10:1039–1050

Choudhuri K, Wiseman D, Brown MH, Gould K, van der Merwe PA (2005) T-cell receptor triggering is critically dependent on the dimensions of its peptide-MHC ligand. Nature 436:578–582

DeMond AL, Mossman KD, Starr T, Dustin ML, Groves JT (2008) T cell receptor micro-cluster transport through molecular mazes reveals mechanism of translocation. Biophys J 94:3286–3292

Depoil D, Fleire S, Treanor BL, Weber M, Harwood NE, Marchbank KL, Tybulewicz VL, Batista FD (2008) CD19 is essential for B cell activation by promoting B cell receptor-antigen microcluster formation in response to membrane-bound ligand. Nat Immunol 9:63–72

Dustin ML (1997) Adhesive bond dynamics in contacts between T lymphocytes and glass supported planar bilayers reconstituted with the immunoglobulin related adhesion molecule CD58. J Biol Chem 272:15782–15788

Dustin ML (2008) Hunter to gatherer and back: immunological synapses and kinapses as variations on the theme of amoeboid locomotion. Annu Rev Cell Dev Biol 24:577–596

Dustin ML, Chan AC (2000) Signaling takes shape in the immune system. Cell 103:283–294

Dustin ML, Colman DR (2002) Neural and immunological synaptic relations. Science 298:785–789

Dustin ML, Cooper JA (2000) The immunological synapse and the actin cytoskeleton: molecular hardware for T cell signaling. Nat Immunol 1:23–29

Dustin ML, Shaw AS (1999) Costimulation: building an immunological synapse. Science 283:649–650

Dustin ML, Springer TA (1988) Lymphocyte function-associated antigen-1 (LFA-1) interaction with intercellular adhesion molecule-1 (ICAM-1) is one of at least three mechanisms for lymphocyte adhesion to cultured endothelial cells. J Cell Biol 107:321–331

Dustin ML, Springer TA (1989) T cell receptor cross-linking transiently stimulates adhesiveness through LFA-1. Nature 341:619–624

Dustin ML, Sanders ME, Shaw S, Springer TA (1987a) Purified lymphocyte function-associated antigen 3 binds to CD2 and mediates T lymphocyte adhesion. J Exp Med 165:677–692

Dustin ML, Selvaraj P, Mattaliano RJ, Springer TA (1987b) Anchoring mechanisms for LFA-3 cell adhesion glycoprotein at membrane surface. Nature 329:846–848

Dustin ML, Singer KH, Tuck DT, Springer TA (1988) Adhesion of T lymphoblasts to epidermal keratinocytes is regulated by interferon gamma and is mediated by intercellular adhesion molecule 1 (ICAM-1). J Exp Med 167:1323–1340

Dustin ML, Ferguson LM, Chan PY, Springer TA, Golan DE (1996a) Visualization of CD2 interaction with LFA-3 and determination of the two-dimensional dissociation constant for adhesion receptors in a contact area. J Cell Biol 132:465–474

Dustin ML, Miller JM, Ranganath S, Vignali DA, Viner NJ, Nelson CA, Unanue ER (1996b) TCR-mediated adhesion of T cell hybridomas to planar bilayers containing purified MHC class II/peptide complexes and receptor shedding during detachment. J Immunol 157:2014–2021

Dustin ML, Bromley SK, Kan Z, Peterson DA, Unanue ER (1997a) Antigen receptor engagement delivers a stop signal to migrating T lymphocytes. Proc Natl Acad Sci USA 94:3909–3913

Dustin ML, Golan DE, Zhu DM, Miller JM, Meier W, Davies EA, van der Merwe PA (1997b) Low affinity interaction of human or rat T cell adhesion molecule CD2 with its ligand aligns adhering membranes to achieve high physiological affinity. J Biol Chem 272:30889–30898

Dustin ML, Olszowy MW, Holdorf AD, Li J, Bromley S, Desai N, Widder P, Rosenberger F, van der Merwe PA, Allen PM, Shaw AS (1998) A novel adapter protein orchestrates receptor patterning and cytoskeletal polarity in T cell contacts. Cell 94:667–677

Dustin ML, Starr T, Coombs D, Majeau GR, Meier W, Hochman PS, Douglass A, Vale R, Goldstein B, Whitty A (2007a) Quantification and modeling of Tripartite CD2-, CD58FC chimera (Alefacept)-, and CD16-mediated cell adhesion. J Biol Chem 282:34748–34757

Dustin ML, Starr T, Varma R, Thomas VK (2007) Supported planar bilayers for study of the immunological synapse. Curr Protoc Immunol, Chapter 18, Unit 18.13

Fischer KD, Kong YY, Nishina H, Tedford K, Marengere LE, Kozieradzki I, Sasaki T, Starr M, Chan G, Gardener S, Nghiem MP, Bouchard D, Barbacid M, Bernstein A, Penninger JM (1998) Vav is a regulator of cytoskeletal reorganization mediated by the T-cell receptor. Curr Biol 8:554–562

Fleire SJ, Goldman JP, Carrasco YR, Weber M, Bray D, Batista FD (2006) B cell ligand discrimination through a spreading and contraction response. Science 312:738–741

Freiberg BA, Kupfer H, Maslanik W, Delli J, Kappler J, Zaller DM, Kupfer A (2002) Staging and resetting T cell activation in SMACs. Nat Immunol 3:911–917

Galbraith CG, Yamada KM, Sheetz MP (2002) The relationship between force and focal complex development. J Cell Biol 159:695–705

Gay D, Coeshott C, Golde W, Kappler J, Marrack P (1986) The major histocompatibility complex-restricted antigen receptor on T cells. IX. Role of accessory molecules in recognition of antigen plus isolated IA. J Immunol 136:2026–2032

Gil D, Schamel WW, Montoya M, Sanchez-Madrid F, Alarcon B (2002) Recruitment of Nck by CD3 epsilon reveals a ligand-induced conformational change essential for T cell receptor signaling and synapse formation. Cell 109:901–912

Gomez TS, Kumar K, Medeiros RB, Shimizu Y, Leibson PJ, Billadeau DD (2007) Formins regulate the actin-related protein 2/3 complex-independent polarization of the centrosome to the immunological synapse. Immunity 26:177–190

Grakoui A, Bromley SK, Sumen C, Davis MM, Shaw AS, Allen PM, Dustin ML (1999) The immunological synapse: a molecular machine controlling T cell activation. Science 285: 221–227

Gunzer M, Schafer A, Borgmann S, Grabbe S, Zanker KS, Brocker EB, Kampgen E, Friedl P (2000) Antigen presentation in extracellular matrix: interactions of T cells with dendritic cells are dynamic, short lived, and sequential. Immunity 13:323–332

Hafeman DG, von Tscharner V, McConnell HM (1981) Specific antibody-dependent interactions between macrophages and lipid haptens in planar lipid monolayers. Proc Natl Acad Sci USA 78:4552–4556

Hollander N, Selvaraj P, Springer TA (1988) Biosynthesis and function of LFA-3 in human mutant cells deficient in phosphatidylinositol anchored proteins. J Immunol 141:4283–4290

Ilani T, Vasiliver-Shamis G, Vardhana S, Bretscher A, Dustin ML (2009) T cell antigen receptor signaling and immunological synapse stability require myosin IIA. Nat Immunol 10:531–539

Izzard CS, Lochner LR (1976) Cell-to-substrate contacts in living fibroblasts: an interference reflexion study with an evaluation of the technique. J Cell Sci 21:129–159

Jacobelli J, Chmura SA, Buxton DB, Davis MM, Krummel MF (2004) A single class II myosin modulates T cell motility and stopping, but not synapse formation. Nat Immunol 5:531–538

Kaizuka Y, Douglass AD, Varma R, Dustin ML, Vale RD (2007) Mechanisms for segregating T cell receptor and adhesion molecules during immunological synapse formation in Jurkat T cells. Proc Natl Acad Sci USA 104:20296–20301

Kaizuka Y, Douglass AD, Vardhana S, Dustin ML, Vale RD (2009) The coreceptor CD2 uses plasma membrane microdomains to transduce signals in T cells. J Cell Biol 185:521–534

Kloboucek A, Behrisch A, Faix J, Sackmann E (1999) Adhesion-induced receptor segregation and adhesion plaque formation: a model membrane study. Biophys J 77:2311–2328

Krummel MF, Sjaastad MD, Wulfing C, Davis MM (2000) Differential clustering of CD4 and CD3ζ during T cell recognition. Science 289:1349–1352

Lee KH, Holdorf AD, Dustin ML, Chan AC, Allen PM, Shaw AS (2002) T cell receptor signaling precedes immunological synapse formation. Science 295:1539–1542

Lee KH, Dinner AR, Tu C, Campi G, Raychaudhuri S, Varma R, Sims TN, Burack WR, Wu H, Wang J, Kanagawa O, Markiewicz M, Allen PM, Dustin ML, Chakraborty AK, Shaw AS (2003) The immunological synapse balances T cell receptor signaling and degradation. Science 302:1218–1222

Liu D, Bryceson YT, Meckel T, Vasiliver-Shamis G, Dustin ML, Long EO (2009) Integrin-dependent organization and bidirectional vesicular traffic at cytotoxic immune synapses. Immunity 31:99–109

Lomnitzer R, Rabson AR (1981) Mechanism of suppression of lymphocyte proliferation by Concanavalin A-activated mononuclear cells. Immunology 43:475–481

Lucas M, Schachterle W, Oberle K, Aichele P, Diefenbach A (2007) Dendritic cells prime natural killer cells by trans-presenting interleukin 15. Immunity 26:503–517

Luo BH, Carman CV, Springer TA (2007) Structural basis of integrin regulation and signaling. Annu Rev Immunol 25:619–647

Marlin SD, Springer TA (1987) Purified intercellular adhesion molecule-1 (ICAM-1) is a ligand for lymphocyte function-associated antigen 1 (LFA-1). Cell 51:813–819

McKeithan TW (1995) Kinetic proofreading in T-cell receptor signal transduction. Proc Natl Acad Sci USA 92:5042–5046

Mempel TR, Henrickson SE, Von Andrian UH (2004) T-cell priming by dendritic cells in lymph nodes occurs in three distinct phases. Nature 427:154–159

Mescher MF (1992) Surface contact requirements for activation of cytotoxic T lymphocytes. J Immunol 149:2402–2405

Metzger H (1992) Transmembrane signaling: the joy of aggregation. J Immunol 149:1477–1487

Milstein O, Tseng SY, Starr T, Llodra J, Nans A, Liu M, Wild MK, van der Merwe PA, Stokes DL, Reisner Y, Dustin ML (2008) Nanoscale increases in CD2-CD48-mediated intermembrane spacing decrease adhesion and reorganize the immunological synapse. J Biol Chem 283:34414–34422

Monks CR, Freiberg BA, Kupfer H, Sciaky N, Kupfer A (1998) Three-dimensional segregation of supramolecular activation clusters in T cells. Nature 395:82–86

Mossman KD, Campi G, Groves JT, Dustin ML (2005) Altered TCR signaling from geometrically repatterned immunological synapses. Science 310:1191–1193

Negulescu PA, Krasieva TB, Khan A, Kerschbaum HH, Cahalan MD (1996) Polarity of T cell shape, motility, and sensitivity to antigen. Immunity 4:421–430

Nguyen K, Sylvain NR, Bunnell SC (2008) T cell costimulation via the integrin VLA-4 inhibits the actin-dependent centralization of signaling microclusters containing the adaptor SLP-76. Immunity 28:810–821

Nolz JC, Gomez TS, Zhu P, Li S, Medeiros RB, Shimizu Y, Burkhardt JK, Freedman BD, Billadeau DD (2006) The WAVE2 complex regulates actin cytoskeletal reorganization and CRAC-mediated calcium entry during T cell activation. Curr Biol 16:24–34

Norcross MA (1984) A synaptic basis for T-lymphocyte activation. Ann Immunol (Paris) 135D:113–134

Oddos S, Dunsby C, Purbhoo MA, Chauveau A, Owen DM, Neil MA, Davis DM, French PM (2008) High-speed high-resolution imaging of intercellular immune synapses using optical tweezers. Biophys J 95:L66–L68

Parthasarathy R, Groves JT (2006) Coupled membrane fluctuations and protein mobility in supported intermembrane junctions. J Phys Chem B 110:8513–8516

Pierres A, Benoliel AM, Bongrand P, van der Merwe PA (1996) Determination of the lifetime and force dependence of interactions of single bonds between surface-attached CD2 and CD48 adhesion molecules. Proc Natl Acad Sci USA 93:15114–15118

Reich Z, Boniface JJ, Lyons DS, Borochov N, Wachtel EJ, Davis MM (1997) Ligand-specific oligomerization of T-cell receptor molecules. Nature 387:617–620

Rothlein R, Dustin ML, Marlin SD, Springer TA (1986) A human intercellular adhesion molecule (ICAM-1) distinct from LFA-1. J Immunol 137:1270–1274

Samelson LE, Patel MD, Weissman AM, Harford JB, Klausner RD (1986) Antigen activation of murine T cells induces tyrosine phosphorylation of a polypeptide associated with the T cell antigen receptor. Cell 46:1083–1090

Sanchez-Madrid F, Krensky AM, Ware CF, Robbins E, Strominger JL, Burakoff SJ, Springer TA (1982) Three distinct antigens associated with human T-lymphocyte-mediated cytolysis: LFA-1, LFA-2, and LFA-3. Proc Natl Acad Sci USA 79:7489–7493

Scatchard G (1949) The attractions of proteins for small molecules and ions. Ann NY Acad Sci 51:660–672

Schlessinger J, Webb WW, Elson EL, Metzger H (1976) Lateral motion and valence of Fc receptors on rat peritoneal mast cells. Nature 264:550–552

Scholer A, Hugues S, Boissonnas A, Fetler L, Amigorena S (2008) Intercellular adhesion molecule-1-dependent stable interactions between T cells and dendritic cells determine CD8+ T cell memory. Immunity 28:258–270

Shao JY, Yu Y, Dustin ML (2005) A model for CD2/CD58-mediated adhesion strengthening. Ann Biomed Eng 33:483–493

Shaw AS, Dustin ML (1997) Making the T cell receptor go the distance: a topological view of T cell activation. Immunity 6:361–369

Shaw S, Luce GE, Quinones R, Gress RE, Springer TA, Sanders ME (1986) Two antigen-independent adhesion pathways used by human cytotoxic T-cell clones. Nature 323:262–264

Shimaoka M, Xiao T, Liu JH, Yang Y, Dong Y, Jun CD, McCormack A, Zhang R, Joachimiak A, Takagi J, Wang JH, Springer TA (2003) Structures of the alpha L I domain and its complex with ICAM-1 reveal a shape-shifting pathway for integrin regulation. Cell 112:99–111

Sims TN, Soos TJ, Xenias HS, Dubin-Thaler B, Hofman JM, Waite JC, Cameron TO, Thomas VK, Varma R, Wiggins CH, Sheetz MP, Littman DR, Dustin ML (2007) Opposing effects of

PKCtheta and WASp on symmetry breaking and relocation of the immunological synapse. Cell 129:773–785

Skokos D, Shakhar G, Varma R, Waite JC, Cameron TO, Lindquist RL, Schwickert T, Nussenzweig MC, Dustin ML (2007) Peptide-MHC potency governs dynamic interactions between T cells and dendritic cells in lymph nodes. Nat Immunol 8:835–844

Smith A, Carrasco YR, Stanley P, Kieffer N, Batista FD, Hogg N (2005) A talin-dependent LFA-1 focal zone is formed by rapidly migrating T lymphocytes. J Cell Biol 170:141–151

Springer TA (1990) Adhesion receptors of the immune system. Nature 346:425–434

Stauffer TP, Meyer T (1997) Compartmentalized IgE receptor-mediated signal transduction in living cells. J Cell Biol 139:1447–1454

Stinchcombe JC, Majorovits E, Bossi G, Fuller S, Griffiths GM (2006) Centrosome polarization delivers secretory granules to the immunological synapse. Nature 443:462–465

Tolar P, Sohn HW, Pierce SK (2005) The initiation of antigen-induced B cell antigen receptor signaling viewed in living cells by fluorescence resonance energy transfer. Nat Immunol 6:1168–1176

Tolar P, Hanna J, Krueger PD, Pierce SK (2009) The constant region of the membrane immunoglobulin mediates B cell-receptor clustering and signaling in response to membrane antigens. Immunity 30:44–55

Tolentino TP, Wu J, Zarnitsyna VI, Fang Y, Dustin ML, Zhu C (2008) Measuring diffusion and binding kinetics by contact area FRAP. Biophys J 95:920–930

Torigoe C, Song J, Barisas BG, Metzger H (2004) The influence of actin microfilaments on signaling by the receptor with high-affinity for IgE. Mol Immunol 41:817–829

Tseng SY, Waite JC, Liu M, Vardhana S, Dustin ML (2008) T cell-dendritic cell immunological synapses contain TCR-dependent CD28-CD80 clusters that recruit protein kinase Ctheta. J Immunol 181:4852–4863

Van Der Merwe PA, Davis SJ (2003) Molecular interactions mediating T cell antigen recognition. Annu Rev Immunol 21:659–684

van der Merwe PA, Barclay AN, Mason DW, Davies EA, Morgan BP, Tone M, Krishnam AKC, Ianelli C, Davis SJ (1994) Human cell-adhesion molecule CD2 binds CD58 (LFA-3) with a very low affinity and an extremely fast dissociation rate but does not bind CD48 or CD59. Biochemistry 33:10149–10160

Varma R, Campi G, Yokosuka T, Saito T, Dustin ML (2006) T cell receptor-proximal signals are sustained in peripheral microclusters and terminated in the central supramolecular activation cluster. Immunity 25:117–127

Watts TH, McConnell HM (1986) High-affinity fluorescent peptide binding to I-Ad in lipid membranes. Proc Natl Acad Sci USA 83:9660–9664

Watts TH, Gaub HE, McConnell HM (1986) T-cell-mediated association of peptide antigen and major histocompatibility complex protein detected by energy transfer in an evanescent wavefield. Nature 320:179–181

Weikl TR, Lipowsky R (2004) Pattern formation during T-cell adhesion. Biophys J 87: 3665–3678

Weis RM, Balakrishnan K, Smith BA, McConnell HM (1982) Stimulation of fluorescence in a small contact region between rat basophil leukemia cells and planar lipid membrane targets by coherent evanescent radiation. J Biol Chem 257:6440–6445

Wherry EJ, Ahmed R (2004) Memory CD8 T-cell differentiation during viral infection. J Virol 78:5535–5545

Wild MK, Cambiaggi A, Brown MH, Davies EA, Ohno H, Saito T, van der Merwe PA (1999) Dependence of T cell antigen recognition on the dimensions of an accessory receptor-ligand complex. J Exp Med 190:31–41

Woolf E, Grigorova I, Sagiv A, Grabovsky V, Feigelson SW, Shulman Z, Hartmann T, Sixt M, Cyster JG, Alon R (2007) Lymph node chemokines promote sustained T lymphocyte motility without triggering stable integrin adhesiveness in the absence of shear forces. Nat Immunol 8:1076–1085

Wu J, Fang Y, Zarnitsyna VI, Tolentino TP, Dustin ML, Zhu C (2008) A coupled diffusion-kinetics model for analysis of contact-area FRAP experiment. Biophys J 95:910–919

Wülfing C, Davis MM (1998) A Receptor/cytoskeletal movement triggered by costimulation during T cell activation. Science 282:2266–2269

Xu C, Gagnon E, Call ME, Schnell JR, Schwieters CD, Carman CV, Chou JJ, Wucherpfennig KW (2008) Regulation of T cell receptor activation by dynamic membrane binding of the CD3epsilon cytoplasmic tyrosine-based motif. Cell 135:702–713

Yokosuka T, Sakata-Sogawa K, Kobayashi W, Hiroshima M, Hashimoto-Tane A, Tokunaga M, Dustin ML, Saito T (2005) Newly generated T cell receptor microclusters initiate and sustain T cell activation by recruitment of Zap70 and SLP-76. Nat Immunol 6:1253–1262

Yokosuka T, Kobayashi W, Sakata-Sogawa K, Takamatsu M, Hashimoto-Tane A, Dustin ML, Tokunaga M, Saito T (2008) Spatiotemporal regulation of T cell costimulation by TCR-CD28 microclusters and protein kinase C theta translocation. Immunity 29:589–601

Zhang F, Marcus WD, Goyal NH, Selvaraj P, Springer TA, Zhu C (2005) Two-dimensional kinetics regulation of alphaLbeta2-ICAM-1 interaction by conformational changes of the alphaL-inserted domain. J Biol Chem 280:42207–42218

Zhu DM, Dustin ML, Cairo CW, Thatte HS, Golan DE (2006) Mechanisms of cellular avidity regulation in CD2-CD58-mediated T cell adhesion. ACS Chem Biol 1:649–658

Zhu DM, Dustin ML, Cairo CW, Golan DE (2007) Analysis of two-dimensional dissociation constant of laterally mobile cell adhesion molecules. Biophys J 92:1022–1034

Zhu J, Luo BH, Xiao T, Zhang C, Nishida N, Springer TA (2008) Structure of a complete integrin ectodomain in a physiologic resting state and activation and deactivation by applied forces. Mol Cell 32:849–861

Immunological Synapses Within Context: Patterns of Cell–Cell Communication and Their Application in T–T Interactions

Junsang Doh and Matthew F. Krummel

Contents

M.F. Krummel (✉)
Department of Pathology and Biological Imaging Development Center, University of California
San Francisco, 513 Parnassus Ave, San Francisco, CA 94143-0511, USA
e-mail: Matthew.Krummel@ucsf.edu

J. Doh
School of Interdisciplinary Bioscience and Bioengineering and Department of Mechanical
Engineering, Pohang University of Science and Technology, 790-784 San31, Hyoja-dong,
Nam-Gu, Pohang, Gyeongbuk, Korea
e-mail: jsdoh@postech.ac.kr

T. Saito and F.D. Batista (eds.), *Immunological Synapse*,
Current Topics in Microbiology and Immunology 340,
DOI 10.1007/978-3-642-03858-7_2, © Springer-Verlag Berlin Heidelberg 2010

Abstract The cell-biology of intercellular communication between T cells and their partners has been greatly advanced over the past 10 years. The key morphological and motility features of cell contact-based communication between T cells and APCs can now be seen as a collection of patterns for cell–cell interactions amongst immune cells more generally, each serving to contribute to the outcome of the contact both locally and globally. Here we review the conservation of these patterns, amongst which is the emergent "immunological synapse," and describe a newly defined example, formed between the adjacent activating T cells. We subsequently seek to put these and the pattern more generally into the framework of system-wide behavior of the immune system. We postulate that the patterns are fine-tuned to provide quorum-like decisions by collections of activating and activated cells that interact over time and space.

1   Introduction

The immune system can be conceived as bearing similarities to a community of human beings inhabiting a city or country; immune cells are of varied origin and abilities (T cells, B cells, natural killer (NK) cells, macrophages, dendritic cells (DCs), etc.), inhabit varied physical spaces in tissues (interdigitating or surveilling various organs, peripheral tissues, and secondary and tertiary lymphoid structures), travel over both short and long distances, interact with one another, and, of course, introduce changes in their environment. The behavior of immune cells, like that of individuals, is partially determined by the features of their physical environment. However, at a deeper level, their behavior is also constrained by their limited means of communication and interaction.

In describing the optimum size for a city – based on maintaining a social cohesion – Aristotle concluded that an entire city should be of a sufficiently small size so that all citizens would be able to hear a single herald in peace or a single general in war [Politics VIII]. Such a stipulation has likely been obviated by dramatic changes in the mechanisms for interaction and communication between individuals (e.g., "broadcast" media such as the newspaper, telephone, internet, etc.). Are there equivalent issues of scale for communication in the immune response?

There are indeed clearly equivalent "broadcast" media such as large releases of soluble cytokines that subsequently permeate organs and organisms and influence multiple cell types. Although there are beneficial "bread crumb"-like trails of chemokines which apparently line epithelial layers and address activated cells to particular tissues, are there global soluble signals to communicate for a system requiring careful recruitment of only specific cells? On the whole, the so-called large "cytokine storms," particularly those of pro-inflammatory mediators such as γIFN, are more highly associated with pathogenic states such as "shock" rather than effective and specific surveillance (Rittirsch et al. 2008). As part of the mandate of the immune system to be specific and only destroy invading organism, it is apparently quite necessary to explicitly address messages, even those of "soluble" mediators so that only certain cells are activated. The "immunological synapse," a recurring pattern of cell–cell junctions for immune-cells represents a portion of the solution for the need for explicit communication. However, as an isolated concept, it does not encompass the total solution for the need for broad communication over a distance.

It is possible to define collections of "solutions" for optimizing human interactions and communication over space. Indeed, such "patterns" are suggested to exist on scales from entire urban design down to considerations of the size of rooms in a house and to be applicable like a "stamp" to treat recurring needs (Alexander et al. 1977). Notably for the analogy to biological systems that arise from defined behaviors of individual players, it is also theorized that design solutions at small scales (quality design of social spaces) are part and parcel of the greater functioning of larger-scales (e.g., entire cities) (Whyte 1988). In a similar manner, the features or patterns that define cell–cell interactions represent the fundamentals toward defining the properties of the immune system as a whole.

In this review, we will address what has emerged as "synapse-based patterns" for cell–cell interactions. We will argue that the "immunological synapse" (IS) as currently described is amongst a collection of a relatively small number of small-scale patterns of motility, morphology, and membrane organization that provide critical features that can permit efficient larger-scale goals to be accomplished: namely self/nonself discrimination, rapid but flexible responses, and group decision making based on the regulated formation of these contacts. We will use an analogous "Pattern" framework as a way to define how the properties of cell–cell contacts provide the adequate specificity, flexibility, and group decision making properties to specific cell types. In particular, we will expand from the T cell–antigen-presenting cell (APC) synapse the synaptic structure that initiated the current intensive study of cell–cell contacts in the immune system, and describe a recently appreciated T–T synaptic contact and the potential quorum sensing that might be facilitated by the application of synapse "patterns" to activating T cells.

2 The Emergent Prototypical Immunological Synapse Dynamics

The contact surface at which T cells recognize and activate in response to peptide fragments in the groove of major histocompatibility complex (MHC) molecules was first proposed to be similar to a neurological synapse by Norcross in 1984 (Norcross 1984). The concept was revived in the late 1990s as a result of the observation of ring-like distributions of integrin lymphocyte function-associated antigen-1 (LFA-1) and their ligands (peripheral-supramolecular activating complexes; pSMACs (Monks et al. 1998)) that surrounded centralized T-cell receptor (TCR)–MHC complexes (central supramolecular activating clusters; cSMACs (Monks et al. 1998)) at T-APC contact sites. Concurrent observations of CD2 clusters (Dustin et al. 1998) and cytoskeletal movement into the contact region (Wulfing and Davis 1998) further solidified the comparison. However, the term gained wide acceptance when used to assess the distributions of TCRs and integrins in simplified model lipid bilayers (Dustin and Colman 2002; Grakoui et al. 1999). It was subsequently argued that these distributions at an adhesive contact were definitively "synaptic" (as opposed to focal adhesions, desmosomes etc.) on the basis of being an adhesive contact with a synaptic space, and characterized by polarized secretion and signaling (Dustin and Colman 2002; Grakoui et al. 1999). With this rapid progress, there emerged a frequent but incorrect interchange of terminology "Synapse," which might best define the cell–cell contact and "cSMAC/pSMAC," which defined a frequently observed organization and differential exclusion of molecules that could be observed within some of those contacts.

When synapse assembly was analyzed in real-time, concurrent with calcium influx downstream of TCR triggering, it became apparent that cell–cell contact was associated with much earlier and smaller TCR–MHC clusters (Krummel et al. 2000), which only later coalesce to the cSMAC/pSMAC structure. Subsequently, receptor-proximal signaling has been demonstrated to be most active in these and even smaller initial "microclusters" but mostly extinguished in the centralized cSMAC structure (Varma et al. 2006; Lee et al. 2002; Mossman et al. 2005), although some recent data suggests that TCRs in the cSMAC may still support signaling in particular circumstances (Cemerski et al. 2008). Recent use of photo-activation of pMHC ligands for the TCR make it clear that early clusters signal within seconds of ligand engagement (Huse et al. 2007) whereas the formation of the cSMAC/pSMAC architecture may take minutes (Krummel et al. 2000; DeMond et al. 2006). A now-modified understanding of a dynamically rearranging synapse includes active remodeling of the membrane domains giving rise to a dispersed cluster- dominated "immature" and subsequent cSMAC-bearing "mature" form (Krummel et al. 2000; Mossman et al. 2005; Campi et al. 2005).

The characterization of immunological synapse dynamics has also been enriched by other parallel developments. First, it has been revealed that cell–cell communication and TCR stimulation at T-APC contacts is frequently associated with short-lived cell–cell contacts rather than prolonged ones. These have not yet proved tractable to study at the molecular level but were first described for T cells interacting with peptide loaded dendritic cells in collagen matrices (Gunzer et al. 2000) where stable interactions are rarely observed but which nevertheless produced T-cell activation. The functionality of short-lived cell–cell interactions is also suggested by the correlation between expression of early-activation antigens following transient contacts in vivo (Mempel et al. 2004) and by the ability of cells to be activated when only given repeatedly interrupted stimuli (Faroudi et al. 2003). While the outcome of these transient interactions may not be complete activation and memory formation (Scholer et al. 2008; Hurez et al. 2003), there is emerging evidence that such interactions provide ample opportunity for specific and polarized cell–cell signaling. In particular, the functional act of cytotoxic T lymphocyte (CTL) killing at T cell–target interactions is achieved with only short-contacts and does not require the formation of a centralized TCR accumulation (Wiedemann et al. 2006; Purbhoo et al. 2004). It is thus important to see the stable IS model, typically including the coalescence of a cSMAC (Grakoui et al. 1999; Krummel et al. 2000; Varma et al. 2006; Mossman et al. 2005; Campi et al. 2005; Dustin et al. 2006), as one example of signaling and direct cell–cell communication, taken from a broader selection of patterns.

A further enrichment of the cSMAC/pSMAC model of cell–cell signaling at the IS is derived from analyses of the contact face morphology and subsequent consideration of the dynamics of membrane apposition for communication at this junction. In glass-supported lipid bilayers where the apposed system has a flattened topology and cannot deform, membrane-membrane interfaces form a very flat and contiguous contact face with the glass-supported surface (Grakoui et al. 1999; Dustin et al. 2006). In completely juxtaposed settings, aggregation of signaling molecules could only occur by movement along the membrane; such movement is indeed observed and typically involves centripetal flow mediated by actin (Varma et al. 2006; Yokosuka et al. 2005). However, the first live-cell imaging of cell–cell based TCR-signaling clusters noted that the process was highly dynamic with clusters forming, dissociating and reforming (Krummel et al. 2000) rather than smoothly moving only inward. Similar non-radial movement was recently observed for larger clusters within an NK-APC synapse, when the synapse was observed specifically "en face" (Oddos et al. 2008). Is this process the same?

An immunological synapse between immune cells and their ligand-bearing partners appears to contain multiple distinct regions of close membrane–membrane apposition which may dynamically remodel in addition to permitting TCR and integrin movements within that juxtaposed membrane space. In support of this, transmission electron microscopy (TEM) analysis of the physiologically relevant contacts suggests that a contiguous flat contact interface is not, in fact, representative of the physiological case for T–DC interactions (Brossard et al. 2005), CTL–target contacts (Stinchcombe et al. 2001), NK–APC (McCann et al. 2003) and typically even in T–B interactions (Krummel MF, unpublished).Within such contacts, the membranes only touch sporadically, with the non-attached regions separated by distances upwards of 50 nm and for stretches of upwards of 1 μm (Brossard et al. 2005; Stinchcombe et al. 2001; McCann et al. 2003). In synpases formed by CTLs and their targets, lytic granules are aligned with these clefts (Stinchcombe et al. 2001). Thus, the physiologically relevant contacts involve significant synaptic clefts formed between regions of closely apposed membrane (see cartoon in Fig. 3), a result that is even more consistent with analogous synapses in neurons than perhaps was appreciated in early studies. Indeed, the functional significance of the synaptic nature of the contact, namely the formation of synaptic spaces for secretion also appears to be supported by the partitioning of secretory domains (Stinchcombe et al. 2001) and vesicles containing IL-2 and γIFN (Huse et al. 2006; Reichert et al. 2001; Kupfer et al. 1994; Kupfer et al. 1991) as well as receptors for these cytokines (Maldonado et al. 2004) at the IS.

3 Functional Patterns of Cell–Cell Communication

It was then prescient for others (Dustin and Colman 2002) to have previously defined "features" of synaptic contacts when relating them to neuronal synapse; including "discreteness," "adhesion," "stability" and "directed" secretion. With our emerging knowledge, it seems timely, however, to look at the current model of an IS as part of a broader pattern that immune cells utilize for cell–cell communication. With less emphasis on the molecular organizations within membrane–membrane junctions of the IS that are to be reviewed by others in this issue, we suggest that the following represent well-established "patterns" of cell–cell communication in the immune system. For each one, we will describe how the pattern appears to provide efficient communication to the system as a whole.

3.1 Dynamic Cellular Assembly and Disassembly

T cell–APC interactions are not permanent structures. Rather, the cell–cell contacts last for seconds to hours but all ultimately result in "abscission" of the T cell from the APC and possible reattachment to other partners (Fig. 1a). In vivo, there is considerable variation in the length of contact and the variability appears to be regulated by the strength of antigenic stimulation (Henrickson et al. 2008; Skokos et al. 2007) as well as T-cell intrinsic factors (Sims et al. 2007). The timing of first arrest is also variable: depending on the route of immunization and adjuvant, the "stop" phase can occur between 2 and 18 h after administration of adjuvant. Some of the timing certainly is influenced by the rate of loading and/or trafficking of the antigen to the lymph node. It is clear that, particularly in high-antigen conditions, soluble peptides administered intravenously can induce cell arrest within minutes (Celli et al. 2007), suggesting there is no obligate lag-phase for arrest. Thus, there is variability in the timing of the pattern, but the generation of multiple but transient cell–cell contacts appears conserved.

This pattern is repeated in CTL–target and NK–target interactions, in which the effector cells may only stay together with the targets for a few minutes prior to moving on to another target. Perhaps this case exemplifies the utility of transient arrest: the ability to interact serially with multiple partners (Wiedemann et al. 2006), which is clearly a benefit to kill most targets. For activating CD4+ T cells, it likely serves to permit T cells to recognize signals on multiple surfaces, potentially choosing the "best" APC encountered (Depoil et al. 2005). Additionally, it is also possible that it allows T cells to "tag" and thereby mature multiple antigen-presenting cells, providing increased specificity for future T cells. This has been proposed to rely upon the chemokine receptor CCR5 and the locally produced CCL3 and CCL4 (Castellino et al. 2006; Hugues et al. 2007).

As a general rule, the pattern of transience in cell–cell contacts increases the number of cells and the area of sites affected by a single cell. In the case of helper

a   Pattern 1: Transient Stability and Intermittent Motility.

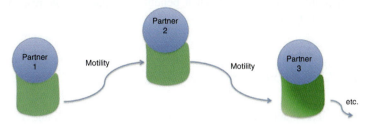

b   Pattern 2: Polarized Secretion Allows Selection of Target Delivery

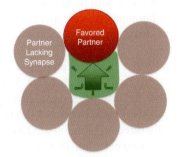

c   Pattern 3: Regulated Adhesion Zone Membrane Morphology Coordinates Numerous
Ongoing Activites.

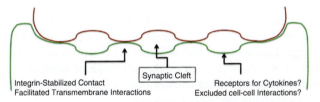

d   Pattern 4: Facilitated Clustering of Transmembrane receptors at Juxtamembrane
Domains Increase Signalosome Efficacy. Global and Local Mechanisms of Enhancement.

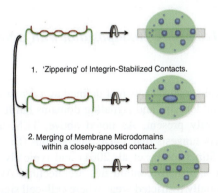

Fig. 1 Basic patterns of immune synapse. (**a**) Dynamic cellular assembly and disassembly. (**b**) Defined but flexible polarity. (**c**) Close membrane-membrane juxtaposition with a synaptic cleft. (**d**) Aggregation and segregation of transmembrane receptors and lipids

T cells, which are limited in numbers but must survey vast regions, it is clear that having multiple contacts may provide clear benefits in expanding the response to include multiple other cells.

3.2   Defined but Flexible Polarity

Synaptic cell–cell contacts allow cells to provide information in the form of signaling or killing events in a specific manner. Polarity of signals generated at cell–cell contacts as well as subsequent secretion into these contacts, then, represents a second highly conserved pattern of immune cell–cell interactions. As shown in Fig. 1b, this pattern permits cells to direct messages to one another while excluding bystanders. As an example, when T cells are engaging a cell presenting peptide–MHC complexes, it has been shown that CD40L is directly accumulated at the IS where it is available to crosslink CD40 (Boisvert et al. 2004). Notably, it has been proposed that this pattern is only true for some signals; vesicles containing γIFN appear to be more synapse localized while other secreted products such as TNF and chemokines may be more broadly directed (Huse et al. 2006). However, given the strict limitation of vesicle–membrane fusion that occurs, there may ultimately prove to be additional restrictions on these latter molecules. As noted above, this pattern provides exquisite spatial specificity for inter-cellular communication by immune cells.

CTL–target and NK–target interactions provide the simplest and most extreme rationale for highly directional secretion towards a particular cell. Such directionality prevents off-target killing of bystanders and restricts delivery of granules to the IS (Stinchcombe et al. 2001). At present, the full range of molecular players achieving this directional specificity are unknown but SNAREs and other proteins of the microtubule cytoskeleton are likely candidates.

3.3   Close Membrane–Membrane Juxtaposition with a Synaptic Cleft

The T cell–APC "immunological synapse" was first defined as a synapse by virtue of the presence of both adhesion domains and signaling domains but it seems that synaptic clefts are also frequently present. As noted above, TEM analysis of physiologically relevant contacts suggests that T–DC interactions (Brossard et al. 2005), CTL–Target contacts (Stinchcombe et al. 2001) and typically even T–B interactions (Krummel MF, unpublished) contain this architecture. As shown in Fig. 1c, there are frequently spatially restricted areas where cell–cell signaling may occur surrounded by membrane domains which may restrict direct membrane contact. The latter domains, however, sample synaptic spaces and provide a region for the accumulation of soluble mediators. Notably, the variable spacing of membranes around the closest point of apposition has been suggested to be important for protein organization in the IS (van der Merwe and Davis 2003; Shaw and Dustin 1997) and MHCs with variable length extracellular domains that result in altered capacities to signal (Choudhuri et al. 2005). However, some "large" molecules that are typically excluded, such as CD43, are not excluded on the basis of extracellular size alone, as tail-less forms can enter the central IS but do not interfere with signaling (Delon et al. 2001).

The presence of multiple domains in the membrane with different degrees of junctional "tightness" reflects variations in lipid composition as well as subcortical actin arrays. In this vein, although this exact architecture may be lacking in glass-supported approximations of cell–cell contacts, the generation of unique zones of membrane in the IS of such systems with differing lateral mobility for specific receptors has been observed in at least one such setting (Douglass and Vale 2005) and the presence of "rafts" (Anderson and Jacobson 2002) as well as protein "islands" in distinct regions (Lillemeier et al. 2006), also occurs at T cell–antigen-coated planar substrate junctions.

This architecture provides flexible regions for signaling receptors, but also regions into which vesicles may easily fuse and permits ongoing actin-organized signalosomes to persist in adjacent regions. While the receptors for cytokines are found in the IS (Maldonado et al. 2004) and cytokines are directed there (Huse et al. 2006; Reichert et al. 2001; Kupfer et al. 1994; Kupfer et al. 1991), the organization of these receptors relative to microclusters of TCRs or to the synaptic space has not been resolved. However, it is clear that regions of CTL granule release do not overlap with regions of TCR accumulation (Stinchcombe et al. 2001), suggesting that the TCR in the most tightly apposed regions of membrane are distinct from synaptic clefts.

3.4 Aggregation and Segregation of Transmembrane Receptors and Lipids

A final pattern that is established in all immunological synapses is the aggregation of receptor complexes and lipid domains (Fig. 1d). Based on observations of topology by TEM, there are likely two scales of clusters and at least two methods of cluster coalescence. Small, initial "micro" clusters likely provide for the formation of higher-ordering signaling arrays or "signalosomes." Clusters of TCRs likely provide a high avidity lattice to capture pMHC complexes on the outside of cells and trap signaling intermediates in their active state on the inside of the membrane. Consistent with this, it has been observed that early microclusters of TCRs are in fact highly enriched for tyrosine-phosphorylation (Varma et al. 2006; Mossman et al. 2005). At the far edges of the synapse, continuous membrane extension and retraction are commonly observed and, at the B–DC synapse, have been observed to be involved in accumulating new ligands for the BCR (Batista et al. 2001).

Distinct from these initial clusters are the centralized clusters, which are most likely, associated with internalization of receptor-complexes (Varma et al. 2006; Mossman et al. 2005). It remains unknown at this point whether coalescence into these larger domains is fundamentally required for internalization of the TCRs or simply occurs most efficiently there. Notably, other participants in signaling intermediates such as CD4 (Krummel et al. 2000) and CD28 (Yokosuka et al. 2008) border centralized TCRs but are not included in the central "cSMAC" (CD4) or segregated from TCR clusters in cSMAC (CD28), consistent with this being an area of less-intense or extinguished signaling.

An unresolved question in the field is the way in which these larger clusters form. As shown for T cells interacting with membranes with reduced lateral protein mobility, it is likely that the formation of these large clusters hastens termination of signaling (Mossman et al. 2005).To this end; the dynamics of coalescence of clusters may involve multiple mechanisms. On the one hand, flat lipid bilayers demonstrate that TCRs can move laterally along the membrane and in a centripetal manner (Varma et al. 2006; Mossman et al. 2005; Yokosuka et al. 2005). In contrast, cluster coalescence in T cell–B cell or NK–APC contacts present a much less concerted effect, although a centralized cSMAC is typically still formed (Krummel et al. 2000; Oddos et al. 2008).

One intriguing possibility, in the confines of a cell–cell interaction, is that multiple mechanisms may act to give the final aggregated structure. While, membrane movement and coalescence of micro clusters in the membrane may drive cluster aggregation within a give domain (Fig. 1d, *middle panel*), the joining of individual membrane–membrane contacts may also be necessary to reorganize contacts in a full synaptic membrane architecture ("zippering," Fig. 1d, *lower panel*).

Regardless, if signaling is amplified by the formation of initial clusters (Varma et al. 2006) but attenuated (Mossman et al. 2005), or, in other circumstances amplified (Cemerski et al. 2008) by cluster coalescence, the fact that membrane proteins move and membranes remodel provides the scaffold upon which the kinetics of signaling and direct sensing of peptide complexes is regulated. This pattern of clustering of receptors at interfaces is in fact conserved across all types of contacts observed between immune cells, and indeed in most cell–cell signaling contexts generally.

4 Four Fundamental Immunological Synapse Patterns Are Observed in the Interactions of Activating T Cells with One Another

So far, we have described immune synapses formed between two cells in which the raison d'etre of the synapse is most associated with priming or cytotoxicity in a specialized cell type (e.g., T cell, B cell, NK cell) by an APC or the functional equivalent. In fact, APC-mediated information transfer plays a central role in the mobilization of multiple arms of immune responses. Thus, it is not surprising that people have primarily focused on the communication between various types of immune cells and APCs. However, immune cell interactions in vivo occur in complex microenvironments where multiple cells dynamically migrate and interact on complicated networks of cells or extracellular matrixes (Bajenoff et al. 2006; Lindquist et al. 2004). It seems necessary, then, to begin to consider more complex multicellular interactions in order to fully understand how the immune system works. In this regard, direct observation of dynamics of immune cells under various immunological settings has been instrumental in revealing various modes of immune cell interactions that have not been fully appreciated before (Cahalan and Parker 2008; Germain et al. 2006).

Among activating T cells, our group and many others (Bajenoff et al. 2006; Sabatos et al. 2008; Hommel and Kyewski 2003; Ingulli et al. 1997; Miller et al. 2004; Bousso and Robey 2003; Tang et al. 2006; Garcia et al. 2007) have observed homotypic interactions (clusters) in antigen-specific T cells during priming in lymph nodes. Previously, homotypic clusters of T cells had been extensively observed as features of T-cell activation during in vitro culture assay, and indeed were shown to be physiologically mediated by LFA-1 (Rothlein et al. 1986; Rothlein and Springer 1986; van Kooyk et al. 1989). When observing these T-cell clusters by real-time methods in vitro and in vivo, not only were these clusters facilitated by integrin-based adhesion, but interactions in the clusters were dynamic, like those of initially contacting T–APC couples, with individual cells entering or leaving contacts with dwell times varying from minutes to hours (Sabatos et al. 2008). This provided evidence for the application of Pattern 1, in which individual T cells may visit one another for directed information exchange. As to other comparisons with the exact topological organization of the T–APC IS, it remains unclear at present whether LFA-1 alone is responsible for the contacts or whether other adhesion receptors may contribute and, indeed, dominate in the later phase. On the whole, it is also unclear at present how specificity is maintained beyond the combined effects of affinity upregulation of LFA-1 (Dustin et al. 1997) and increased expression of intercellular adhesion molecule-1 (ICAM-1) (Tohma et al. 1992) induced by TCR signaling. Nonetheless, the transient stability pattern appears to provide specificity, as unactivated T cells did not participate in these multicellular clusters and had short interaction times (typically less than 1 min) during encounters in vivo (Sabatos et al. 2008).

APCs are not strictly necessary for the transient nucleation of T-cell clusters; T cells stimulated by anti-CD3/CD28 or phorbol 12-myristate 13-acetate (PMA)/ionomycin formed similarly arrayed and dynamic multicellular clusters. This was apparently borne out by observations of T–T contacts distal to DC cell bodies, giving rise to the model for these interactions shown in Fig. 2. However, given the density of the DC network in lymph nodes (Lindquist et al. 2004), it is impossible to say with certainty that DC contacts were not occurring.

In addition to "transient stability" (Pattern 1), further characterization of cell–cell interfaces in the T-cell aggregates revealed that this emerging cell–cell contact

Fig. 2 A model of homotypic
cluster formation of
activating T cells during
in vivo priming. Naïve T cells
are activated by antigen
presenting dendritic cells
after several hours of stable
interactions. Then, they
regain motility, but swarm
around their priming sites
rather than migrate away.
During this dynamic
swarming phase, they form
dynamic homotypic clusters

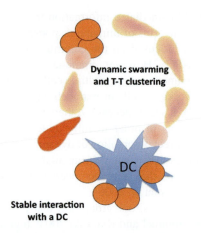

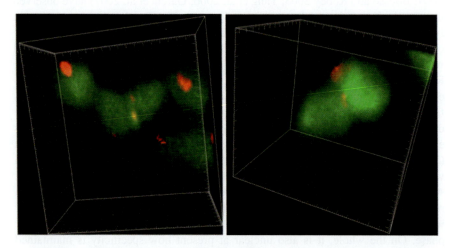

Fig. 3 MTOC polarization toward T-cell synapse in vivo. *Green*: OT-II T cell, *red*: pericentrin.
CFSE-labeled OT-II T cells were injected to C57BL/6 mice, and subsequently immunized with
ovalbumin protein emulsified in complete Freund's adjuvalent. Draining lymph nodes were
isolated 20 h after immunization, embedded in optimal cutting temperature compound, and frozen
under liquid nitrogen. The frozen lymph nodes were sectioned by a cryostat with 80 μm thick and
pericentrin was stained fluorophore-conjugated antibodies. Images of pericentrin-stained lymph
node sections were acquired using confocal microscope and processed by Imaris

region matches each of the other communication patterns described in Chap. 3.
This includes the observation that secretory vesicles of T cells are frequently
polarized toward neighboring T cells, indicating directed secretion of soluble
factors between two adjacent T cells (Pattern 2). More in-depth assessment of
cell polarity demonstrated pronounced polarization of pericentrin, an MTOC associated protein, toward adjacent activating T cells. We have also been able to detect
this polarized pericentrin localization in T cells activating directly in the lymph
node (Fig. 3) although we've only isolated these with low frequency due to

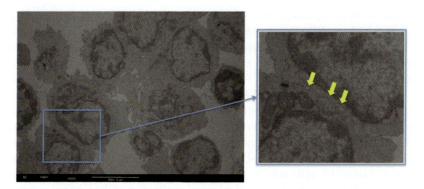

Fig. 4 Ultrastructure of T–T synapses. BALB/c wild type T cells were stimulated by PMA/ionomycin for 18 h, and their clusters were analyzed by transmission electron microscopy

technical limitations of tissue section staining. Along with secretory vesicle polarization shown by TEM, this indicates directional secretion of soluble factors from one cell to another cell through the synaptic space. Extending this to specific cytokines, we demonstrated that polarized vesicles near T–T interfaces contained interlukin-2, a cytokine produced by T cells during the early phase of activation and plays a critical role in T-cell activation, proliferation, differentiation, survival, and even apoptosis (Gaffen and Liu 2004; Kim et al. 2006).

Membrane ultrastructures of interfaces formed between activating T cells analyzed by TEM also exhibited canonical synaptic structure (Pattern 3); tight membrane apposition of two adjacent T cells with multiple clefts, similar to the multifocal synapse structure formed between naïve CD4+ T cells and dendritic cells (Brossard et al. 2005) and that between CTL and targets (Stinchcombe et al. 2001) or NK and their APC (McCann et al. 2003) (Fig. 4). Also, we were able to use "catch" reagents to localize the sites of uptake of T cell secreted IL-2. This demonstrated that IL-2 was indeed directed across and accumulated in these synaptic gaps in the catch assay. Notably, directional secretion of IL-2 is beneficial for T cells in the clusters in IL-2 reception compared with isolated T cells, due to the higher local IL-2 concentration at the synaptic junction – both in terms of the amount of IL-2 accumulated and in terms of the "focusing" of the cytokine into apparent "patches" within the cell–cell contact.

Finally, consistent with the application of Pattern 4, we demonstrated the formation of signaling complexes of IL-2 receptors at the T–T synapses; Intracellular pools of IL-2, IL-2 receptors (IL-2Rs), and signaling components of IL-2R accumulated near the interfaces formed between activating T cells.

Additionally, the synaptic structure appears to alter signaling in a fundamental way for IL-2 signaling. IL-2 binding to IL-2R induces phosphorylation of STAT-5 by Janus kinase 1 (JAK1) and JAK3 which are associated with β and γ subunits of IL-2 receptor, respectively (Lin and Leonard 2000). Phosphorylated STAT-5 (pSTAT-5) is known to dimerize and subsequently translocate to the nucleus for the transcription of target genes. We fluorescently stained pSTAT-5 to measure the strength of IL-2 signaling, and substantial amounts of T cells in the clusters exhibited higher pSTAT-5 staining than isolated T cells, indicating enhanced IL-2 signaling in the T-cell clusters. Interestingly, pSTAT-5 localized near interfaces of cell–cell contact as well as nuclei, and staining of pSTAT-5 near synaptic junctions revealed bright puncta. When overlaid with intracellular pools of IL-2 by dual staining, the majority of pSTAT-5 puncta were either co-localized or adjacent to IL-2 staining of neighboring cells, suggesting that pSTAT-5 accumulation near synaptic region was a result of directional IL-2 secretion. This observation agrees well with the finding that IL-2 signaling during anti-viral CD4+ priming was mostly paracrine, not autocrine (Long and Adler 2006), and indeed synaptic spaces formed between activated T cells may be the place where IL-2 paracrine delivery occurs.

Together, this provides a newly discovered application of the synapse patterns in activating T cells, following TCR stimulation. Unlike the more prototypical (T-APC, B-DC, NK-Target) examples involved in the initial priming of the cells by antigen–receptor ligand bearing cells, it suggests a specialized platform for cytokine mediated interactions.

5 Signaling Implication of T–T contacts for IL-2 Receptor Structure and Function

What does the discovery of "synaptic T–T IL-2 signaling" in particular contribute to our understanding of this cytokine and its function? It is clear from multiple studies that IL-2 can be added "in solution" and will function this way (Laurence et al. 2007; Liao et al. 2008), suggesting that it is not technically necessary that the secretion starts out being directional. Then, is it possible that there are major differences between cytokine signaling via synaptic junction and cytokine signaling by the binding of cytokines from the bulk? It is straightforward to imagine the enhancement of cytokine signaling via directed secretion of cytokines and polarization of cytokine receptors to the synaptic region by increasing local concentration of cytokines. In fact, that was the case when the local cytokine level was measured by cell-based IL-2 capture assay, and cytokine signaling strength was measured by the level of phosphorylation of STAT-5 (Sabatos et al. 2008). Also, through synaptic secretion and uptake, the majority of cytokines secreted by one cell would be captured by the other cell and little cytokine would be released outside of the synaptic space, resulting in increased specificity/efficiency on a per-molecule basis. However, the functional significance of this array may extend beyond this simple "efficiency" aspect and is indicated, as discussed in the observation of phosphorylated STAT-5 on the membrane in addition to within the nucleus, the latter being the prevailing result from experiments using soluble cytokines. To understand this, it is necessary to review the known mechanisms of IL-2 receptor signaling.

IL-2 receptor is composed of three distinct polypeptide chain subunits; IL-2Rα (CD25), IL-2Rβ (CD122, also IL-15Rβ), and common γc (CD132, also a signaling receptor of many other cytokines such as IL-4, IL-7, IL-9, IL-15, and IL-27) (Waldmann 2006). Combinations of three subunits constitute receptors with three different affinities; low affinity receptor IL-2Rα (K_d ~ 10 nM), intermediate affinity heterodimeric receptor IL-2Rβγc (K_d ~ 1 nM), and high affinity heterotrimeric receptor IL-2Rαβγc (K_d ~ 10 pM) (Gaffen and Liu 2004; Kim et al. 2006). IL-2Rα is significantly upregulated upon activation, to at least an order of magnitude higher than the expression level of IL-2Rβγc (Robb et al. 1987), and has very short cytoplasmic domain. Thus, it is suggested that the main role of IL-2Rα is to enhance cytokine binding by forming high affinity heterotrimeric receptors with IL-2Rβγc, or by first capturing IL-2 from the extracellular environment, due to its high abundance and fast on-rate, and subsequently forming a heterotrimeric receptor with IL-2Rβγc (Stauber et al. 2006; Wang et al. 2005). IL-2Rβ and γc are members of type I cytokine receptor super family and play a central role in IL-2 signaling (Gaffen 2001). Cytokine binding to IL-2Rβγc triggers phosphorylation of the receptor and JAK1 and JAK3, which are associated with the cytoplasmic tails of IL-2Rβ and γc, respectively. Phosphorylation of the receptor induces the association of STAT-5, a key transcription factor of IL-2 signaling, with the phosphorylated receptor and subsequent phosphorylation of STAT-5. Then, pSTAT-5 dissociates from the receptor, dimerizes, and translocates to the nucleus to activate multiple genes. At T–T junctions, when the three polypeptide chains of IL-2 receptors were stained, distinct patterns of receptor distribution were observed; IL-2Rα distribution was mostly uniform, while substantial local enrichment of γc in synaptic regions was frequently observed. (IL-2Rβ staining was too dim to be detected.) This, a priori, suggests a variable stoichiometry of the three-chains across the cell–cell interface; as mentioned above, expression level of IL-2Rα is at least ten-fold higher than that of IL-2Rβγc.

Under what conditions of receptor–ligand occupancy might this result be explained? It could just reflect the local accumulation of trimeric IL-2R near synaptic interfaces and enhanced paracrine signaling of IL-2 as a result (upper panel of Fig. 5). However, one interesting possibility is that IL-2 captured by one T cell's IL-2Rα may interact with IL-2Rβγc of another T cell through a T–T synapse (middle panel of Fig. 5). This type of cytokine transpresentation has been well documented for IL-15, a cytokine with significant similarities to IL-2; IL-15 bound to the IL-15Rα (K_d ~ 10 pM) of monocytes or dendritic cells can trigger signaling to NK cells or CD8+ memory T cells, which constitutively express IL-15Rβγc (Dubois et al. 2002). Given the structural similarity of IL-2Rα and IL-15Rα, IL-2Rα also can present receptor-bound IL-2 to neighboring cells (Chirifu et al. 2007). Indeed there is evidence that IL-2 transpresentation occurs between IL-2Rα expressing cells and IL-2Rβγc expressing cells (Eicher and Waldmann 1998). Since the binding affinity of IL-2 for IL-2Rα is about 1,000-fold lower than the binding affinity of IL-15 for IL-15Rα, IL-2 transpresentation might require specialized synaptic junctions such as T–T synapses.

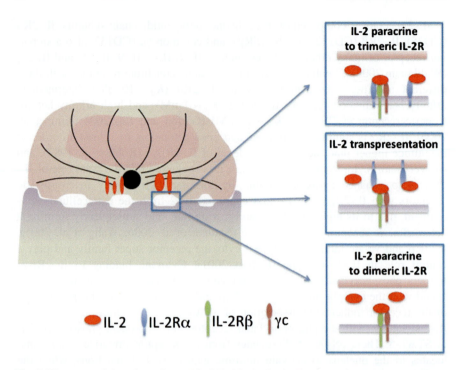

Fig. 5 Three potential configurations of IL-2/IL-2R binding at T–T synaptic junction. IL-2 directionally secreted to the synapses formed between activating T cells can be bound to the heterotrimeric receptor IL-2Rαβγc (*upper*), or be bound first by IL-2Rα of one T cell and subsequently presented to the other T cell (*middle*), or be bound to the heterodimeric receptor IL-2Rβγc and trigger receptor signaling in the absence of IL-2Rα (*lower*)

IL-2 bound to IL-2Rαβγc was shown to be subsequently internalized and degraded with IL-2Rβγc, while IL-2Rα is dissociated from quaternary complexes in endosomes and recycled to cell surfaces (Hemar et al. 1995). If an IL-2 molecule bound to IL-2Rα of one cell can interact with IL-2Rβγc on the other cell, the duration of IL-2 signaling by the IL-2Rβγc expressing cell might be substantially extended by the suppression of receptor internalization and degradation. Therefore, local accumulation of pSTAT-5 near the synaptic junction may be an evidence of extended duration of IL-2 signaling by transpresentation of IL-2.

Additionally, IL-2 transpresentation may be beneficial to "less"-activated T cells with lower IL-2Rα expression than adjacent "more"-activated T cells that can transpresent IL-2. In this way, successfully activated T cells may assist new clones which arrive at the priming site later, or have weaker TCR affinity, or are specific to less abundant foreign antigens. As a result, diversity of TCR repertoire against foreign pathogens can be increased and immune evasion by mutation or antigen presentation disruption can be minimized.

Transpresentation of IL-2 may not be necessary for cooperation among activating T cells, though. Directionally secreted IL-2 to synaptic spaces could directly bind intermediate affinity receptor IL-2Rβγc and signal through IL-2Rβγc without binding IL-2Rα (lower panel of Fig. 5). Again, this is beneficial for T cells with low expression levels of IL-2Rα. It is important to note that under model antigen ovalbumin immunization, the activating clusters of T cells were mostly composed of antigen specific transgenic T cells and participation of wild type T cells in the clusters was minimal. This indicates that T-cell synapses would not assist activation of antigen non-specific T cells (Sabatos et al. 2008).

Finally, we note that many receptor–ligand pairs are engaged at the synaptic junction formed between activating T cells. One example is the interaction of LFA-1 with ICAM-1 and ICAM-2, which plays a critical role in the formation and maintenance of the synapse, but may also trigger some signaling to T cells. It is possible that T–T synapses may mediate crosstalk between IL-2R signaling and other receptor signaling pathways by promoting various receptor–ligand interactions.

6   Additional Roles of T–T Synaptic Contact

In the previous chapters, we described a novel immune synapse formed between activating CD4+ T cells, mostly at the molecular and cellular levels. In this chapter, we will discuss further the potential roles of T–T synapses in modulating immune responses under various physiological circumstances. Also, we will extend the discussion of T–T synapses from homotypic clusters of activating CD4+ T cells to multicellular clusters composed of multiple subsets of T cells.

6.1   *Physiological Circumstances of T-Cell Cluster Formation and Its Role in Secondary Responses*

Only tiny fractions of T cells recognize antigens from a specific pathogen. Therefore, if all the T cells in the lymph node are randomly migrating in search of antigens, the possibility of multiple activating T cells intermingling within the same lymph node would be extremely low. However, it has been recently shown that in inflamed lymph nodes, when T cells (either CD4+ or CD8+) recognize DCs presenting their target antigens, both T cells and DCs secrete chemokiness CCL3 and CCL4 to recruit CCR5 expressing T cells (Castellino et al. 2006; Hugues et al. 2007). This chemokine driven migration of activating T cells might enable multicellular cluster formation of activating T cells, even low physiological precursor frequencies.

CCL3/CCL4 secreted by activating T cells can recruit both CD4+ and CD8+ T cells. Thus, activating CD4+ T cells and CD8+ T cells may intermingle via synaptic interactions. Synaptic delivery of IL-2 during priming of CD8+ T cells could drive then IL-2 paracrine signaling critical for the expansion of CD8+ memory T cell upon secondary challenge (Williams et al. 2006).

Increases in precursor frequencies would also increase the probability of synaptic T–T interactions; memory responses and alloreactive T-cell activation leading to transplantation rejection are two examples of physiological high precursor frequencies. In fact, substantial clustering of memory T cells in lymph nodes was observed during the secondary challenge of lymphocytic choriomeningitis virus (R.S. Friedman, J. Hu, M.F.K., and M. Mattloubian). The clusters we observed may ultimately play a more prominent role once precursor levels are higher or in response to pathogens that stimulate a large fraction of T cells in the primary activation.

6.2   "Quorum Sensing" by the Immune System for Activation and Differentiation of the Effectors

Can information sharing across a synaptic junction confer the capacity for quorum decision making in populations of T cells, such that the response ultimately focuses on the correct response? Even under identical stimulation conditions, cytokine secretion profiles at the single cell level are quite diverse, and typically only a subpopulation of T cells produces certain cytokines. A detailed mechanism or exact reason for this heterogeneity is not clear yet, but the heterogeneity of activating T cells may require their cooperation for optimal activation and differentiation by sharing resources. IL-2 is indeed a critical factor for survival, proliferation, and differentiation of T cells, whose mRNA transcription occurs in only subpopulation of activating T cells (Saparov et al. 1999). If collaboration is necessary, there might be a "critical number" of T cells for full activation and differentiation, something akin to bacterial "quorum sensing." There are evidences that increases in precursor frequencies may inhibit full activation and differentiation of T cells due to the internal competition among T cells for the acquisition of limited amount of resources in vivo (Bar et al. 2008; Hataye et al. 2006). These results appear to contradict our "quorum sensing" hypothesis, but it can be reconciled if there are "optimal" ranges of initial precursor frequencies – below which T cells are poorly activated due to lack of cooperation, and above which T cells are poorly activated due to internal competition. Alternatively, clonal competition may occur among identical clones or clones specific against identical epitopes, while cooperativity among T cells may take place among activating T cells specific for different epitopes from identical pathogens.

6.3   Polarization of Helper T-Cell Differentiation via Synaptic Cytokine Sharing

CD4+ helper T cells differentiate into various subsets of effectors depending on the cytokine milieu they are exposed to for the effective clearance of diverse pathogens

(Constant and Bottomly 1997; Bettelli et al. 2008). Key cytokines for Th differentiation and their genetic regulation have been extensively studied, but how those cytokines coordinate the differentiation of T cells in vivo has still remained elusive. We propose that immune synapses formed between T cells serve as platforms to spread differentiated phenotypes of effector T cells by directional secretion of key cytokines. It has been shown that some cytokines critical for Th skewing such as IL-2, γIFN, and IL-10 are directionally secreted (Huse et al. 2006), and some of their receptors are also polarized toward the immune synapses (Maldonado et al. 2004), suggesting that synaptic secretion of those cytokines via T–T synapse may happen, and indeed may play a critical role in the propagation of phenotypes of already polarized T cells participating in the synapses. However, IL-4, a critical cytokine for Th2 differentiation and also for differentiation of T cells to a newly discovered IL-9- and IL-10-producing subset (Dardalhon et al. 2008; Veldhoen et al. 2008), is secreted multidirectionally. Additionally, many pro- and anti-inflammatory cytokines critical for Th differentiation and reprogramming at the periphery are not, or may not be delivered directionally. Therefore, it is likely that combinations of synaptic and non-synaptic secretion of cytokines would guide proper differentiation of activating and activated T cells depending on the circumstances.

6.4   T–T Interactions during the Cessation of the Immune Response: The Facilitation of Fas/TNF Interactions Leading to Apoptosis?

Immune synapses formed, even transiently, between T cells may also down-modulate the response by facilitating engagements of TNF-receptor family members, inducing apoptosis to each other. It is well-established that cell–cell contacts by activating T cells can lead to activation-induced cell death (AICD) (Lenardo 1991), frequently via Fas/FasL or TNF receptor engagements (Sytwu et al. 1996). It is thus tempting to speculate that the pattern we have observed for T–T engagements both in vitro and in vivo will play regulatory roles in permitting or facilitating the down regulation of the response by this mechanism. To this end, it is worth noting that synaptic contacts have been shown to recruit other TNF-family-member transmembrane proteins to the T–APC synapse (Boisvert et al. 2004).

6.5   Treg Exclusion in T–T Contacts

It was recently reported that regulatory T cells take up IL-2 more rapidly than activating T cells even though their IL-2Rα expression levels are comparable (Pandiyan et al. 2007). Since IL-2 is a critical survival factor for activating T cells, IL-2 deprivation in activating CD4+ T cells due to rapid IL-2 uptake by

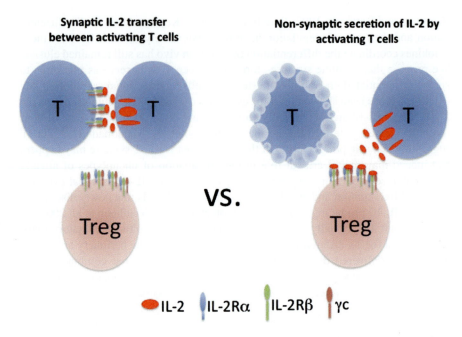

Fig. 6 Effect of synaptic secretion of IL-2 on IL-2 dependent survival of activating T cells. If IL-2 is secreted via synaptic interface, it will be successfully transferred to the neighboring activating T cells (*left*). In contrast, if IL-2 is secreted in non-synaptic manner, most of IL-2 secreted to the bulk will be taken up by adjacent Tregs, and neighboring T cells may undergo apoptosis due to the starvation of IL-2 (*right*)

adjacent Treg may cause the death of activating T cells. Synaptic secretion of IL-2 among activating CD4+ T cells may be important in situations where activating T cells and regulatory T cells compete for limited amount of IL-2 (Fig. 6). If combined with the recently reported negative feedback regulation of IL-2 secretion (Villarino et al. 2007), synaptic secretion of IL-2 in multicellular clusters of activating T cells may allow for optimal secretion of IL-2 "just enough" for T cells in the clusters, so that IL-2 uptake/signaling by neighboring Treg may be minimal. According to our observation, regulatory T cells make only transient contact with CD4+ T cells during priming in lymph nodes, indicating that regulatory T cells will not take part in multicellular clusters of activating T cells (Tang et al. 2006).

7   Creating System-Wide Decisions Through Collective and Spatiotemporal Information Sharing

It should be clear from the discussion of the application of synapse patterns at T–T junctions that such contacts are not neutral for the functioning of the immune response. In the case of the T–T junction, we have discussed numerous implications of the pattern for the outcome of the T-cell response. These can be summarized by the following criteria that would seem critical for the integrity of the immune system.

7.1 Cell-Based Vectorial Spreading of Information

High motility between contact formations allows the immune system to use individual immune cells as "vectors" to carry information from one contact to another. Modifications to the cells' signaling potential from one contact is thus purveyed, possibly over a great distance, and transmitted as a secretory or transmembrane signal, at the next.

7.2 Selection of a System of Appropriate Cell Types

Implicit in Pattern 2 is the idea that a given cell may choose to secrete only into a single cell at any one time. This also implies that it is capable of choosing the "type" of cell (APC, T, NK, Macrophage, etc.) into which it will secrete. Thus, a wide variety of synapse opportunities permits the activated cell to discriminate and activate specific cell types.

7.3 A Very Steep Gradient of Cues at Each Encounter Point

Pattern 3 dictates a very steep gradient of the most important cues surrounding activated cells. While some secreted molecules might "spill" from the synaptic space, the concentration would be dramatically higher in the inter-cellular clefts. In this light it is interesting that chemokines, which attract cells to a region, appear not to follow Pattern 2 (i.e., may be non-directionally secreted). However, the ultimate ability of each attracted cell to reap signaling benefits from following a chemokine cue is still maintained, possibly by selection for the dwell-time in contacts once contact is achieved. By analogy to the single Herald of Aristotle, it is as if non-citizens (cells) can still hear the herald but only citizens have the right to vote (to make a substantial synapse bearing the features of Patterns 2–4).

7.4 Repeated Selection for Specificity and Mutual Enhancement

Since each T, NK, or B cell that moves and re-engages has already been selected for its recognition of foreign antigen, it transmits to each APC or target a signal that corresponds to the strength of the signal. Thus, T cells are not only first activated based on their ability to recognize the pMHC complex alongside the arsenal of costimulatory signals that a local APC may provide – it also carries along the ability to retransmit the degree of stimulation to APCs based on their ability to interact. In the case of secondary T–APC contacts, this may again rely on the presence of pMHC complexes on the second APC to influence the synapse duration and therefore the accumulation of focal signaling clusters (Pattern 4). In the case of T–T contacts, more primordial "activation" may serve as the basis of mutual adhesion and lead to specific transmission of information to cells bearing appropriate cell-surface signatures. This permits enhancement of the response over a period of time while selecting against cells whose specificity for the insult is not as significant.

8   Concluding Remarks

Two final notes bear stating. Firstly, these patterns are malleable with regard to microenvironment. Some parts of the patterns may be inhibited by prevailing conditions – for example the tumor microenvironment could allow contact surfaces while preventing polarization of secretion (Allows patterns 1, 3, and 4 while inhibiting 2). Secondly, to understand the building blocks and their implications is to be able to consider therapeutics. It may be that successful particle-based therapeutics may be designed to "seed" synapses of various kinds and for various stages of cell activation.

Therefore, it is the quality of these interactions that actually defines the efficacy of the system as a whole. In the case of human beings, the quality of interactions defines the growth and prosperity of the human community; destructive interactions lead to erosion of structure and the social fabric whereas positive interactions lead to cooperative growth and prosperity. In the case of the immune system, the quality of cell–cell interactions defines the successful survival of the larger organism in a world crowded with parasites and pathogens.

Acknowledgments JD was supported by the Korea Science and Engineering Foundation (KOSEF) NCRC grant funded by the Korea government (MEST) (No. R15-2004-033-06002-0) and a grant of the Korea Healthcare technology R&D Project, Ministry for Health, Welfare and Family Affairs, Republic of Korea (Grant No. A084147). MFK was supported by funding from the Sandler family fund, the JDRF and the Leukemia and Lymphoma Society. We thank Peter Beemiller for the critical reading, and Miju Kim for assistance with graphics.

References

Alexander C, Ishikawa S, Silverstein M (1977) A pattern language: towns, buildings, construction. Oxford University Press, New York

Anderson RGW, Jacobson K (2002) Cell biology – a role for lipid shells in targeting proteins to caveolae, rafts, and other lipid domains. Science 296(5574):1821–1825

Bajenoff M et al (2006) Stromal cell networks regulate lymphocyte entry, migration, and territoriality in lymph nodes. Immunity 25(6):989–1001

Bar JJ, Khanna KM, Lefrancois L (2008) Endogenous naive CD8(+) T cell precursor frequency regulates primary and memory responses to infection. Immunity 28(6):859–869

Batista FD, Iber D, Neuberger MS (2001) B cells acquire antigen from target cells after synapse formation. Nature 411(6836):489–494

Bettelli E et al (2008) Induction and effector functions of T(H)17 cells. Nature 453 (7198):1051–1057

Boisvert J, Edmondson S, Krummel MF (2004) Immunological synapse formation licenses CD40-CD40L accumulations at T-APC contact sites. J Immunol 173(6):3647–3652

Bousso P, Robey E (2003) Dynamics of CD8(+) T cell priming by dendritic cells in intact lymph nodes. Nat Immunol 4(6):579–585

Brossard C et al (2005) Multifocal structure of the T cell – dendritic cell synapse. Eur J Immunol 35(6):1741–1753

Cahalan MD, Parker I (2008) Choreography of cell motility and interaction dynamics imaged by two-photon microscopy in lymphoid organs. Annu Rev Immunol 26:585–626

Campi G, Varma R, Dustin ML (2005) Actin and agonist MHC-peptide complex-dependent T cell receptor microclusters as scaffolds for signaling. J Exp Med 202(8):1031–1036

Castellino F et al (2006) Chemokines enhance immunity by guiding naive CD8(+) T cells to sites of CD4 T cell-dendritic cell interaction. Nature 440(7086):890–895

Celli S, Lemaitre F, Bousso P (2007) Real-time manipulation of T cell-dendritic cell interactions in vivo reveals the importance of prolonged contacts for CD4(+) T cell activation. Immunity 27 (4):625–634

Cemerski S et al (2008) The balance between T cell receptor signaling and degradation at the center of the immunological synapse is determined by antigen quality. Immunity 29 (3):414–422

Chirifu M et al (2007) Crystal structure of the IL-15-IL-15R alpha complex, a cytokine-receptor unit presented in trans. Nat Immunol 8(9):1001–1007

Choudhuri K et al (2005) T-cell receptor triggering is critically dependent on the dimensions of its peptide-MHC ligand. Nature 436(7050):578–582

Constant SL, Bottomly K (1997) Induction of TH1 and TH2 CD4+ T cell responses: the alternative approaches. Annu Rev Immunol 15:297–322

Dardalhon V et al (2008) IL-4 inhibits TGF-beta-induced Foxp3(+) T cells and, together with TGF-beta, generates IL-9(+) IL-10(+) Foxp3(-) effector T cells. Nat Immunol 9 (12):1347–1355

Delon J, Kaibuchi K, Germain RN (2001) Exclusion of CD43 from the immunological synapse is mediated by phosphorylation-regulated relocation of the cytoskeletal adaptor moesin. Immunity 15(5):691–701

DeMond AL et al (2006) Control of antigen presentation with a photoreleasable agonist peptide. J Am Chem Soc 128(48):15354–15355

Depoil D et al (2005) Immunological synapses are versatile structures enabling selective T cell polarization. Immunity 22(2):185–194

Douglass AD, Vale RD (2005) Single-molecule microscopy reveals plasma membrane microdomains created by protein-protein networks that exclude or trap signaling molecules in T cells. Cell 121(6):937–950

Dubois S et al (2002) IL-15R alpha recycles and presents IL-15 in trans to neighboring cells. Immunity 17(5):537–547

Dustin ML, Colman DR (2002) Neural and immunological synaptic relations. Science 298 (5594):785–789

Dustin ML et al (1997) Antigen receptor engagement delivers a stop signal to migrating T lymphocytes. Proc Natl Acad Sci USA 94(8):3909–3913

Dustin ML et al (1998) A novel adaptor protein orchestrates receptor patterning and cytoskeletal polarity in T-cell contacts. Cell 94(5):667–677

Dustin ML et al (2006) T cell-dendritic cell immunological synapses. Curr Opin Immunol 18 (4):512–516

Eicher DM, Waldmann TA (1998) IL-2R alpha on one cell can present IL-2 to IL-2R beta/gamma (c) on another cell to augment IL-2 signaling. J Immunol 161(10):5430–5437

Faroudi M et al (2003) Cutting edge: T lymphocyte activation by repeated immunological synapse formation and intermittent signaling. J Immunol 171(3):1128–1132

Gaffen SL (2001) Signaling domains of the interleukin 2 receptor. Cytokine 14(2):63–77

Gaffen SL, Liu KD (2004) Overview of interleukin-2 function, production and clinical applications. Cytokine 28(3):109–123

Garcia Z et al (2007) Competition for antigen determines the stability of T cell-dendritic cell interactions during clonal expansion. Proc Natl Acad Sci USA 104(11):4553–4558

Germain RN et al (2006) Dynamic imaging of the immune system: progress, pitfalls and promise. Nat Rev Immunol 6(7):497–507

Grakoui A et al (1999) The immunological synapse: a molecular machine controlling T cell activation. Science 285(5425):221–227

Gunzer M et al (2000) Antigen presentation in extracellular matrix: interactions of T cells with dendritic cells are dynamic, short lived, and sequential. Immunity 13(3):323–332

Hataye J et al (2006) Naive and memory CD4(+) T cell survival controlled by clonal abundance. Science 312(5770):114–116

Hemar A et al (1995) Endocytosis of interleukin-2 receptors in human T-lymphocytes – distinct intracellular-localization and fate of the receptor alpha-chain, beta-chain, and gamma-chain. J Cell Biol 129(1):55–64

Henrickson SE et al (2008) T cell sensing of antigen dose governs interactive behavior with dendritic cells and sets a threshold for T cell activation. Nat Immunol 9(3):282–291

Hommel M, Kyewski B (2003) Dynamic changes during the immune response in T cell-antigen-presenting cell clusters isolated from lymph nodes. J Exp Med 197(3):269–280

Hugues S et al (2007) Dynamic imaging of chemokine-dependent CD8(+) T cell help for CD8(+) T cell responses. Nat Immunol 8(9):921–930

Hurez V et al (2003) Restricted clonal expression of IL-2 by naive T cells reflects differential dynamic interactions with dendritic cells. J Exp Med 198(1):123–132

Huse M et al (2006) T cells use two directionally distinct pathways for cytokine secretion. Nat Immunol 7(3):247–255

Huse M et al (2007) Spatial and temporal dynamics of T cell receptor signaling with a photo-activatable agonist. Immunity 27(1):76–88

Ingulli E et al (1997) In vivo detection of dendritic cell antigen presentation to CD4(+) T cells. J Exp Med 185(12):2133–2141

Kim HP, Imbert J, Leonard WJ (2006) Both integrated and differential regulation of components of the IL-2/IL-2 receptor system. Cytokine Growth Factor Rev 17(5):349–366

Krummel MF et al (2000) Differential clustering of CD4 and CD3 zeta during T cell recognition. Science 289(5483):1349–1352

Kupfer A, Mosmann TR, Kupfer H (1991) Polarized expression of cytokines in cell conjugates of helper T cells and splenic B cells. Proc Natl Acad Sci USA 88(3):775–779

Kupfer H, Monks CR, Kupfer A (1994) Small splenic B cells that bind to antigen-specific T helper (Th) cells and face the site of cytokine production in the Th cells selectively proliferate: immunofluorescence microscopic studies of Th-B antigen-presenting cell interactions. J Exp Med 179(5):1507–1515

Laurence A et al (2007) Interleukin-2 signaling via STAT5 constrains T helper 17 cell generation. Immunity 26(3):371–381

Lee KH et al (2002) T cell receptor signaling precedes immunological synapse formation. Science 295(5559):1539–1542

Lenardo MJ (1991) Interleukin-2 programs mouse alpha-beta-lymphocytes-T for apoptosis. Nature 353(6347):858–861

Liao W et al (2008) Priming for T helper type 2 differentiation by interleukin 2-mediated induction of interleukin 4 receptor alpha-chain expression. Nat Immunol 9(11):1288–1296

Lillemeier BF et al (2006) Plasma membrane-associated proteins are clustered into islands attached to the cytoskeleton. Proc Natl Acad Sci USA 103(50):18992–18997

Lin JX, Leonard WJ (2000) The role of Stat5a and Stat5b in signaling by IL-2 family cytokines. Oncogene 19(21):2566–2576

Lindquist RL et al (2004) Visualizing dendritic cell networks in vivo. Nat Immunol 5 (12):1243–1250

Long MX, Adler AJ (2006) Cutting edge: paracrine, but not autocrine, IL-2 signaling is sustained during early antliviiral. CD4 T cell response. J Immunol 177(7):4257–4261

Maldonado RA et al (2004) A role for the immunological synapse in lineage commitment of CD4 lymphocytes. Nature 431(7008):527–532

McCann FE et al (2003) The size of the synaptic cleft and distinct distributions of filamentous actin, ezrin, CD43, and CD45 at activating and inhibitory human NK cell immune synapses. J Immunol 170(6):2862–2870

Mempel TR, Henrickson SE, von Andrian UH (2004) T-cell priming by dendritic cells in lymph nodes occurs in three distinct phases. Nature 427(6970):154–159

Miller MJ et al (2004) Imaging the single cell dynamics of CD4(+) T cell activation by dendritic cells in lymph nodes. J Exp Med 200(7):847–856

Monks CRF et al (1998) Three-dimensional segregation of supramolecular activation clusters in T cells. Nature 395(6697):82–86

Mossman KD et al (2005) Altered TCR signaling from geometrically repatterned immunological synapses. Science 310(5751):1191–1193

Norcross MA (1984) A synaptic basis for T-lymphocyte activation. Ann Immunol (Paris) 135D:113–134

Oddos S et al (2008) High-speed high-resolution imaging of intercellular immune synapses using optical tweezers. Biophys J 95:L66–L68

Pandiyan P et al (2007) CD4(+) CD25(+) Foxp3(+) regulatory T cells induce cytokine deprivation-mediated apoptosis of effector CD4(+) T cells. Nat Immunol 8(12):1353–1362

Purbhoo MA et al (2004) T cell killing does not require the formation of a stable mature immunological synapse. Nat Immunol 5(5):524–530

Reichert P et al (2001) Cutting edge: in vivo identification of TCR redistribution and polarized IL-2 production by naive CD4 T cells. J Immunol 166(7):4278–4281

Rittirsch D, Flierl MA, Ward PA (2008) Harmful molecular mechanisms in sepsis. Nat Rev Immunol 8(10):776–787

Robb RJ et al (1987) Interleukin 2 binding molecule distinct from the Tac protein: analysis of its role in formation of high-affinity receptors. Proc Natl Acad Sci USA 84:2002–2006

Rothlein R, Springer TA (1986) The requirement for lymphocyte function-associated antigen 1 in homotypic leukocyte adhesion stimulated by phorbol ester. J Immunol 163(5):1132–1149

Rothlein R et al (1986) A human intercellular adhesion molecule (ICAM-1) distinct from LFA-1. J Immunol 137(4):1270–1274

Sabatos CA et al (2008) A synaptic basis for paracrine interleukin-2 signaling during homotypic T cell interaction. Immunity 29(2):238–248

Saparov A et al (1999) Interleukin-2 expression by a subpopulation of primary T cells is linked to enhanced memory/effector function. Immunity 11(3):271–280

Scholer A et al (2008) Intercellular adhesion molecule-1-dependent stable interactions between T cells and dendritic cells determine CD8(+) T cell memory. Immunity 28(2):258–270

Shaw AS, Dustin ML (1997) Making the T cell receptor go the distance: a topological view of T cell activation. Immunity 6(4):361–369

Sims TN et al (2007) Opposing effects of PKC theta and WASp on symmetry breaking and relocation of the immunological synapse. Cell 129(4):773–785

Skokos D et al (2007) Peptide-MHC potency governs dynamic interactions between T cells and dendritic cells in lymph nodes. Nat Immunol 8(8):835–844

Stauber DJ et al (2006) Crystal structure of the IL-2 signaling complex: paradigm for a hetero-trimeric cytokine receptor. Proc Natl Acad Sci USA 103(8):2788–2793

Stinchcombe JC et al (2001) The immunological synapse of CTL contains a secretory domain and membrane bridges. Immunity 15(5):751–761

Sytwu HK, Liblau RS, McDevitt HO (1996) The roles of Fas/APO-1 (CD95) and TNF in antigen-induced programmed cell death in T cell receptor transgenic mice. Immunity 5(1):17–30

Tang QZ et al (2006) Visualizing regulatory T cell control of autoimmune responses in nonobese diabetic mice. Nat Immunol 7(1):83–92

Tohma S, Ramberg JE, Lipsky PE (1992) Expression and distribution of CD11a/CD18 and CD54 during human T cell-B cell interactions. J Leukoc Biol 52:97–103

van der Merwe PA, Davis SJ (2003) Molecular interactions mediating T cell antigen recognition. Annu Rev Immunol 21:659–684

van Kooyk Y et al (1989) Enhancement of LFA-1-mediated cell adhesion by triggering through CD2 or CD3 on T lymphocytes. Nature 342(6251):811–813

Varma R et al (2006) T cell receptor-proximal signals are sustained in peripheral microclusters and terminated in the central supramolecular activation cluster. Immunity 25(1):117–127

Veldhoen M et al (2008) Transforming growth factor-beta "reprograms" the differentiation of T helper 2 cells and promotes an interleukin 9-producing subset. Nat Immunol 9(12):1341–1346

Villarino AV et al (2007) Helper T cell IL-2 production is limited by negative feedback and STAT-dependent cytokine signals. J Exp Med 204(1):65–71

Waldmann TA (2006) The biology of interleukin-2 and interleukin-15: implications for cancer therapy and vaccine design. Nat Rev Immunol 6(8):595–601

Wang XQ, Rickert M, Garcia KC (2005) Structure of the quaternary complex of interleukin-2 with its alpha, beta, and gamma(c) receptors. Science 310(5751):1159–1163

Whyte WH (1988) City: rediscovering the center. Doubleday, New York

Wiedemann A et al (2006) Cytotoxic T lymphocytes kill multiple targets simultaneously via spatiotemporal uncoupling of lytic and stimulatory synapses. Proc Natl Acad Sci USA 103(29):10985–10990

Williams MA, Tyznik AJ, Bevan MJ (2006) Interleukin-2 signals during priming are required for secondary expansion of CD8(+) memory T cells. Nature 441(7095):890–893

Wulfing C, Davis MM (1998) A receptor/cytoskeletal movement triggered by costimulation during T cell activation. Science 282(5397):2266–2269

Yokosuka T et al (2005) Newly generated T cell receptor microclusters initiate and sustain T cell activation by recruitment of Zap70 and SLP-76. Nat Immunol 6(12):1253–1262

Yokosuka T et al (2008) Spatiotemporal regulation of T cell costimulation by TCR-CD28 microclusters and protein kinase C theta translocation. Immunity 29(4):589–601

Molecular and Cellular Dynamics at the Early Stages of Antigen Encounter: The B-Cell Immunological Synapse

Yolanda R. Carrasco

Contents

Abstract The recent development and application of sophisticated technology in the study of the initial stages of the B-cell immune response has lead to a tremendous revolution in the field. The use of real-time confocal microscopy, total interference reflection fluorescence (TIRF) microscopy and in vitro models has revealed the molecular details of the antigen recognition process by B cells. Moreover, experimental models that allow tracking of antigen in vivo in concert with multiphoton microscopy have provided critical information as to the how, where, and when naïve B cells encounter antigen in vivo. This review focuses on the latest data regarding the early phase of the humoral immune response at molecular and cellular levels.

Y.R. Carrasco
Department of Immunology and Oncology, National Centre of Biotechnology/CSIC, Darwin 3, UAM-Campus de Cantoblanco Madrid E-28049, Spain
e-mail: ycarrasco@cnb.csic.es

T. Saito and F.D. Batista (eds.), *Immunological Synapse*,
Current Topics in Microbiology and Immunology 340,
DOI 10.1007/978-3-642-03858-7_3, © Springer-Verlag Berlin Heidelberg 2010

1   Introduction

B cells are essential effectors of the adaptive immune response to pathogens. They are responsible for pathogen neutralization and clearance by the production of antigen-specific antibodies. The prompt onset of the humoral immune response is thus crucial in the fight against invaders. This process depends mainly on the ability of naïve B cells to hunt for antigen in secondary lymphoid organs (SLO). The capacity of the B cell to recognize antigen in its native conformation through the B-cell receptor (BCR) confers an important advantage that accelerates this process.

A large proportion of antigen encounters in vivo responsible for eliciting the B-cell immune response are in a membrane-bound form. Antigen recognition on a target membrane leads to the establishment of a stable long-lasting interaction between the B cell and the antigen-presenting cell (APC), known as Immunological Synapse (IS) (Batista et al. 2001; Carrasco et al. 2004). The IS was initially described on T cells (Grakoui et al. 1999; Monks et al. 1998) and later also on natural killer (NK) cells (Davis et al. 1999). Its main feature is the molecular rearrangement of ligand/receptors in distinct domains named as supramolecular activation clusters (SMACs) at the contact zone. In particular, the "mature IS" presents a central cluster of antigen receptor (central SMAC, cSMAC), BCR/ antigen in the case of B cells, surrounded by a peripheral ring of the adhesion molecules LFA-1/ICAM-1 (peripheral SMAC, pSMAC) (Carrasco et al. 2004). In vitro studies point to the critical role of IS formation for B-cell activation (Carrasco et al. 2004; Fleire et al. 2006); latest results suggest the in vivo existence of this supramolecular structure (Carrasco and Batista 2007). The actual role of the IS is highly debated; initially envisaged as the platform for intracellular BCR signalling, nowadays it is viewed as the stand for efficient BCR-mediated antigen internalization that leads to optimal B-cell activation through the recruitment of T-cell help.

The presence and potential roles of the "B cell IS" have been extensively discussed previously (Batista et al. 2007; Carrasco and Batista 2006a; Harwood and Batista 2008). Hence, in the current chapter, I will focus on very recent data concerning the molecular dynamics of the antigen recognition process and IS formation by B cells. In addition, I will discuss latest findings that have provided insights into the strategy of naïve B cells for maximizing the efficiency of antigen searching in vivo. I will also comment on novel data derived from imaging studies performed at the very early stages of naïve B-cell antigen recognition and activation in vivo.

2   Molecular Dynamics of B-Cell Antigen Recognition and IS Formation

2.1   A Two-Phase Response Leads to B-Cell Synapse Formation

The recognition of membrane-bound antigen through the BCR triggers a two-phase cellular response (Fleire et al. 2006) (Fig. 1). First the B cell spreads over the surface of the antigen-presenting membrane, reaching a maximum around the 5 first minutes of contact, and gathers antigen into small clusters via BCR interaction. Then, a longer contraction phase follows which drives the collection of BCR/ antigen microclusters at the centre of the cell-to-cell contact site. This spreading-contraction response ends with the formation of the IS (Fig. 1).

The two-phase response shapes the B-cell activation process by promoting a maximum efficiency in antigen gathering and accumulation (Fleire et al. 2006). The spreading facilitates BCR-signalling dissemination, therefore B-cell activation, and allows affinity discrimination of antigens (Fleire et al. 2006). The abundance of antigen and the affinity of the BCR for it are master regulators of the spreading-contraction response. High affinity and/or density of antigen promote maximum membrane spreading and, thereby, the accumulation of increased amounts of antigen at the cSMAC. In addition, it requires both the initiation of BCR-mediated signalling and the reorganization of the B-cell cytoskeleton. In this regard, the tyrosine kinases Lyn and Syk, and the signalling molecules PLCγ2 and Vav

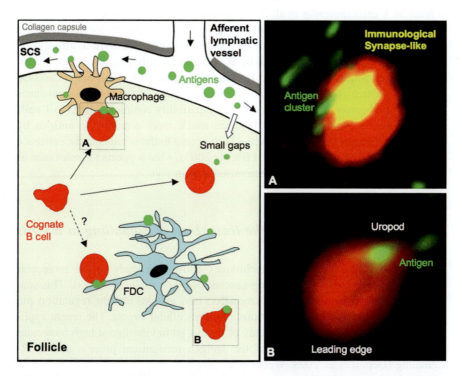

Fig. 1 A spreading-contraction response drives Immunological Synapse (IS) formation. The cartoon summarizes the two-phase response triggered after BCR-engagement. The encounter of membrane-tethered antigen on the surface of the APC activates BCR-signalling and, therefore, B-cell spreading (phase 1). During this phase the B cell maximizes antigen gathering by increasing the contact surface with the APC. BCR/antigen microclusters are also formed, core of the microsignalosomes assembly. In the phase 2 the B-cell contracts, concentrates the antigen at the centre of the B cell–APC contact, internalizes it, and establishes the IS

(GEF for Rho GTPases) have been proved to be key for B-cell spreading (Weber et al. 2008). The small GTPase Rac2 and Rap GTPases also control the dramatic morphological changes and cytoskeletal reorganization required for this cellular response (Arana et al. 2008; Lin et al. 2008).

The B-cell IS presents the two main features of the mature IS, initially described on T cells (Grakoui et al. 1999; Monks et al. 1998), a cSMAC of BCR/antigen surrounded by a pSMAC of the adhesion molecules LFA-1/ICAM-1 (Carrasco et al. 2004). In addition, B cells can also recruit the VLA-4/VCAM-1 pair of adhesion molecules to the mature IS (Carrasco and Batista 2006b). This complex molecular segregation of receptors implies severe cytoskeletal rearrangements on the B cells; F-actin polarizes towards the IS and forms a ring where the integrins anchored to establish the pSMAC. It has been shown that the members of the Vav family of proteins Vav1 and Vav2, and the GTPases Rac2, but not Rac1 and Rap1 are key players in the assembly of the F-actin platform at the B-cell IS (Arana et al. 2008; Lin et al. 2008). The cSMAC lacks F-actin, but it has been suggested an important role for microtubules in the active vesicle trafficking that takes place at this SMAC at least on T cells (Serrador et al. 2004; Stinchcombe et al. 2006).

But, what is the role of the IS? In vitro studies showed that IS formation allows B-cell triggering under antigen-limiting conditions (low density/low affinity), is important for affinity discrimination by B cells, and finally permits more efficient B-cell antigen acquisition, essential for later recruitment of T-cell help (Carrasco et al. 2004; Fleire et al. 2006). This remarkable feature of the B-cell IS enhances processing and presentation on major histocompatibility complex (MHC) to T cells when antigen is limited. B cells, thus, are much more sensitive to antigen by triggering IS formation. As I will discuss later, recent findings indicate the existence of the B-cell IS in vivo (Carrasco and Batista 2007), what supports the relevance of this molecular structure for B-cell activation also in vivo.

2.2   Microsignalosomes as the Basic Unit of Signalling in B Cells

Single-cell fluorescence imaging techniques allows the study of the molecular dynamics of receptors and signalling cascades in their cellular context. This spatially resolved biochemistry in real time offers new insights into the regulation and function of ligand–receptor interactions and intracellular events. The recent application of TIRF microscopy to the study of B cells let to visualize at high molecular resolution the very early events of the antigen recognition process and BCR-signalling (Depoil et al. 2008; Weber et al. 2008).

The data show that the engagement of membrane-tethered antigen drives the formation of BCR microclusters containing IgM and IgD (Depoil et al. 2008) (Fig. 1). These microclusters contain around a 100 BCRs, and lack the presence of the inhibitory phosphatase CD45. The BCR-microclusters are *hot spots* of signalling molecule recruitment, as they are enriched on tyrosine phosphorilated proteins. Nevertheless, initial BCR clustering seems to be signalling independent and occurs by diffusion trapping (Depoil et al. 2008). A recent spatiotemporal characterization of the early signalling events after BCR engagement shows the sequential action of the tyrosin kinases Lyn and Syk on B-cell spreading, and the recruitment of Syk to the BCR-microclusters (Weber et al. 2008). The signalling molecules PLCγ2 and Vav are also later recruited, and together with Btk and Blnk play a key role in the dissemination of the intracellular signalling and in the spreading cellular response, as previously mentioned (Weber et al. 2008). Still it is necessary to define the molecular effectors and/or mechanisms that turn the microcluster-signal in the cytoskeletal rearrangements that drive the B-cell spreading-contraction response after antigen encounter.

Thus, the organization of immunoreceptors into microclusters is seen as "an exquisite and flexible way to regulate their signalling activity" (reviewed in (Harwood and Batista 2008)). Individual microclusters permit the dynamic recruitment of other clusters containing positive or negative regulators that may modulate the immunoreceptor signalling. Furthermore, being *hot spots* of signalling, the microclusters have been re-named as "microsignalosomes" and are considered as the basic unit of signalling in B cells, as also reported on T cells (Campi et al. 2005; Varma et al. 2006; Yokosuka et al. 2005). All together, these recent findings point at the concept of microsignalosomes as the common entity for signalling among lymphocytes.

2.3   The Importance of the Context

The presentation of antigen on a cell membrane implies the presence of a molecular context with the capacity to modulate the process of antigen recognition and activation of B cells. Previous studies point to an important role of the "*adhesive context*" on the B-cell response (Carrasco and Batista 2006b; Carrasco et al. 2004). The adhesion molecules ICAM-1 and VCAM-1, ligands of the LFA-1 and VLA-4 integrins, respectively, are highly expressed on the surface of FDC, DC and macrophages. These proteins promote the interaction of B cells with potential antigen presenting cells (Koopman et al. 1991; Kushnir et al. 1998). Furthermore, the recognition of antigen in their presence lowers the threshold for B-cell activation (Carrasco and Batista 2006b; Carrasco et al. 2004). This is mainly achieved by promoting B-cell adhesion through LFA-1 and VLA-4 expressed on the B-cell surface, in synergy with BCR antigen engagement. The increased adhesion enlarges the contact area of the B cell with the APC and, thus, facilitates antigen engagement and synapse formation. The signalling cascade initiated upon BCR engagement that leads to integrin activation and adhesion involves src-family tyrosine kinases, Vav1 and Vav2, PLCγ2, PI3K and the small GTPase Rac2, but not Rac1 (Arana et al. 2008; Spaargaren et al. 2003).

The presence of co-receptors and their ligands in the molecular context of antigen recognition modulates also B-cell activation. A recent study of the very early events of B-cell antigen recognition and activation demonstrate an unpredicted and critical role for the co-receptor CD19 in enhancing BCR signalling in response to membrane-tethered antigen (Depoil et al. 2008). CD19 seems to act as a membrane adaptor protein with the capacity of association with many signalling molecules such as Vav, PI3K and the tyrosin kinase Lyn. The transient recruitment of CD19 to BCR-antigen microclusters promotes signal amplification by bringing signalling molecules to the contact surface; as a result, the number of microclusters increases and, therefore, it promotes B-cell activation. Inhibitory co-receptors are also players on this supramolecular organization. FcγRIIB is a potent negative regulator of B-cell activation when it is colligated to the BCR through antigen-containing immune complexes (Sohn et al. 2008). The authors suggest that this is achieved through the destabilization of the BCR association with lipid rafts, therefore, the impairment of early BCR-signalling and synapse formation (Sohn et al. 2008).

2.4 Antigen Presenting Cells

Different cell types present native antigen tethered on their surface to B cells. For example, follicular dendritic cells (FDC) retain antigen in the form of immune complex through Fc receptors and complement receptors on their surface and present it to B cells (Haberman and Shlomchik 2003; Kosco-Vilbois 2003). Several evidences show the capacity of Dendritic Cells (DC) to capture and retain native antigen, transport it to SLO and present it to B cells (Balazs et al. 2002; Berney et al. 1999; Colino et al. 2002; Wykes et al. 1998). My very recent work and two other groups have shown how SLO resident macrophages capture antigen arriving via the lymph from peripheral tissues and present it to B cells in the primary follicle (Carrasco and Batista 2007; Junt et al. 2007; Phan et al. 2007). So far, the molecular mechanism or mechanisms by which DC and macrophages present intact antigen to B cells are practically unknown.

Therefore, in vivo antigen presentation to B cells may take place by different routes; possibly the use of one or another, or more than one, is going to be determined by aspects such as the physical properties of the antigen itself, its amount, as well as its entrance route into SLO. As it will be discussed in the next section, recent reports address these questions in vivo. The set up of experimental models to track antigen in vivo alongside the use of multiphoton microscopy have shed light on this quite obscure topic.

3 Cellular Dynamics at the Onset of the B-Cell Response In Vivo

3.1 The Naïve B-Cell Migration Pattern: Searching for Antigen

Naïve B-cells survey for specific antigen the SLO, where pathogens and other potential antigens are driven. The strategy of naïve B cells to maximize the efficiency of this search is based on their continuous recirculation between spleen, lymph nodes and other structures that form part of the secondary lymphoid tissue network. Naïve B cells enter lymph nodes from the blood through the high endothelial venules (HEV), and migrate across the T-cell zone to localize in the follicular area, where they can spend up to 24 h before exiting through the efferent lymphatics, return to the blood, and repeat the same process (Cyster 2005; Okada and Cyster 2006). This homeostatic migration of naïve B cells is orchestrated by members of the chemokine and chemokine receptor families, in particular CXCL13/CXCR5, and by the lysophospholipid sphingosine-1-phosphate (S1P) and its receptor $S1P_1$.

Once naïve B cells arrive in the follicular area, they move at an average speed of 6 μm/min, as observed by multiphoton microscopy studies (Miller et al. 2002; Okada et al. 2005). Follicular B-cell basal motility depends on chemokine receptor signalling (Han et al. 2005), probably on the CXCL13/CXCR5 pair. This dynamic behaviour allows naïve B cells to explore the entire follicular area, thus increasing their chances to find specific antigen. The FDC network in the follicles serves as a scaffold for follicular B-cell movement (Bajenoff et al. 2006). FDC are the main CXCL13 producers in the lymphoid tissue (Cyster 2005), and express high levels of Fc and complement receptors that they use to capture and display antigen to B cells (Szakal et al. 1989; Tew et al. 1997). Naïve B cells would thus encounter antigens along the paths on which they move. The synergy between these two mechanisms, the dynamic behaviour of naïve B cells within follicles and antigen retention on the substrate for B-cell movement, maximize the efficiency of the naïve B cell search for specific antigen.

After a period of random movement in the follicle, naïve B cells return to circulation to continue the search in other SLO. The egress of follicular B cells is regulated by $S1P/S1P_1$ (Matloubian et al. 2004). S1P is abundant in blood, in contrast with its low levels in lymphoid tissue. It is suggested that the diminished presence of this ligand in lymphoid tissue allows up-regulation of $S1P_1$ receptor levels at the cell membrane (Okada and Cyster 2006; Pham et al. 2008); as a consequence, naïve B cells would sense and respond to S1P, overcome retention signals and exit the lymphoid tissue.

3.2 Early Steps in Antigen Recognition and Activation of Naïve B Cells

Naïve B cells organize in follicular structures within the SLO. The follicle has long been considered the main site for B-cell antigen encounter, with the FDC network as the surface that displays antigen, in the form of immune complexes (Tew et al. 1997). Nonetheless, there was no bona fide evidence for the relevance of follicular structures and the FDC network in the initial stages of B-cell priming. Moreover, the role of FDC in the B-cell response has been intensely debated (Haberman and

Shlomchik 2003; Kosco-Vilbois 2003). The development and recent application of new imaging technology, in particular confocal microscopy and real-time multi-photon microscopy, has provided crucial mechanistic insights into this topic. Using distinct experimental models to track antigen in vivo (low molecular weight antigen, antigen coated-particles, antigen-containing immune complexes, antigen coated-viruses), four groups underlined the primary follicle as the location for antigen encounter by naïve B cells, stressing the boundary between the follicle and the subcapsular sinus (SCS) as the main B-cell priming site within the whole follicular area (Carrasco and Batista 2007; Junt et al. 2007; Pape et al. 2007; Phan et al. 2007) (Fig. 2). A macrophage subset located at the lymph node SCS has a critical role in the capture and transport of antigen from the SCS into the follicle and, thus, in the presentation of antigen to follicular B cells (Junt et al. 2007) (Fig. 2).

The follicles are the main spot for concentration of the diverse repertoire of naïve B cells. The strategic location of follicles close to the antigen-draining zones of SLO (SCS in lymph nodes, marginal zone (MZ) in spleen) allows rapid B cell access to incoming antigens. By these two means, concentration and location, naïve B cells ensure efficient detection of cognate antigens.

3.2.1 Tracking Antigen Recognition In Vivo

The tracking of particulate antigen in vivo allows quantitative studies of the initial stages of B-cell antigen recognition. By just 60 min after administration of

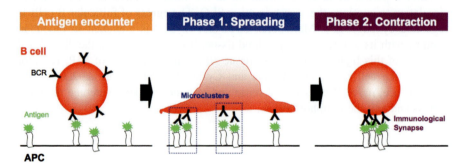

Fig. 2 Priming of naïve B cells in draining lymph node follicles. Panel on the left shows a cartoon that summarizes where naïve B cells can encounter specific antigen within the follicle. SCS macrophages have an important role in presenting antigen to naïve B cells, but probably also FDC. In addition, naïve B cells would encounter small antigen that diffuses through the small gaps of the SCS floor. The two different dynamic stages described for antigen-loaded B cells are also highlighted (*dashed line boxes*) in the cartoon: (**a**) Naïve B cell of rounded cell shape, mainly stopped, and attached to the antigen-binding site. A cluster of antigen is detected at one side of the B cell (Immunological Synapse-like); (**b**) Naïve B cell showing a polarized, migratory cell shape, actively migrating and carrying antigen in the uropod. Panels on the right show multiphoton microscopy images of both B-cell dynamic stages (**a**) and (**b**); naïve B cells and antigen are shown in *red* and in *green*, respectively

antigen-coated particles, almost 50% of follicular cognate B cells have encountered and captured antigen; frequency increases with time, and by 24 h nearly all cognate B cells in the follicle have encountered antigen, become activated, and migrate to the B cell–T cell boundary, seeking T-cell help (Carrasco and Batista 2007). At very early time points (up to 4 h after antigen administration), antigen-loaded B cells localize only in the upper half of the follicles, indicating that particulate antigen encounter occurs mainly near the SCS (Fig. 2). Moreover, the quantity of particulate antigen per specific B cell increases with time, suggesting that B cells acquire antigen in sequential encounters within the follicle before migrating to the B cell–T cell border (Carrasco and Batista 2007). The whole process is accelerated when low molecular weight antigen is used (Pape et al. 2007). The majority of follicular cognate B cells acquire antigen by 10 min after administration; again, initial encounter with small antigens takes place near the SCS (Fig. 2).

The brief period post-administration required for antigen detection and capture by specific naïve B cells also suggests that B-cells residing in the follicle at the time of antigen arrival constitute the majority of the antibody response. In the distinct models analyzed (Carrasco and Batista 2007; Junt et al. 2007; Pape et al. 2007; Phan et al. 2007), antigen was administered only once and was consumed mainly by the cognate B cells in the follicle at that time. B cells entering the follicle probably have a role in persistent infections, in which antigen would arrive continuously to the follicle, as well as in later phases of the antibody response.

Although the four reports highlight the boundary between the follicle and the SCS as a key site for B-cell priming, their observations also suggest additional possibilities. In the absence of large numbers of cognate B cells, antigen is deposited on the FDC surface (Carrasco and Batista 2007); in addition, non-cognate B cells capture antigen from the SCS macrophages by a complement receptor-dependent pathway and deliver it to FDC (Phan et al. 2007). These findings suggest that in normal conditions of B-cell clonal abundance, the follicular FDC network may also be a location for naïve B-cell antigen encounter (Fig. 2).

3.2.2   In Vivo B-Cell Dynamics

Multiphoton microscopy has allowed real time, in situ visualization and study of B-cell dynamics during the initial stages of antigen encounter in draining lymph node follicles. As discussed above, follicular naïve B cells move by "random walk" at an average velocity of 4–6 μm/min (Miller et al. 2002; Okada et al. 2005). Two distinct forms of behaviour are observed relative to naïve B-cell localization within the follicle (Carrasco and Batista 2007). While naïve B cells are highly motile deep in the follicle, they move more slowly and describe short tracks in the zone near the SCS. This may allow careful scanning of the SCS macrophages, the crucial route of antigen entry into the draining lymph node. The signal(s) that promote this different behaviour are unknown, but it could be due to the distinct substrates of movement (macrophages vs. FDC), to different chemotactic signals (a chemokine other than CXCL13), or to both.

Antigen exposure changes the dynamics of cognate B cells by gradually decreasing their movement within the follicle (Carrasco and Batista 2007; Okada et al. 2005). At the earliest time points in the antigen recognition process, antigen-loaded B cells show two distinct forms of behaviour or stages at the single cell level (Carrasco and Batista 2007) (Fig. 2). In one case, naïve B cells are highly motile, showing a polarized, migratory shape and bearing the antigen in the uropod; these cells are found mainly deep in the follicle. In the second case, the naïve B cells are rounded and are confined to a small area of movement in which they can stay for prolonged periods (>15 min); they appear to be attached to the antigen-binding site, which forms a cluster at one side of the cell. These B cells localize mainly at the boundary between the follicle and the SCS. Antigen recognition thus further reduces B cell movement in the area near the SCS.

3.2.3   B-Cell IS In Vivo

The rounded B-cell shape, its prolonged confinement to a small area with almost no movement, and in particular, the formation of an antigen cluster to which it attaches, are all hallmark features of the B-cell IS (Batista et al. 2001; Carrasco et al. 2004) (Fig. 2). In addition, some B cells showed in vivo a spreading-contraction response in order to gather antigen coated particles into a cluster (Carrasco and Batista 2007). The multiphoton microscopy findings detailed above perfectly fit with the in vitro data and, thus, indicate the in vivo existence of the B-cell IS (Carrasco and Batista 2007). Despite the crucial roles of the IS for in vitro B-cell activation (discussed below), its relevance for B-cell activation in vivo remains to be addressed.

4   Concluding Remarks

Talking in molecular terms, the in vitro studies have reached a striking progress in the understanding of the initial stages of membrane-tethered antigen recognition and B-cell activation. The IS formation is critical for increasing the sensibility of B cells to antigen. The spreading-contraction response triggered after BCR engagement that heads IS assembly, maximizes the gathering and collection of antigen. The observation in vivo of a synapse-like structure upon B-cell antigen encounter stresses the relevance of these in vitro findings. In addition, the antigen-induced BCR-microclusters emerge as the sites for initiation of B-cell signalling and core of microsignalosomes construction from which the signalling propagates. Still important issues remain to be addressed. The on-going use of single-cell imaging techniques in the study of the molecular mechanisms underlying the early events of B-cell activation will continue to impart knowledge in the years to come.

Going bigger, the recent findings discussed here have shed light on the "how, where and when" in vivo naïve B cell encounter antigen. The follicle-SCS boundary in lymph nodes emerges as a key B-cell antigen recognition site and the follicles as the location for B-cell priming. The SCS macrophages are a device for capturing antigen that arrives via the lymph and transfers it to the follicle; they are also important for presenting antigen to naïve B cells. Spleen MZ macrophages may have a similar function, in this case facilitating the presentation of blood-borne antigens to follicular naïve B cells. Finally, the quickness of naïve B-cell recognition after antigen administration suggests that B cells are initial sensors and effectors of the adaptive immune response. In conclusion, a more defined picture is now emerging of the initial steps of the B-cell response; though the studies discussed here focus their attention in the lymph nodes, it is possible that we will find a similar scenario in the other SLO. The development of experimental models that allow real time, in situ antigen tracking and visualization of the early stages of the B-cell immune response in vivo has been vital for these advances. It will be exciting to see the data that arise from the use and improvement of these models, for answering the many still-open questions about the nature of the B-cell immune response.

Acknowledgements I thank Ignacio Moreno de Alborán and Carlos Ardavín for a critical reading of the manuscript, and also Catherine Mark for editorial assistance. Y.R.C. is supported by a Ramón y Cajal contract from the Spanish Ministry of Science. The Department of Immunology and Oncology was founded and is supported by the Spanish National Research Council (CSIC) and by Pfizer.

References

Arana E, Vehlow A, Harwood NE, Vigorito E, Henderson R, Turner M, Tybulewicz VL, Batista FD (2008) Immunity 28:88–99

Bajenoff M, Egen JG, Koo LY, Laugier JP, Brau F, Glaichenhaus N, Germain RN (2006) Immunity 25:989–1001

Balazs M, Martin F, Zhou T, Kearney J (2002) Immunity 17:341–352

Batista FD, Iber D, Neuberger MS (2001) Nature 411:489–494

Batista FD, Arana E, Barral P, Carrasco YR, Depoil D, Eckl-Dorna J, Fleire S, Howe K, Vehlow A, Weber M, Treanor B (2007) Immunol Rev 218:197–213

Berney C, Herren S, Power CA, Gordon S, Martinez-Pomares L, Kosco-Vilbois MH (1999) J Exp Med 190:851–860

Campi G, Varma R, Dustin ML (2005) J Exp Med 202:1031–1036

Carrasco YR, Batista FD (2006a) Curr Opin Immunol 18:286–291

Carrasco YR, Batista FD (2006b) EMBO J 25:889–899

Carrasco YR, Batista FD (2007) Immunity 27:160–171

Carrasco YR, Fleire SJ, Cameron T, Dustin ML, Batista FD (2004) Immunity 20:589–599

Colino J, Shen Y, Snapper CM (2002) J Exp Med 195:1–13

Cyster JG (2005) Annu Rev Immunol 23:127–159

Davis DM, Chiu I, Fassett M, Cohen GB, Mandelboim O, Strominger JL (1999) Proc Natl Acad Sci USA 96:15062–15067

Depoil D, Fleire S, Treanor BL, Weber M, Harwood NE, Marchbank KL, Tybulewicz VL, Batista FD (2008) Nat Immunol 9:63–72

Fleire SJ, Goldman JP, Carrasco YR, Weber M, Bray, D, Batista FD (2006) Science 312:738–741

Grakoui A, Bromley SK, Sumen C, Davis MM, Shaw AS, Allen PM, Dustin ML (1999) Science 285:221–227

Haberman AM, Shlomchik MJ (2003) Nat Rev Immunol 3:757–764

Han SB, Moratz C, Huang NN, Kelsall B, Cho H, Shi CS, Schwartz O, Kehrl JH (2005) Immunity 22:343–354

Harwood NE, Batista FD (2008) Immunity 28:609–619

Junt T, Moseman EA, Iannacone M, Massberg S, Lang PA, Boes M, Fink K, Henrickson SE, Shayakhmetov DM, Di Paolo NC, van Rooijen N, Mempel TR, Whelan SP, von Andrian UH (2007) Nature 450:110–114

Koopman G, Parmentier HK, Schuurman HJ, Newman W, Meijer CJ, Pals ST (1991) J Exp Med 173:1297–1304

Kosco-Vilbois MH (2003) Nat Rev Immunol 3:764–769

Kushnir N, Liu L, MacPherson GG (1998) J Immunol 160:1774–1781

Lin KB, Freeman SA, Zabetian S, Brugger H, Weber M, Lei V, Dang-Lawson M, Tse KW, Santamaria R, Batista FD, Gold MR (2008) Immunity 28:75–87

Matloubian M, Lo CG, Cinamon G, Lesneski MJ, Xu Y, Brinkmann V, Allende ML, Proia RL, Cyster JG (2004) Nature 427:355–360

Miller MJ, Wei SH, Parker I, Cahalan MD (2002) Science 296:1869–1873

Monks CR, Freiberg BA, Kupfer H, Sciaky N, Kupfer A (1998) Nature 395:82–86

Okada T, Cyster JG (2006) Curr Opin Immunol 18:278–285

Okada T, Miller MJ, Parker I, Krummel MF, Neighbors M, Hartley SB, O'Garra A, Cahalan MD, Cyster JG (2005) PLoS Biol 3:e150

Pape KA, Catron DM, Itano AA, Jenkins MK (2007) Immunity 26:491–502

Pham TH, Okada T, Matloubian M, Lo CG, Cyster JG (2008) Immunity 28:122–133

Phan TG, Grigorova I, Okada T, Cyster JG (2007) Nat Immunol 8:992–1000

Serrador JM, Cabrero JR, Sancho D, Mittelbrunn M, Urzainqui A, Sanchez-Madrid F (2004) Immunity 20:417–428

Sohn HW, Pierce SK, Tzeng SJ (2008) J Immunol 180:793–799

Spaargaren M, Beuling EA, Rurup ML, Meijer HP, Klok MD, Middendorp S, Hendriks RW, Pals ST (2003) J Exp Med 198:1539–1550

Stinchcombe JC, Majorovits E, Bossi G, Fuller S, Griffiths GM (2006) Nature 443:462–465

Szakal AK, Kosco MH, Tew JG (1989) Annu Rev Immunol 7:91–109

Tew JG, Wu J, Qin D, Helm S, Burton GF, Szakal AK (1997) Immunol Rev 156:39–52

Varma R, Campi G, Yokosuka T, Saito T, Dustin ML (2006) Immunity 25:117–127

Weber M, Treanor B, Depoil D, Shinohara H, Harwood NE, Hikida M, Kurosaki T, Batista FD (2008) J Exp Med 205:853–868

Wykes M, Pombo A, Jenkins C, MacPherson GG (1998) J Immunol 161:1313–1319

Yokosuka T, Sakata-Sogawa K, Kobayashi W, Hiroshima M, Hashimoto-Tane A, Tokunaga M, Dustin ML, Saito T (2005) Nat Immunol 6:1253–1262

Inhibitory and Regulatory Immune Synapses

Philipp Eissmann and Daniel M. Davis

Contents

Abstract Cell contact-dependent inhibition and regulation of immune responses play an essential role in balancing the need for rapid and efficient responses to a wide variety of pathological challenges, while at the same time maintaining self-tolerance. Much attention has been given to immune synapses that lead to the activation of, for example, cell-mediated cytotoxicity, and here we compare the supramolecular dynamics of synapses that lead to inhibition or regulatory functions. We focus on natural killer cells where such different synapses have been best studied. An emergent principle is that inhibition or regulatory responses are commonly achieved by selective recruitment of signalling proteins to the synapse and exclusion of membrane-proximal intracellular proteins needed for activation. We also discuss evidence that an inhibitory synapse triggers or maintains effector cells in a migratory configuration, which serves to break the synapse before the steps needed for effector cell activation can be completed. This model implies that the concept of kinetic-proofreading, previously used to describe activation of

D.M. Davis (✉) and P. Eissmann
Division of Cell and Molecular Biology, Imperial College London, Sir Alexander Fleming Building, South Kensington, London SW7 2AZ, UK
e-mail: d.davis@imperial.ac.uk

T. Saito and F.D. Batista (eds.), *Immunological Synapse*,
Current Topics in Microbiology and Immunology 340,
DOI 10.1007/978-3-642-03858-7_4, © Springer-Verlag Berlin Heidelberg 2010

individual T-cell receptors, can also apply in determining the outcome of intercellular conjugation.

1 Introduction

Many of the key cell surface molecules involved in immune cell surveillance have been identified and an important new scientific frontier is to understand where and when each protein–protein interaction occurs to regulate cell functions. Thus, imaging has a major role to play in contemporary cell biology and one interesting theme to emerge is that immune cell communication is often accompanied by the segregation of proteins into micrometre-scale domains at an intercellular contact or immune synapse (IS) (Davis 2006). More recently, it has been shown that kinases, adaptors and antigen receptors accumulate at synapses within micron- or sub-micron-scaled structures termed microclusters. T- and B-cell receptor signalling, for example, is initiated in such microclusters (Bunnell et al. 2002; Campi et al. 2005; Yokosuka et al. 2005) and these signals are terminated as microclusters move from the periphery to the centre of the IS (Harwood and Batista 2008; Seminario and Bunnell 2008; Varma et al. 2006; Yokosuka et al. 2005). In natural killer (NK) cells, phosphorylation of inhibitory killer cell immunoglobulin (Ig)-like receptors (KIR) is restricted to microclusters (Treanor et al. 2006) implicating that inhibitory signalling is also restricted to microclusters. The emerging new paradigm is that interactions between immune cell kinases, adaptors and other proteins are at least in part controlled by the dynamics of supramolecular assemblies rather than isolated protein–protein interactions that are commonly depicted in textbook diagrams of immune receptor signalling pathways. While this has been widely discussed for immune cell activation, here we review what happens at an IS where inhibitory or regulatory signals dominate.

2 Definition of Inhibitory Immune Synapses

It is well established that inhibitory receptor functions are crucial to maintaining self-tolerance and control responses spatially and temporally while allowing rapid and efficient responses when appropriate (Long 1999). This is particularly evident from the data associating inhibitory receptor dysfunction, or genetic variations in inhibitory receptor expression, with susceptibility to a variety of diseases, including autoimmunity, viral infection and cancer (Chouaib et al. 2002; Pritchard and Smith 2003; Rajagopalan and Long 2005). Broadly, inhibitory receptors can be divided into two classes based on the presence or absence of cytoplasmic immunoreceptor tyrosine-based inhibition motifs (ITIMs). Inhibition by ITIM-containing receptors is initiated by tyrosine phosphorylation and recruitment of Src homology 2 (SH2) domain-containing phosphatases SHP-1 and/or SHP-2 or the

SH2 domain-containing inositol phosphatase (SHIP) (Daeron et al. 2008; Long 2008). Engagement of inhibitory receptors changes the micrometre-scale organization of proteins at the IS, compared to activating interactions to form a so-called "inhibitory immune synapse" (Davis and Dustin 2004). An inhibitory synapse is not merely a transient intercellular contact at which little happens. Such transient interactions may occur when T cells briefly interact with target cells or APCs that lack a relevant peptide/MHC and they do not involve assembly of an IS. Rather, an inhibitory synapse can be defined as an intercellular contact at which the encounter causes proteins to segregate into micrometre-scale domains and where directed signalling serves to terminate or prevent immune cell activation.

Such inhibitory immune synapses were first proposed for NK cells conjugated to EBV-transformed B cells that were protected from lysis by expression of class I MHC protein recognized by inhibitory NK-cell receptors (Davis et al. 1999). It is broadly accepted that expression of class I MHC protein facilitates self-tolerance by NK cells and that conversely, viral-infected or tumour cells can become susceptible to lysis by NK cells via decreased expression of self class I MHC protein (Karre et al. 1986). Commonly referred to as the "missing self-hypothesis" (Ljunggren and Karre 1990), this provides a conceptual framework in which the importance of an inhibitory IS is well-documented.

Recently, ligation of inhibitory receptors has been shown to assemble distinct synaptic structures in many other immune cell interactions, including those involving T cells, B cells and macrophages (Dietrich et al. 2001; Fourmentraux-Neves et al. 2008; Guerra et al. 2002; Henel et al. 2006; Schneider et al. 2008; Sohn et al. 2008; Tsai and Discher 2008). For example, subpopulations of T cells express inhibitory receptors of the KIR family, the C-type lectin-like heterodimer CD94/NKG2A, the Ig-like transcript (ILT) 2 or members of the CD28:B7 Ig superfamily, such as CTLA-4 (CD154) (Peggs et al. 2008; Ugolini and Vivier 2000). Engagement of these receptors negatively regulates signalling through the T-cell antigen receptor (Chouaib et al. 2002; Peggs et al. 2008; McMahon and Raulet 2001; Snyder et al. 2002; Ugolini and Vivier 2000; van Bergen et al. 2004) and influences the supramolecular organization of the IS (Dietrich et al. 2001; Fourmentraux-Neves et al. 2008; Guerra et al. 2002; Henel et al. 2006; Schneider et al. 2008). The B cell inhibitory receptor FcγRIIB similarly disrupts formation of an activating synapse in response to membrane bound antigen (Sohn et al. 2008). The formation of a phagocytic contact between macrophages and red blood cells is inhibited by binding of the inhibitory receptor SIRPα (CD172a) to its ligand CD47 (Tsai and Discher 2008). These data extend the concept of the inhibitory synapse to other cellular interactions and demonstrate its broad relevance.

3 Formation of Inhibitory Synapses

The inhibitory NK-cell IS is the best studied inhibitory IS and may be considered "prototypic" (see Fig. 1 for a summary of molecular processes at the inhibitory NK-cell IS). Inhibition of NK-cell activity through engagement of inhibitory

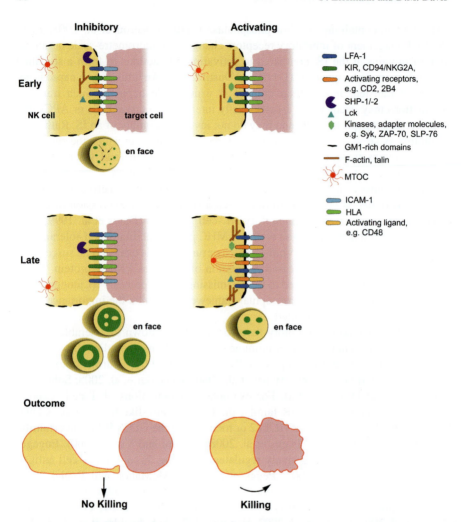

Fig. 1 Comparison of the inhibitory and cytolytic NK-cell IS. Contacts between NK cells and target cells that are protected from NK cell attack result in the formation of an inhibitory synapse with recruitment of inhibitory receptors bound to their respective MHC ligands (Davis et al. 1999; Eriksson et al. 1999b). Initially, inhibitory receptors appear in small clusters that move from the periphery to the centre of the IS to form larger aggregates during IS maturation (Oddos et al. 2008). Concomitantly, the phosphatases SHP-1 and SHP-2 and the kinase Lck accumulate. In the early inhibitory IS, cytoskeletal proteins talin and F-actin and GM1-rich microdomains are detectable (Masilamani et al. 2006; Treanor et al. 2006; Vyas et al. 2002, 2004). Lck, F-actin, talin and GM1-rich microdomains are excluded from the inhibitory IS at later time points, while SHP-1 and SHP-2 remain (Vyas et al. 2002, 2004). Inhibitory receptors segregate from integrins and arrange in different patterns across the synapse being either homogeneously distributed, ring shaped, or containing multiple exclusions (Almeida and Davis 2006; Carlin et al. 2001; Davis et al. 1999; Vyas et al. 2004). Activating receptors, e.g., CD2 and 2B4, are present within the inhibitory IS (Schleinitz et al. 2008). Finally, the NK cell detaches from the target and moves away. Target cells that display reduced expression of class I MHC protein or increased expression of activating NK cell

receptors is essential to provide protection of "self" (Ljunggren and Karre 1990) because, in contrast to T- and B-cells, NK-cell activation does not depend on antigen receptors and is independent of prior sensitization or priming. Inhibitory receptors expressed on human NK cells include the ITIM-containing class I MHC protein binding KIRs and CD94/NKG2A (Lanier 2005). These inhibitory receptors and their ligands rapidly cluster at an inhibitory IS (Davis et al. 1999; Dietrich et al. 2001; Egen and Allison 2002; Eriksson et al. 1999b; Fourmentraux-Neves et al. 2008; Henel et al. 2006; Standeven et al. 2004). Interestingly, clustering of KIR and its class I MHC protein ligands is largely a spontaneous process triggered by binding alone. Accumulation of these proteins does not require receptor signalling or ligation of adhesion molecules (Fassett et al. 2001; Faure et al. 2003) and is largely independent of actin reorganization or ATP-driven cellular processes (Almeida and Davis 2006; Carlin et al. 2001; Davis et al. 1999; Standeven et al. 2004). Indeed, insect cell transfectants expressing class I MHC protein, considered to not express any other ligands for NK cells, can trigger efficient clustering and tyrosine phosphorylation of KIR at the NK-cell IS (Faure et al. 2003). Intriguingly, clustering and phosphorylation of KIR does require the presence of divalent cations such as Zn^{2+} (Davis et al. 1999; Fan et al. 2000; Fassett et al. 2001; Rajagopalan and Long 1998; Rajagopalan et al. 1995; Vales-Gomez et al. 2001), although the molecular basis for this remains unclear. It still remains to be established if efficient spontaneous clustering of inhibitory NK-cell receptors and ligands is essential for their function but it is tempting to speculate that the rapid spontaneous clustering of inhibitory receptors and ligands is important in keeping NK-cell responses tightly controlled. In contrast, however, recruitment of the inhibitory receptor CTLA-4 to the T-cell IS is proportional to the strength of the TCR stimulus (Egen and Allison 2002). This difference may reflect an interesting distinction in the functions and/or mechanisms by which these different inhibitory receptors operate but this requires further investigation.

The supramolecular organization of class I MHC protein across an inhibitory NK-cell IS can form a single cluster, a ring, or a cluster containing multiple regions where class I MHC protein is excluded (Almeida and Davis 2006; Carlin et al. 2001; Oddos et al. 2008). These configurations are dynamic and interchangeable (Almeida and Davis 2006). However, these patterns are less clear for peripheral blood NK-cell clones compared to larger immortal NK-cell lines and thus, it seems unlikely that class I MHC protein being organized in a single or multiple foci, for example, has any direct influence on the outcome of the cell–cell interaction (Almeida and Davis 2006). Instead, recent evidence points to the extent of co-localisation or segregation

←───

Fig. 1 (continued) ligands will activate NK cell cytotoxicity. Early stages of the cytolytic IS are characterized by actin reorganization, the accumulation of GM1-rich microdomains and the recruitment of kinases and adapter molecules including Lck, Syk, ZAP-70 and SLP-76 (Orange et al. 2003; Vyas et al. 2001, 2002, 2004). During maturation, f-actin reorganizes to form a ring in the periphery of the IS, while the MTOC and lytic granules polarize towards the centre (Culley et al. 2009; McCann et al. 2003; Orange et al. 2003; Orange et al. 2002; Vyas et al. 2001). Inhibitory receptors can still be present in cytolytic IS but cluster in multifocal patterns (Almeida and Davis 2006; Schleinitz et al. 2008)

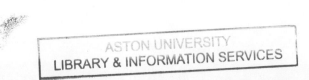

between different receptor/ligand pairs within the organized IS being the important issue. For example, the level of expression of HLA-C on target cells determined its supramolecular organization and the extent of segregation from ICAM-1 (CD54) at the NK-cell IS (Almeida and Davis 2006). Strikingly, for individual peripheral blood NK clones, specific thresholds in the level of target cell HLA-C needed to cause segregation of HLA-C from ICAM-1 at the IS, directly correlated with the threshold needed to functionally inhibit cytotoxicity (Almeida and Davis 2006). Thus, the organization of HLA-C at the IS, determined by its level of expression, may directly influence NK-cell inhibition by regulating the proximity of activating and inhibitory receptors. This would be consistent with earlier studies, using mAb cross-linking, demonstrating that co-clustering of activating and inhibitory receptors was required for inhibition (Blery et al. 1997).

What causes the segregation of different receptor/ligand pairs across the inhibitory NK-cell IS remains unproven. In the "kinetic-segregation model" for T cell receptor triggering it has been proposed that proteins can be organized according to the size of their extracellular domains (Davis and van der Merwe 2006). Accordingly at the inhibitory NK-cell IS, it has been demonstrated that larger proteins, e.g., CD43, are excluded from the IS (McCann et al. 2003). Moreover, the size of KIR-MHC protein is significantly smaller than that of LFA-1 (CD11a/C18)-ICAM-1, which is consistent with their segregation being driven by size differences (Davis 2002; Davis and van der Merwe 1996, 2006; McCann et al. 2002; Springer 1990). Such a model would also explain why the extent of segregation between these proteins was greater when their expression levels were increased (Almeida and Davis 2006). However, a prediction of this model would be that the size of the synaptic cleft would match the size of different proteins where they clustered. In contrast, at least after fixation for examination by electron microscopy, the size of the synaptic cleft varies considerably and apparently randomly, seemingly able to accommodate a range of protein sizes in close proximity (McCann et al. 2003). Thus, it is important to study in more detail whether the size of proteins influences their organization at the NK-cell IS and if so, it must be clarified whether this affects protein segregation at the level of microclusters and/or larger-scale segregation across the synapse.

While some receptor/ligand pairs can accumulate spontaneously, active receptor signalling also plays a crucial role in the organization of inhibitory synapses. Functional ITIM tyrosines and the catalytic activity of SHP-1 are required for disruption of the actin cytoskeleton and exclusion of GM1-rich microdomains from NK-cell or cytotoxic T-cell synapses (Fassett et al. 2001; Guerra et al. 2002; Lou et al. 2000; Masilamani et al. 2006). Proteins associated with GM1-rich microdomains play an essential role in the initial phosphorylation of activating NK-cell receptors (Inoue et al. 2002; Watzl and Long 2003). Thus, one way in which inhibitory NK-cell receptors can be effective, is by blocking the actin-cytoskeleton dependent recruitment of signalling proteins within GM1-rich microdomains to the IS (Endt et al. 2007; Fassett et al. 2001; Fourmentraux-Neves et al. 2008; Guerra et al. 2002; Lou et al. 2000; Masilamani et al. 2006; Sanni et al. 2004; Sohn et al. 2008; Tsai and Discher 2008; Vyas et al. 2002; Vyas et al. 2004; Watzl and Long 2003). Consistent with this model, activating receptors CD2 and 2B4 (CD244) are not inhibited from being recruited to an inhibitory NK-cell IS (Schleinitz et al. 2008), but rather are likely to be impaired in their ability to signal there. Similarly in B cells, for example, the inhibitory receptor FcγRIIB blocks association of the BCR with lipid raft-like domains and also prevents subsequent accumulation of BCR-enriched microclusters in the centre of the synapse (Sohn et al. 2008). In T cells, the inhibitory receptor CTLA-4 inhibits formation of ZAP-70 microclusters (Schneider et al. 2008). Taken together, this suggests a common principle in that inhibitory synapses still accumulate activating receptors and ligands, but specifically exclude the membrane-proximal intracellular proteins needed for activation.

4 Balancing Synapses with Kinapses and Kinetic Proofreading at the Cellular Level

The term kinapse has recently been proposed to describe junctions involving moving T cells that allow signals to be integrated (Dustin 2008a, b). Kinapses lack the degree of stability characteristic for synapses and cell polarity is maintained in the direction of cell movement, rather than being orientated to face the intercellular contact. It is well established that ligation of the TCR delivers a stop signal to T cells (Dustin et al. 1997) that precedes synapse formation (Lee et al. 2002). NK cells similarly crawl over the surface of target cells, notably with higher motility for inhibitory contacts (Burshtyn et al. 2000; Davis et al. 1999; Eriksson et al. 1999a). Likewise, ligation of activating NK-cell receptors provides a stop signal that results in symmetrical spreading of NK cells over their targets, while ligation of inhibitory receptors provides a reverse-stop signal that breaks the symmetry of spreading and encourages NK-cell migration (Culley et al. 2009). Similarly, the inhibitory receptor CTLA-4 reverses the TCR-mediated stop signal (Schneider et al. 2006). Thus, an inhibitory synapse may be considered as a transient symmetrical synapse driving an effector cell to revert to its migratory kinapse configuration. PKCθ and WASp were found to favour T cells forming a kinapse or synapse, respectively (Sims et al. 2007). It would be interesting to determine if inhibitory NK-cell IS exploit these pathways in driving cells to a kinapse configuration. Indeed, inhibitory signals in NK cells are known to directly regulate cytoskeletal processes involving WASp (Krzewski et al. 2006) and Vav (Stebbins et al. 2003).

It is well established that cytolytic NK cell synapses go through sequential steps that lead to the directed release of lytic granules (Davis 2002, 2009; Davis and Dustin 2004; Krzewski and Strominger 2008; Orange 2008; Wulfing et al 2003). Thus, the process of cellular activation can be considered as directly analogous to the model of kinetic-proofreading for triggering individual TCR signals (McKeithan 1995). Specifically, there are a number of steps that two cells in contact must go through before lytic granules are released or other effector functions realized. These include a multitude of cellular processes, such as calcium flux, integrin-mediated tight adhesion, MTOC reorientation, translocation of granules to the synapse and many others. These steps introduce a series of time delays from initial intercellular contact until the effector function is realized, e.g. lytic granules are released. Thus, an inhibitory synapse serves to shorten the half-life of the intercellular conjugate and break the IS before these steps can be completed, preventing effector functions.

5 Unzipping the Synapse

There has been extensive research on the assembly of the IS yet relatively little attention has been given to its disassembly. Thousands of individual protein–protein interactions exist across the IS such that the disassembly of this contact cannot be trivial. Perhaps most acutely, when inhibition dominates the outcome of surveillance, e.g. at the inhibitory NK-cell IS, protein–protein interactions accumulated at the synapse must be rapidly removed or broken so that NK cells can readily move on to survey other target cells. Similarly, for cytolytic interactions involving CTL or NK cells, it is unclear how the effector cells efficiently move away from dead or dying target cells. Efficient disassembly of the synapse is important to allow cells to move between target cells and must be necessary, for example, for CTL or NK cells to sequentially kill several target cells (Bhat and Watzl 2007; Martz 1976). It has been demonstrated that some receptors are endocytosed from the IS upon ligation, e.g., the T-cell receptor (TCR) (Cemerski et al. 2008; Lee et al. 2003), but it has not been directly tested whether or not these events are important in the disassembly of the IS. Indeed, it is unclear how many protein-protein interactions would need to be removed from an IS to allow cells to move apart. Alternatively, it can be envisaged that exocytosis of the synaptic membrane from the target cells or APCs could contribute to the disassembly of the IS. This could relate to the common process of intercellular transfer of surface proteins between immune cells that can occur by several specific mechanisms (Davis 2007; LeMaoult et al. 2007). More broadly, the extent to which specific signalling events control termination of the synapse has been little studied. It is well understood that inside-out signalling leads to a high-affinity conformation of LFA-1 that in turn contributes to intercellular conjugation and assembly of the IS (Luo et al. 2007). However, it has been far less-studied whether or not specific signals could return LFA-1 to a lower affinity state and contribute to the disassembly of the synapse.

6 Regulatory Synapses

In addition to the autonomous interaction of NK cells with infected or transformed cells, research has expanded in recent years to study the cross-talk between NK cells and other immune cells, including monocytes, macrophages, dendritic cells and T cells. These interactions can augment or initiate NK-cell responses to pathological challenges and can also shape adaptive immune responses, e.g., by triggering DC maturation (Andoniou et al. 2008; Fernandez et al. 1999; Moretta et al. 2006; Newman and Riley 2007; Raulet 2004; Strowig et al. 2008). Contact-dependent reciprocal stimulation plays an important role during these interactions and several studies have therefore investigated the organization of these intercellular contacts termed regulatory synapses (Borg et al. 2004; Brilot et al. 2007; Nedvetzki et al. 2007; Pallandre et al. 2008).

7 The Regulatory NK-Cell Synapse

Regulatory NK-cell synapses are long lasting and accumulate activating receptors, cytokine receptors and adhesion molecules (Borg et al. 2004; Brilot et al. 2007; Nedvetzki et al. 2007; Semino et al. 2005). Figure 2 summarizes current knowledge of the molecular arrangements at such regulatory NK-cell synapses. In contrast to an inhibitory IS, cytoskeletal components, f-actin, fascin and talin as well as GM1-rich microdomains all accumulate at the regulatory IS (Borg et al. 2004; Brilot et al. 2007; Nedvetzki et al. 2007; Semino et al. 2005). Inhibitory receptors do still cluster at such IS and accumulate adjacent to clusters of cytokine receptors, surrounded by a ring of LFA-1 and talin (Brilot et al. 2007). Cytokines and cytokine receptors accumulate at the regulatory NK-cell IS (Borg et al. 2004; Brilot et al. 2007; Semino et al. 2005). IL-18 is directionally secreted across the synapse between NK cells and immature DCs (iDCs) and stimulates secretion of HMGB1 by NK cells, which in turn is necessary to induce DC maturation (Semino et al. 2005). Mature DCs (mDCs) polarize preassembled stores of IL-12 towards the NK-cell IS (Borg et al. 2004) and NK cells accumulate the high affinity subunit of the IL-15 receptor, IL-15Rα, at the IS (Brilot et al. 2007). Polarization of cytokines towards the regulatory NK-cell IS implicates an importance of synapse formation for directed cytokine secretion. This is likely to be important in a wide range of immune cell interactions. For example, co-culture experiments using a transwell membrane recently determined that IL-18 is delivered to NK cells in a contact dependent manner by Kupffer (liver macrophage-like) cells (Tu et al. 2008). As determined for T cells, a general principle is that some cytokines and chemokines are secreted multi-directionally from effector cells, to have a broad impact on inflammation, while others are secreted directionally via the IS where specific intercellular communication is required (Brilot et al. 2007).

8 Triggering Cytokine Secretion Versus Cytolysis

There is evidence that immature DCs are susceptible to lysis by NK cells and acquire protection from lysis by maturation (Moretta et al. 2006; Strowig et al. 2008). Killing of iDCs can be triggered via the natural cytotoxicity receptor NKp30

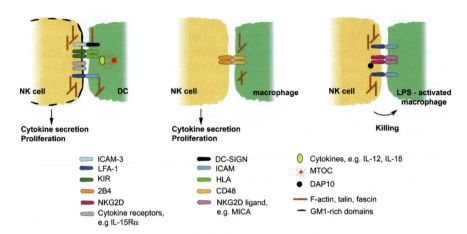

Fig. 2 The regulatory NK-cell IS. The interaction of NK cells with DCs or macrophages can induce NK cell proliferation or cytokine secretion, without triggering cytotoxicity. The resulting IS has therefore been termed regulatory (Borg et al. 2004; Brilot et al. 2007; Nedvetzki et al. 2007; Pallandre et al. 2008). DCs polarize the MTOC and cytokines including IL-12 and IL-18 towards the IS (Borg et al. 2004). In NK cells, the IL-15Rα subunit is recruited to the contact site where it segregates from inhibitory NK-cell receptors (Brilot et al. 2007). Furthermore, adhesion molecules and their ligands, e.g. LFA-1, DC-SIGN and ICAM-3, polarize towards the cell interface (Borg et al. 2004; Brilot et al. 2007). Both, NK cells and DCs show reorganization of the actin-cytoskeleton, with cytoskeletal proteins including f-actin, talin and fascin accumulating at the synapse (Borg et al. 2004; Brilot et al. 2007). Additionally, GM1-rich microdomains enrich within the NK cell membrane in the contact area (Borg et al. 2004). Macrophages stimulate NK cell proliferation and cytokine secretion and prime NK cell cytotoxicity against susceptible target cells. This is largely dependent on the engagement of the 2B4 receptor, which is recruited to the centre of such regulatory synapses. In these contacts F-actin accumulates at the synapse from within macrophages, but not NK cells. Macrophages exposed to a high dose of LPS upregulate ligands for the NK cell receptor NKG2D and are subsequently killed by NK cells. These cytolytic NK cell–macrophage synapses accumulate NKG2D and the signalling adapters DAP10 and CD3ζ at the centre of the IS, while ICAM-1 locates to the periphery. F-actin accumulates at the contact area from within the NK cells, but not in the macrophages (Nedvetzki et al. 2007)

(CD337) (Ferlazzo et al. 2002; Spaggiari et al. 2001) while increased expression of class I MHC protein during DC maturation provides protection from NK-cell lysis (Carbone et al. 1999; Ferlazzo et al. 2002). Whether macrophages induce a cyto-lytic or regulatory NK-cell IS depends on the activation state of the macrophage in terms of the strength of TLR-4 stimulation (Nedvetzki et al. 2007). Macrophages that are stimulated with a low dose of LPS form regulatory synapses, characterized by the recruitment of the NK-cell receptor 2B4, while stimulation with a high dose of LPS induces upregulation of NKG2D (CD314) ligands on macrophages that triggers NKG2D-mediated killing (Nedvetzki et al. 2007).

It is particularly intriguing that 2B4 is recruited to the regulatory NK-cell-macrophage IS and is important for triggering cytokine secretion (Nedvetzki et al. 2007), while at other synapses, e.g., during interactions with tumour cell targets, 2B4 ligation triggers cytotoxicity (Bhat et al. 2006). Mechanisms must be in place to determine the function of 2B4-mediated activation. One possibility is that this depends on the synergy with other activating receptors. Indeed, only specific combinations of activating receptors can induce granule exocytosis in human NK cells (Bryceson et al. 2006). Receptors not specifically associated with NK-cell activation can be important in determining the NK cell response. For example, the chemokine CX3CL1 influences the distribution of KIR at the NK cell–DC synapse and is able to prevent phosphorylation of its ITIMs (Pallandre et al. 2008). Of particular interest, 2B4 has been shown to directly interact with a variety of signalling molecules (Eissmann et al. 2005) and to mediate activation of granule exocytosis or cytokine secretion (Kubin et al. 1999; Nakajima et al. 1999; Tangye et al. 1999), as well as inhibition (Parolini et al. 2000; Sivori et al. 2002). Thus, the availability of downstream signalling proteins at the IS may determine the outcome of 2B4 stimulation in NK cells. In this case, regulatory synapses would function by selectively recruiting certain membrane-proximal adaptors or kinases, analogous to the restricted recruitment of signalling proteins seen at inhibitory synapses.

Overall, it is clear that there is an important role for the IS in balancing activation, regulation and inhibition of immune responses. Much of what has been achieved so far is a direct result of the inter-disciplinary approach that immunologists have taken relatively recently to probe molecular recognition by individual cells. The continuing development and application of new techniques that allow intercellular communication to be probed with superior spatial and temporal resolution will enable scientists to resolve many of the outstanding issues highlighted throughout this review. Already, numerous recent super-resolution imaging techniques have the potential to directly report the spatial and temporal relationships of the key molecules (Fernandez-Suarez and Ting 2008). Perhaps most exciting is that as we continue to probe immune cell recognition with superior resolution, unexpected signalling and integration mechanisms that were not apparent at conventional diffraction-limited resolution will surely be revealed.

Acknowledgements We thank current members of our laboratory and F.J. Culley, M.A. Purbhoo, F.V. de Abreu, P.M.W. French, M.A.A. Neil and A.I. Magee for useful discussions. We thank N. Powell for assistance with preparing the figures. Research in our laboratory is funded by The Medical Research Council, The Biotechnology and Biological Sciences Research Council, The Wellcome Trust, a Lister Institute Research Prize and a Wolfson Royal Society Research Merit Award (to DMD).

References

Almeida CR, Davis DM (2006) Segregation of HLA-C from ICAM-1 at NK cell immune synapses is controlled by its cell surface density. J Immunol 177:6904–6910

Andoniou CE, Coudert JD, Degli-Esposti MA (2008) Killers and beyond: NK-cell-mediated control of immune responses. Eur J Immunol 38:2938–2942

Bhat R, Watzl C (2007) Serial killing of tumor cells by human natural killer cells – enhancement by therapeutic antibodies. PLoS ONE 2:e326

Bhat R, Eissmann P, Endt J, Hoffmann S, Watzl C (2006) Fine-tuning of immune responses by SLAM-related receptors. J Leukoc Biol 79:417–424

Blery M, Delon J, Trautmann A, Cambiaggi A, Olcese L, Biassoni R, Moretta L, Chavrier P, Moretta A, Daeron M et al (1997) Reconstituted killer cell inhibitory receptors for major histocompatibility complex class I molecules control mast cell activation induced via immunoreceptor tyrosine-based activation motifs. J Biol Chem 272:8989–8996

Borg C, Jalil A, Laderach D, Maruyama K, Wakasugi H, Charrier S, Ryffel B, Cambi A, Figdor C, Vainchenker W et al (2004) NK cell activation by dendritic cells (DCs) requires the formation of a synapse leading to IL-12 polarization in DCs. Blood 104:3267–3275

Brilot F, Strowig T, Roberts SM, Arrey F, Munz C (2007) NK cell survival mediated through the regulatory synapse with human DCs requires IL-15Ralpha. J Clin Invest 117:3316–3329

Bryceson YT, March ME, Ljunggren HG, Long EO (2006) Activation, coactivation, and costimulation of resting human natural killer cells. Immunol Rev 214:73–91

Bunnell SC, Hong DI, Kardon JR, Yamazaki T, McGlade CJ, Barr VA, Samelson LE (2002) T cell receptor ligation induces the formation of dynamically regulated signaling assemblies. J Cell Biol 158:1263–1275

Burshtyn DN, Shin J, Stebbins C, Long EO (2000) Adhesion to target cells is disrupted by the killer cell inhibitory receptor. Curr Biol 10:777–780

Campi G, Varma R, Dustin ML (2005) Actin and agonist MHC-peptide complex-dependent T cell receptor microclusters as scaffolds for signaling. J Exp Med 202:1031–1036

Carbone E, Terrazzano G, Ruggiero G, Zanzi D, Ottaiano A, Manzo C, Karre K, Zappacosta S (1999) Recognition of autologous dendritic cells by human NK cells. Eur J Immunol 29:4022–4029

Carlin LM, Eleme K, McCann FE, Davis DM (2001) Intercellular transfer and supramolecular organization of human leukocyte antigen C at inhibitory natural killer cell immune synapses. J Exp Med 194:1507–1517

Cemerski S, Das J, Giurisato E, Markiewicz MA, Allen PM, Chakraborty AK, Shaw AS (2008) The balance between T cell receptor signaling and degradation at the center of the immunological synapse is determined by antigen quality. Immunity 29:414–422

Chouaib S, Thiery J, Gati A, Guerra N, El Behi M, Dorothee G, Mami-Chouaib F, Bellet D, Caignard A (2002) Tumor escape from killing: role of killer inhibitory receptors and acquisition of tumor resistance to cell death. Tissue Antigens 60:273–281

Culley FJ, Johnson M, Evans JH, Kumar S, Crilly R, Casasbuenas J, Schnyder T, Mehrabi M, Deonarain MP, Ushakov DS et al (2009) Natural killer cell signal integration balances synapse symmetry and migration. PLoS Biol 7:e1000159

Daeron M, Jaeger S, Du Pasquier L, Vivier E (2008) Immunoreceptor tyrosine-based inhibition motifs: a quest in the past and future. Immunol Rev 224:11–43

Davis DM (2002) Assembly of the immunological synapse for T cells and NK cells. Trends Immunol 23:356–363

Davis DM (2006) Intrigue at the immune synapse. Sci Am 294:48–55

Davis DM (2007) Intercellular transfer of cell-surface proteins is common and can affect many stages of an immune response. Nat Rev Immunol 7:238–243

Davis DM (2009) Mechanisms and functions for the duration of intercellular contacts made by lymphocytes. Nat Rev Immunol 9:543–555

Davis DM, Dustin ML (2004) What is the importance of the immunological synapse? Trends Immunol 25:323–327

Davis SJ, van der Merwe PA (1996) The structure and ligand interactions of CD2: implications for T-cell function. Immunol Today 17:177–187

Davis SJ, van der Merwe PA (2006) The kinetic-segregation model: TCR triggering and beyond. Nat Immunol 7:803–809

Davis DM, Chiu I, Fassett M, Cohen GB, Mandelboim O, Strominger JL (1999) The human natural killer cell immune synapse. Proc Natl Acad Sci USA 96:15062–15067

Dietrich J, Cella M, Colonna M (2001) Ig-like transcript 2 (ILT2)/leukocyte Ig-like receptor 1 (LIR1) inhibits TCR signaling and actin cytoskeleton reorganization. J Immunol 166:2514–2521

Dustin ML (2008a) Hunter to gatherer and back: immunological synapses and kinapses as variations on the theme of amoeboid locomotion. Annu Rev Cell Dev Biol 24:577–596

Dustin ML (2008b) T-cell activation through immunological synapses and kinapses. Immunol Rev 221:77–89

Dustin ML, Bromley SK, Kan Z, Peterson DA, Unanue ER (1997) Antigen receptor engagement delivers a stop signal to migrating T lymphocytes. Proc Natl Acad Sci USA 94:3909–3913

Egen JG, Allison JP (2002) Cytotoxic T lymphocyte antigen-4 accumulation in the immunological synapse is regulated by TCR signal strength. Immunity 16:23–35

Eissmann P, Beauchamp L, Wooters J, Tilton JC, Long EO, Watzl C (2005) Molecular basis for positive and negative signaling by the natural killer cell receptor 2B4 (CD244). Blood 105:4722–4729

Endt J, McCann FE, Almeida CR, Urlaub D, Leung R, Pende D, Davis DM, Watzl C (2007) Inhibitory receptor signals suppress ligation-induced recruitment of NKG2D to GM1-rich membrane domains at the human NK cell immune synapse. J Immunol 178:5606–5611

Eriksson M, Leitz G, Fallman E, Axner O, Ryan JC, Nakamura MC, Sentman CL (1999a) Inhibitory receptors alter natural killer cell interactions with target cells yet allow simultaneous killing of susceptible targets. J Exp Med 190:1005–1012

Eriksson M, Ryan JC, Nakamura MC, Sentman CL (1999b) Ly49A inhibitory receptors redistribute on natural killer cells during target cell interaction. Immunology 97:341–347

Fan QR, Long EO, Wiley DC (2000) Cobalt-mediated dimerization of the human natural killer cell inhibitory receptor. J Biol Chem 275:23700–23706

Fassett MS, Davis DM, Valter MM, Cohen GB, Strominger JL (2001) Signaling at the inhibitory natural killer cell immune synapse regulates lipid raft polarization but not class I MHC clustering. Proc Natl Acad Sci USA 98:14547–14552

Faure M, Barber DF, Takahashi SM, Jin T, Long EO (2003) Spontaneous clustering and tyrosine phosphorylation of NK cell inhibitory receptor induced by ligand binding. J Immunol 170:6107–6114

Ferlazzo G, Tsang ML, Moretta L, Melioli G, Steinman RM, Munz C (2002) Human dendritic cells activate resting natural killer (NK) cells and are recognized via the NKp30 receptor by activated NK cells. J Exp Med 195:343–351

Fernandez NC, Lozier A, Flament C, Ricciardi-Castagnoli P, Bellet D, Suter M, Perricaudet M, Tursz T, Maraskovsky E, Zitvogel L (1999) Dendritic cells directly trigger NK cell functions: cross-talk relevant in innate anti-tumor immune responses in vivo. Nat Med 5:405–411

Fernandez-Suarez M, Ting AY (2008) Fluorescent probes for super-resolution imaging in living cells. Nat Rev Mol Cell Biol 9:929–943

Fourmentraux-Neves E, Jalil A, Da Rocha S, Pichon C, Chouaib S, Bismuth G, Caignard A (2008) Two opposite signaling outputs are driven by the KIR2DL1 receptor in human CD4+ T cells. Blood 112:2381–2389

Guerra N, Michel F, Gati A, Gaudin C, Mishal Z, Escudier B, Acuto O, Chouaib S, Caignard A (2002) Engagement of the inhibitory receptor CD158a interrupts TCR signaling, preventing dynamic membrane reorganization in CTL/tumor cell interaction. Blood 100:2874–2881

Harwood NE, Batista FD (2008) New insights into the early molecular events underlying B cell activation. Immunity 28:609–619

Henel G, Singh K, Cui D, Pryshchep S, Lee WW, Weyand CM, Goronzy JJ (2006) Uncoupling of T-cell effector functions by inhibitory killer immunoglobulin-like receptors. Blood 107:4449–4457

Inoue H, Miyaji M, Kosugi A, Nagafuku M, Okazaki T, Mimori T, Amakawa R, Fukuhara S, Domae N, Bloom ET et al (2002) Lipid rafts as the signaling scaffold for NK cell activation: tyrosine phosphorylation and association of LAT with phosphatidylinositol 3-kinase and phospholipase C-gamma following CD2 stimulation. Eur J Immunol 32:2188–2198

Karre K, Ljunggren HG, Piontek G, Kiessling R (1986) Selective rejection of H-2-deficient lymphoma variants suggests alternative immune defence strategy. Nature 319:675–678

Krzewski K, Strominger JL (2008) The killer's kiss: the many functions of NK cell immunological synapses. Curr Opin Cell Biol 20:597–605

Krzewski K, Chen X, Orange JS, Strominger JL (2006) Formation of a WIP-, WASp-, actin-, and myosin IIA-containing multiprotein complex in activated NK cells and its alteration by KIR inhibitory signaling. J Cell Biol 173:121–132

Kubin MZ, Parshley DL, Din W, Waugh JY, Davis-Smith T, Smith CA, Macduff BM, Armitage RJ, Chin W, Cassiano L et al (1999) Molecular cloning and biological characterization of NK cell activation-inducing ligand, a counterstructure for CD48. Eur J Immunol 29:3466–3477

Lanier LL (2005) NK cell recognition. Annu Rev Immunol 23:225–274

Lee KH, Holdorf AD, Dustin ML, Chan AC, Allen PM, Shaw AS (2002) T cell receptor signaling precedes immunological synapse formation. Science 295:1539–1542

Lee KH, Dinner AR, Tu C, Campi G, Raychaudhuri S, Varma R, Sims TN, Burack WR, Wu H, Wang J et al (2003) The immunological synapse balances T cell receptor signaling and degradation. Science 302:1218–1222

LeMaoult J, Caumartin J, Carosella ED (2007) Exchanges of membrane patches (trogocytosis) split theoretical and actual functions of immune cells. Hum Immunol 68:240–243

Ljunggren HG, Karre K (1990) In search of the "missing self": MHC molecules and NK cell recognition. Immunol Today 11:237–244

Long EO (1999) Regulation of immune responses through inhibitory receptors. Annu Rev Immunol 17:875–904

Long EO (2008) Negative signaling by inhibitory receptors: the NK cell paradigm. Immunol Rev 224:70–84

Lou Z, Jevremovic D, Billadeau DD, Leibson PJ (2000) A balance between positive and negative signals in cytotoxic lymphocytes regulates the polarization of lipid rafts during the development of cell-mediated killing. J Exp Med 191:347–354

Luo BH, Carman CV, Springer TA (2007) Structural basis of integrin regulation and signaling. Annu Rev Immunol 25:619–647

Martz E (1976) Multiple target cell killing by the cytolytic T lymphocyte and the mechanism of cytotoxicity. Transplantation 21:5–11

Masilamani M, Nguyen C, Kabat J, Borrego F, Coligan JE (2006) CD94/NKG2A inhibits NK cell activation by disrupting the actin network at the immunological synapse. J Immunol 177:3590–3596

McCann FE, Suhling K, Carlin LM, Eleme K, Taner SB, Yanagi K, Vanherberghen B, French PM, Davis DM (2002) Imaging immune surveillance by T cells and NK cells. Immunol Rev 189:179–192

McCann FE, Vanherberghen B, Eleme K, Carlin LM, Newsam RJ, Goulding D, Davis DM (2003) The size of the synaptic cleft and distinct distributions of filamentous actin, ezrin, CD43, and CD45 at activating and inhibitory human NK cell immune synapses. J Immunol 170: 2862–2870

McKeithan TW (1995) Kinetic proofreading in T-cell receptor signal transduction. Proc Natl Acad Sci USA 92:5042–5046

McMahon CW, Raulet DH (2001) Expression and function of NK cell receptors in CD8+ T cells. Curr Opin Immunol 13:465–470

Moretta L, Ferlazzo G, Bottino C, Vitale M, Pende D, Mingari MC, Moretta A (2006) Effector and regulatory events during natural killer-dendritic cell interactions. Immunol Rev 214:219–228

Nakajima H, Cella M, Langen H, Friedlein A, Colonna M (1999) Activating interactions in human NK cell recognition: the role of 2B4-CD48. Eur J Immunol 29:1676–1683

Nedvetzki S, Sowinski S, Eagle RA, Harris J, Vely F, Pende D, Trowsdale J, Vivier E, Gordon S, Davis DM (2007) Reciprocal regulation of human natural killer cells and macrophages associated with distinct immune synapses. Blood 109:3776–3785

Newman KC, Riley EM (2007) Whatever turns you on: accessory-cell-dependent activation of NK cells by pathogens. Nat Rev Immunol 7:279–291

Oddos S, Dunsby C, Purbhoo MA, Chauveau A, Owen DM, Neil MAA, Davis DM, French PMW (2008) High-speed high-resolution imaging of intercellular immune synapses using optical tweezers. Biophys J 95:L66–L68

Orange JS (2008) Formation and function of the lytic NK-cell immunological synapse. Nat Rev Immunol 8:713–725

Orange JS, Ramesh N, Remold-O'Donnell E, Sasahara Y, Koopman L, Byrne M, Bonilla FA, Rosen FS, Geha RS, Strominger JL (2002) Wiskott-Aldrich syndrome protein is required for NK cell cytotoxicity and colocalizes with actin to NK cell-activating immunologic synapses. Proc Natl Acad Sci USA 99:11351–11356

Orange JS, Harris KE, Andzelm MM, Valter MM, Geha RS, Strominger JL (2003) The mature activating natural killer cell immunologic synapse is formed in distinct stages. Proc Natl Acad Sci USA 100:14151–14156

Pallandre JR, Krzewski K, Bedel R, Ryffel B, Caignard A, Rohrlich PS, Pivot X, Tiberghien P, Zitvogel L, Strominger JL et al (2008) Dendritic cell and natural killer cell cross-talk: a pivotal role of CX3CL1 in NK cytoskeleton organization and activation. Blood 112:4420–4424

Parolini S, Bottino C, Falco M, Augugliaro R, Giliani S, Franceschini R, Ochs HD, Wolf H, Bonnefoy JY, Biassoni R et al (2000) X-linked lymphoproliferative disease. 2B4 molecules displaying inhibitory rather than activating function are responsible for the inability of natural killer cells to kill Epstein-Barr virus-infected cells. J Exp Med 192:337–346

Peggs KS, Quezada SA, Allison JP (2008) Cell intrinsic mechanisms of T-cell inhibition and application to cancer therapy. Immunol Rev 224:141–165

Pritchard NR, Smith KG (2003) B cell inhibitory receptors and autoimmunity. Immunology 108:263–273

Rajagopalan S, Long EO (1998) Zinc bound to the killer cell-inhibitory receptor modulates the negative signal in human NK cells. J Immunol 161:1299–1305

Rajagopalan S, Long EO (2005) Understanding how combinations of HLA and KIR genes influence disease. J Exp Med 201:1025–1029

Rajagopalan S, Winter CC, Wagtmann N, Long EO (1995) The Ig-related killer cell inhibitory receptor binds zinc and requires zinc for recognition of HLA-C on target cells. J Immunol 155:4143–4146

Raulet DH (2004) Interplay of natural killer cells and their receptors with the adaptive immune response. Nat Immunol 5:996–1002

Sanni TB, Masilamani M, Kabat J, Coligan JE, Borrego F (2004) Exclusion of lipid rafts and decreased mobility of CD94/NKG2A receptors at the inhibitory NK cell synapse. Mol Biol Cell 15:3210–3223

Schleinitz N, March ME, Long EO (2008) Recruitment of activation receptors at inhibitory NK cell immune synapses. PLoS ONE 3:e3278

Schneider H, Downey J, Smith A, Zinselmeyer BH, Rush C, Brewer JM, Wei B, Hogg N, Garside P, Rudd CE (2006) Reversal of the TCR stop signal by CTLA-4. Science 313:1972–1975

Schneider H, Smith X, Liu H, Bismuth G, Rudd CE (2008) CTLA-4 disrupts ZAP70 microcluster formation with reduced T cell/APC dwell times and calcium mobilization. Eur J Immunol 38:40–47

Seminario MC, Bunnell SC (2008) Signal initiation in T-cell receptor microclusters. Immunol Rev 221:90–106

Semino C, Angelini G, Poggi A, Rubartelli A (2005) NK/iDC interaction results in IL-18 secretion by DCs at the synaptic cleft followed by NK cell activation and release of the DC maturation factor HMGB1. Blood 106:609–616

Sims TN, Soos TJ, Xenias HS, Dubin-Thaler B, Hofman JM, Waite JC, Cameron TO, Thomas VK, Varma R, Wiggins CH et al (2007) Opposing effects of PKCtheta and WASp on symmetry breaking and relocation of the immunological synapse. Cell 129:773–785

Sivori S, Falco M, Marcenaro E, Parolini S, Biassoni R, Bottino C, Moretta L, Moretta A (2002) Early expression of triggering receptors and regulatory role of 2B4 in human natural killer cell precursors undergoing in vitro differentiation. Proc Natl Acad Sci USA 99:4526–4531

Snyder MR, Muegge LO, Offord C, O'Fallon WM, Bajzer Z, Weyand CM, Goronzy JJ (2002) Formation of the killer Ig-like receptor repertoire on CD4+CD28null T cells. J Immunol 168:3839–3846

Sohn HW, Pierce SK, Tzeng SJ (2008) Live cell imaging reveals that the inhibitory FcgammaRIIB destabilizes B cell receptor membrane-lipid interactions and blocks immune synapse formation. J Immunol 180:793–799

Spaggiari GM, Carosio R, Pende D, Marcenaro S, Rivera P, Zocchi MR, Moretta L, Poggi A (2001) NK cell-mediated lysis of autologous antigen-presenting cells is triggered by the engagement of the phosphatidylinositol 3-kinase upon ligation of the natural cytotoxicity receptors NKp30 and NKp46. Eur J Immunol 31:1656–1665

Springer TA (1990) Adhesion receptors of the immune system. Nature 346:425–434

Standeven LJ, Carlin LM, Borszcz P, Davis DM, Burshtyn DN (2004) The actin cytoskeleton controls the efficiency of killer Ig-like receptor accumulation at inhibitory NK cell immune synapses. J Immunol 173:5617–5625

Stebbins CC, Watzl C, Billadeau DD, Leibson PJ, Burshtyn DN, Long EO (2003) Vav1 dephosphorylation by the tyrosine phosphatase SHP-1 as a mechanism for inhibition of cellular cytotoxicity. Mol Cell Biol 23:6291–6299

Strowig T, Brilot F, Munz C (2008) Noncytotoxic functions of NK cells: direct pathogen restriction and assistance to adaptive immunity. J Immunol 180:7785–7791

Tangye SG, Lazetic S, Woollatt E, Sutherland GR, Lanier LL, Phillips JH (1999) Cutting edge: human 2B4, an activating NK cell receptor, recruits the protein tyrosine phosphatase SHP-2 and the adaptor signaling protein SAP. J Immunol 162:6981–6985

Treanor B, Lanigan PM, Kumar S, Dunsby C, Munro I, Auksorius E, Culley FJ, Purbhoo MA, Phillips D, Neil MA et al (2006) Microclusters of inhibitory killer immunoglobulin-like receptor signaling at natural killer cell immunological synapses. J Cell Biol 174:153–161

Tsai RK, Discher DE (2008) Inhibition of "self" engulfment through deactivation of myosin-II at the phagocytic synapse between human cells. J Cell Biol 180:989–1003

Tu Z, Bozorgzadeh A, Pierce RH, Kurtis J, Crispe IN, Orloff MS (2008) TLR-dependent cross talk between human Kupffer cells and NK cells. J Exp Med 205:233–244

Ugolini S, Vivier E (2000) Regulation of T cell function by NK cell receptors for classical MHC class I molecules. Curr Opin Immunol 12:295–300

Vales-Gomez M, Erskine RA, Deacon MP, Strominger JL, Reyburn HT (2001) The role of zinc in the binding of killer cell Ig-like receptors to class I MHC proteins. Proc Natl Acad Sci USA 98:1734–1739

van Bergen J, Thompson A, van der Slik A, Ottenhoff TH, Gusekloo J, Koning F (2004) Phenotypic and functional characterization of CD4 T cells expressing killer Ig-like receptors. J Immunol 173:6719–6726

Varma R, Campi G, Yokosuka T, Saito T, Dustin ML (2006) T cell receptor-proximal signals are sustained in peripheral microclusters and terminated in the central supramolecular activation cluster. Immunity 25:117–127

Vyas YM, Mehta KM, Morgan M, Maniar H, Butros L, Jung S, Burkhardt JK, Dupont B (2001) Spatial organization of signal transduction molecules in the NK cell immune synapses during MHC class I-regulated noncytolytic and cytolytic interactions. J Immunol 167:4358–4367

Vyas YM, Maniar H, Dupont B (2002) Cutting edge: differential segregation of the SRC homology 2-containing protein tyrosine phosphatase-1 within the early NK cell immune synapse distinguishes noncytolytic from cytolytic interactions. J Immunol 168:3150–3154

Vyas YM, Maniar H, Lyddane CE, Sadelain M, Dupont B (2004) Ligand binding to inhibitory killer cell Ig-like receptors induce colocalization with Src homology domain 2-containing protein tyrosine phosphatase 1 and interruption of ongoing activation signals. J Immunol 173:1571–1578

Watzl C, Long EO (2003) Natural killer cell inhibitory receptors block actin cytoskeleton-dependent recruitment of 2B4 (CD244) to lipid rafts. J Exp Med 197:77–85

Wulfing C, Purtic B, Klem J, Schatzle JD (2003) Stepwise cytoskeletal polarization as a series of checkpoints in innate but not adaptive cytolytic killing. Proc Natl Acad Sci USA 100: 7767–7772

Yokosuka T, Sakata-Sogawa K, Kobayashi W, Hiroshima M, Hashimoto-Tane A, Tokunaga M, Dustin ML, Saito T (2005) Newly generated T cell receptor microclusters initiate and sustain T cell activation by recruitment of Zap70 and SLP-76. Nat Immunol 6:1253–1262

The Immunological Synapse, TCR Microclusters, and T Cell Activation

Tadashi Yokosuka and Takashi Saito

Contents

T. Saito (✉)
WPI Immunology Frontier Research Center, Suita, Osaka 565-0081, Japan
e-mail: saito@rcai.riken.jp

T. Yokosuka
Laboratory for Cell Signaling, RIKEN Research Center for Allergy and Immunology,
1-7-22 Suehiro-cho, Tsurumi-ku, Yokohama 230-0045, Japan
e-mail: yokosuka@rcai.riken.jp

T. Saito and F.D. Batista (eds.), *Immunological Synapse*,
Current Topics in Microbiology and Immunology 340,
DOI 10.1007/978-3-642-03858-7_5, © Springer-Verlag Berlin Heidelberg 2010

Abstract T cell activation begins with the interaction between an antigen-specific T cell and an antigen-presenting cell (APC). This interaction results in the formation of the immunological synapse, which had been considered to be responsible for antigen recognition and T cell activation. Recent advances in imaging analysis have provided new insights into T cell activation. The T cell receptor (TCR) microclusters, TCRs, kinases, and adaptors are generated upon antigen recognition at the interfaces between the T cells and the APCs and serve as a fundamental signaling unit for T cell activation. CD28-mediated costimulation is also found to be regulated by the formation of microclusters. Therefore, the dynamic regulations of TCR and CD28 microcluster formation, migration, and interaction are the key events for the initiation of T cell-mediated immune responses. Comprehensive analyses of the composition and characteristics of the TCR microcluster have identified its dynamic features. This review will outline new discoveries of the microclusters and its related concept in T cell activation.

1   Introduction

T cells play a pivotal role in orchestrating the immune system. T cell responses are induced by antigen recognition through the T cell receptors (TCRs), which bind antigen peptide–major histocompatibility (MHCp) complexes on antigen-presenting cells (APCs). It was known that upon interaction between the T cells and the APCs, TCRs and other accessory molecules accumulated at the interface between the two cell types (Norcross 1984; Paul et al. 1987). Just ten years ago, the immunological synapse was defined as a special molecular architecture for recognition and signaling, where the receptors and adhesion molecules could be structurally and kinetically organized for the initial and sustained T cell activation (Monks et al. 1998; Grakoui et al. 1999). The concept of the immunological synapse beautifully correlated with what was known about T cell antigen recognition and activation; however, this model could not explain early activation events, which can occur within 1 min. A much smaller signaling unit was predicted to form prior to the mature immunological synapse formation. Indeed, the TCR microcluster was discovered as a signaling cluster containing receptors, accessory molecules, and downstream signaling molecules (Bunnell et al. 2002; Campi et al. 2005; Yokosuka et al. 2005; Saito and Yokosuka 2006). Microclusters dynamically change the localization and the assembled molecules at the immunological synapse and induce initial and sustained TCR signaling as well as costimulation signals (Depoil et al. 2008; Yokosuka et al. 2008). This model is now known to describe the signaling of other lymphocytes, including B cells, natural killer (NK) cells, and natural killer T (NKT) cells (Davis and Dustin 2004). In this review, we discuss the signaling clusters for T cell activation from the viewpoint of the microclusters as the minimum signaling unit that can be visualized and propose a new model of T cell activation.

2   The Immunological Synapse

2.1   Discovery of the Immunological Synapse

T cells recognize cognate antigen by interacting with APCs to form immunological synapses (Huppa and Davis 2003). The term "synapse" was first used in the immune system by Norcross in 1984 in a prescient theoretical paper describing the accumulation and function of various molecules at the T cell–APC interface (Norcross 1984), and, ten years later, Paul revived this term (Paul and Seder 1994). Similar to the CD4$^+$ T cell–APC synapse, Kupfer noticed the reorientation of the microtubule-organizing center (MTOC) and Golgi apparatus toward the cytotoxic T lymphocyte (CTL)–target cell interface as an early event in CTL killing. Later, his group reported membrane and cytoskeletal reorientation at the junction between a T cell–B cell conjugate, leading to the important discovery of the supramolecular activation cluster (SMAC), a highly patterned clustering and segregation of cell surface molecules, particularly antigen receptors and adhesion molecules (Monks et al. 1997; Monks et al. 1998). Dustin and his colleagues superbly demonstrated the kinetics of immunological synapse formation using the McConnell's planar bilayer system (McConnell et al. 1986; Grakoui et al. 1999). The immunological synapse has been identified not only in the T cell–APC conjugates but also at the interface between B cell–membrane-bound antigen (Fleire et al. 2006), NK cell–target cell (Orange 2008), and NKT cell–CD1d-expressing cell (McCarthy et al. 2007). On the other hand, as we discuss later in Sect. 5, there has been known variability in functional heterogeneity of the immunological synapse, particularly of the central-SMAC (c-SMAC). Some T cell lines, thymocytes, as well as T cells upon weak stimulus do not show SMAC formations.

2.2   Architecture of the Immunological Synapse

The immunological synapse is traditionally characterized by a "bull's eye" structure, c-SMAC, and peripheral-SMAC (p-SMAC) (Monks et al. 1998; Huppa and Davis 2003; Dustin 2009) (Fig. 1). The major components of the c-SMAC are key molecules for T cell signaling, such as TCR/CD3–MHCp, CD28 – or cytotoxic T-lymphocyte antigen-4 (CTLA-4) – CD80/CD86, and protein kinase C θ (PKCθ). In contrast, the p-SMAC is composed of cytoskeleton-related or adhesion molecules structurally supporting the immunological synapse, such as leukocyte function-associated antigen-1 (LFA-1)/talin – intracellular adhesion molecule-1 (ICAM-1) and CD2–CD48/CD58. The distal-SMAC (d-SMAC) was defined later as a region enriched in molecules with long extracellular domains, such as CD45 (Freiberg et al. 2002) and CD43 (Allenspach et al. 2001; Delon et al. 2001; Revy et al. 2001; Roumier et al. 2001; Stoll et al. 2002). The alignment of these receptors was originally determined by the size of the ectodomain, supported by the kinetic

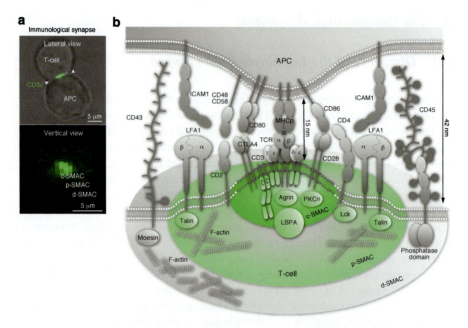

Fig. 1 Architecture of the conventional immunological synapse. The immunological synapse is traditionally depicted by a "bull's eye" structure between a T cell and an antigen-presenting cell (APC) (Monks et al. 1998; Grakoui et al. 1999; Davis and Dustin 2004). (**a**) The CD3 core is clearly identified at the stable conjugation between a T cell and an APC by fluorescence-labeled anti-CD3ε antibodies (*lateral view, top*). The immunological synapse is divided to central-supramolecular activation cluster (c-SMAC), peripheral- (p-) SMAC, and distal- (d-) SMAC in the vertical view (*bottom*). (**b**) The alignment of the receptors and the adhesion molecules are considered to be ordered by size of ectodomain (Davis and van der Merwe 2006); T cell receptor (TCR)/CD3 complex – MHC-peptide (MHCp), CD28/protein kinase C θ (PKCθ) – CD80/86, cytotoxic T-lymphocyte antigen 4 (CTLA-4) – CD80/CD86, Agrin, and lysobisphosphatidic acid (LBPA) in the c-SMAC; CD2–CD48/CD58, leukocyte function-associated antigen-1 (LFA-1)/talin–intracellular adhesion molecule 1 (ICAM-1), F-actin, and CD4/Lck in the p-SMAC; and CD43/moesin, CD45, and F-actin in the d-SMAC (Davis and Dustin 2004)

segregation model (Davis and van der Merwe 2006). It was thought that the c-SMAC mediates antigen recognition and subsequent T cell activation, whereas the p-SMAC supports T cell–APC conjugation and maintains the architecture of the immunological synapse.

3 TCR Microclusters and the Immunological Synapse

3.1 Discovery of TCR Microclusters

It was known for many years that TCR cross linking caused the multimerization of TCR/CD3 complexes and induced T cell activation. Although it was suggested that even a single MHCp (Irvine et al. 2002) could trigger a transient calcium response in T cells, tetrameric MHCp was a potent stimulus for sustained activation (Boniface et al. 1998). Receptor clustering following recruitment of signaling molecules was first imaged for FcεRI on mast cells, where the clusters recruited Syk and phospholipase C (PLC) γ1 (Stauffer and Meyer 1997), and a study using live HeLa cells showed stimulation-induced membrane recruitment of zeta-chain-associated protein kinase 70 kDa (ZAP-70) and CD3ζ (Sloan-Lancaster et al. 1998). Thereafter, using the antigen-presenting lipid bilayers, an outermost ring of TCR–MHCp at the T cell–bilayer interface and its subsequent translocation toward the center were demonstrated (Grakoui et al. 1999). However, the time course of c-SMAC formation does not fit to that of the early signaling such as tyrosine phosphorylation and intracellular Ca^{2+} flux. Thus, special clustering other than c-SMAC may be induced prior to c-SMAC formation. Davis and Krummel first observed small clustering of CD3ζ at the interface between a T cell and a B cell lymphoma prior to c-SMAC formation. These CD3ζ clusters were initially synchronized with the onset of the calcium response and stabilized at the center of the interface (Krummel et al. 2000; Krummel and Davis 2002). Samelson and Bunnell used anti-CD3-coated coverslips and Jurkat T cells introduced by various fluorescence-tagged molecules and discovered the generation and dynamic movement of the clustering of TCRs, their downstream molecules, and the phosphoproteins (Bunnell et al. 2002), which they called "signaling clusters" as soon as T cells attached to the coverslips. Finally, we have established the combined technology of total internal reflection fluorescence microscopy (TIRFM) and antigen-presenting lipid bilayers and developed a new understanding of "TCR microclusters" as a minimal unit mediating both initial and sustained TCR signaling (Campi et al. 2005; Yokosuka et al. 2005; Saito and Yokosuka 2006).

3.2   Dynamics of TCR Microcluster Formation

TCR microclusters are first generated as transient structures composed of 30–300 TCRs at the initial contact region of the T cell–APC or T cell–bilayer interface (Yokosuka et al. 2005; Varma et al. 2006). They are sequentially formed at the new contact regions of the interface during the first few minutes during cell spreading. The number of visible TCR microclusters is 100–300 per cell and increases upon stimulation with high-dose antigens or strong agonists, as is the size of the microclusters (Yokosuka et al. 2005). After maximum spreading, all TCR microclusters translocate toward the center of the interface to form the c-SMAC of the conventional immunological synapse (Fig. 2).

How TCR microclusters translocate to form the c-SMAC is not clear yet (Mossman et al. 2005). Actin cytoskeleton-mediated translocation is a possible candidate (Billadeau et al. 2007). An actin-rich ring was generated at the peripheral boundary of the T cell–anti-CD3-coated coverslip and continuously remodeled by TCR engagement (Bunnell et al. 2001), and the actin polymerization inhibitor

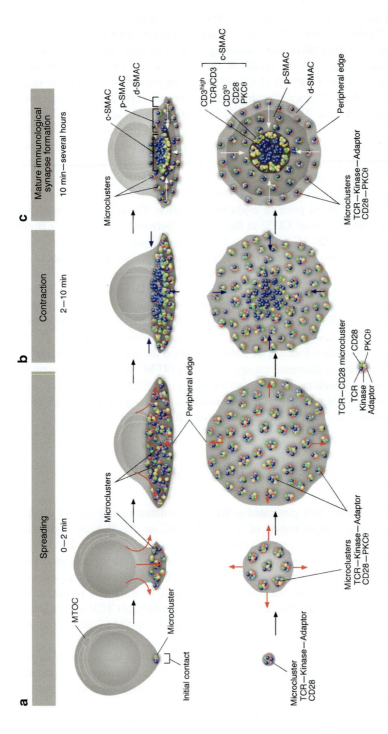

Fig. 2 Dynamic process of antigen recognition and T cell activation by TCR microclusters. Upon the recognition of antigens, a T cell sequentially changes its shape along three steps: spreading, contraction, and immunological synapse formation (Saito and Yokosuka 2006; Yokosuka and Saito 2009). (**a**) When a T cell attaches an antigen-presenting lipid bilayer, TCRs and CD28 form the same clusters as "TCR–CD28 microclusters." Following the first attachment, the T cell continues to spread, generating new TCR microclusters at the peripheral edge. TCR microclusters recruit both kinases and adaptors in TCR-proximal

blocked TCR microcluster translocation (Varma et al. 2006). It was proposed that continuous actin flow generated from outside to inside at the interface is critical for the centripetal translocation of TCR microclusters and the segregation from LFA-1 (Vicente-Manzanares and Sanchez-Madrid 2004; Kaizuka et al. 2007). Recently, myosin IIA was suggested to function in TCR microcluster translocation (Ilani et al. 2009). Critical roles for actin rearrangement have also been shown in the CD3ζ–microfilament association (Rozdzial et al. 1995) and the T cell response. Furthermore, various cytoskeleton-related molecules has been shown to be involved in the regulation of the immunological synapse (Vicente-Manzanares and Sanchez-Madrid 2004; Billadeau et al. 2007): Wiskott–Aldrich syndrome protein (WASp) and WASP-interacting protein (WIP) (Sasahara et al. 2002; Barda-Saad et al. 2004), Abelson interactor (Abi) (Zipfel et al. 2006), ezrin-radixin-moesin-binding phophoprotein EBP50 (Itoh et al. 2002), the leukocyte-specific homolog of cortactin HS1 (Gomez et al. 2006), WASP-family verprolin homologous protein 2 (WAVE2) (Nolz et al. 2006), the receptor tyrosine kinase c-Abl (Huang et al. 2008), and the hematopoietic specific actin- and Arp2/3 complex-binding protein Coronin-1A (Mugnier et al. 2008).

4 TCR Microcluster as a Signalosome for T cell Activation

4.1 Microcluster Composition

Biochemical studies have identified dozens of signal transducing molecules and their assembly for TCR downstream signaling. However, these pathways do not necessarily reflect the spatial and temporal regulation in real-time in cells. TCR–MHCp binding triggers both assembly of these molecules and formation of TCR microclusters; it is critical for our understanding of the process to identify which signaling molecules are involved. Using anti-CD3-coated coverslips, Samelson's group obtained images of microcluster-localizing molecules that included kinases, adaptors, and effector molecules (Seminario and Bunnell 2008). We and others have shown the assembly of most of these molecules within TCR microclusters in normal T cells on a planar membrane (Campi et al. 2005; Yokosuka et al. 2005;

←

Fig. 2 (continued) signaling and induce tyrosine phosphorylation and intracellular calcium flux, resulting in the initial T cell activation. CD28 specifically recruits protein kinase C θ (PKCθ) at TCR microclusters. (b) After reaching the maximum spreading, the T cell starts to contract. TCR microclusters centripetally migrate and fuse with each other to form a large aggregation of the receptors. However, kinases and adaptors dissociate from TCR microclusters. (c) Ten minutes later, TCR microclusters finally form a central supramolecular activation cluster (c-SMAC), which is divided into two regions with the different CD3 density. The CD3-high (CD3^{hi}) region is a single clod of TCRs, but in contrast the CD3-low (CD3^{lo}) region contains CD28, which effectively retains PKCθ at the relatively outer region of the c-SMAC, suggesting T cell sustained signaling. New functional TCR–CD28 microclusters are continuously generated at the peripheral edge and translocated toward the c-SMAC, which may support PKCθ recruitment to the plasma membrane and maintain both the TCR-proximal signaling and the shape of the immunological synapse

Saito and Yokosuka 2006; Varma et al. 2006; Yokosuka et al. 2008; Yokosuka and Saito 2009) (Fig. 3). By analyzing colocalization of the signaling molecules with TCR microclusters, the following molecules were localized with initial microclusters; ZAP-70, phosphatydilinositol-3 kinase (PI3K), linker for activation of T cells (LAT), growth factor receptor-bound protein 2 (Grb2), Grb2-related adaptor protein (Gads), Src homology 2 domain-containing leukocyte-specific phosphoprotein of 76 kDa (SLP-76), non-catalytic region of tyrosine kinase (Nck), the guanine nucleotide exchange factor Vav, PLCγ1, PKCθ, and F-actin and its relating molecule WASp (Bunnell et al. 2002; Barda-Saad et al. 2004; Singer et al. 2004; Campi et al. 2005; Yokosuka et al. 2005; Braiman et al. 2006; Balagopalan et al. 2007; Seminario and Bunnell 2008; Yokosuka et al. 2008).

Do phospholipid metabolites of the plasma membrane contribute to the clustering of intracellular molecules? Activated PLCγ1 generates inositol triphosphate (IP3) and diacylglycerol (DAG), which induces intracellular calcium flux and membrane recruitment of the cysteine-rich domain (CRD)-containing molecules, respectively. Phosphoinositide 3-kinase (PI3K) produces phosphatidylinositol 3,4,5-trisphosphate (PIP3), which recruits pleckstrin homology (PH)-domain-containing molecules such as PLCγ1, Akt, Vav, and Itk. Both CRD and PH-domain fluorescent probes (Costello et al. 2002; Spitaler et al. 2006) do not accumulate in TCR microclusters, whereas PLCγ1 and PI3K do, suggesting that the generation of these second mediators might be essential but not sufficient for these signaling pathway through TCR clustering.

Assembly of these signaling molecules in TCR microclusters is transient and occurs in the newly generated microclusters. Every TCR microcluster initially contains almost the same components, but most of the kinases and adaptors dissemble from the microclusters before reaching the c-SMAC, and appear to be internalized by endocytosis. A critical question is whether signaling molecules internalized without TCR are still active in signal transduction. In this regard, analysis of SLP-76 clusters in Jurkat T cells suggested active signaling as the intracellular compartments. These SLP-76-containing microclusters were relatively stable, localized with LAT and Gads, internalized into the subcellular compartment, and eventually induce sustained activation signals (Bunnell et al. 2006). Similar subcellular signalosomes were reported for Ras signaling at Golgi and in an autophagosome-like structure in B cells (Mor and Philips 2006). However, because clusters of SLP-76 or ZAP-70 in normal T cells were not detectable after their dissociation from TCR microclusters on antigen-presenting lipid bilayers, it remains to be determined whether these molecules continue to induce active signals intracellularly in normal T cells.

4.2   Evidence of Microclusters as Signalosome

The most critical feature of the TCR microcluster is that it functions as the signalosome for T cell activation by recruiting the most proximal TCR signaling

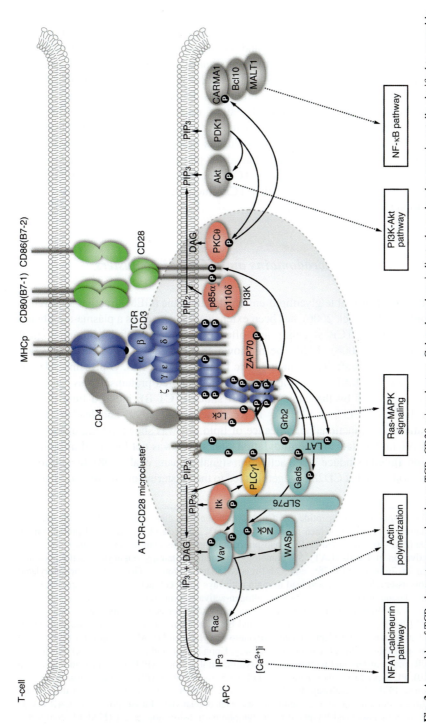

Fig. 3 Assembly of TCR–downstream molecules as TCR–CD28 microclusters. Colored markers indicate the molecules experimentally clarified to assemble as initial TCR–CD28 microclusters (Campi et al. 2005; Yokosuka et al. 2005; Yokosuka et al. 2008; Yokosuka and Saito 2009). Colorless molecules are simply accumulated at the immunological synapse but not at the microclusters. Ligation of T cell receptor (TCR) by

molecules to induce activation within the microclusters. From the earliest time point, each TCR microcluster contains TCRs, kinases, and adaptors (Campi et al. 2005; Yokosuka et al. 2005; Saito and Yokosuka 2006). The evidence that each TCR microcluster can transmit activation signals was obtained in two ways. One was the detection of phosphoproteins such as phospho-CD3ζ and phospho-ZAP-70 within the microclusters, and the other was the fact that the kinetics of the intracellular calcium flux paralleled that of microcluster formation. Thus, the TCR microcluster, not the c-SMAC, functions as a signalosome for T cell activation. After c-SMAC formation, microclusters are continuously generated at the periphery of the interface, and are stained for phospho-tyrosine or phospho-ZAP-70. Blocking the generation of new TCR microclusters resulted in inhibition of T cell activation, demonstrating that TCR microclusters are required for T cell activation (Varma et al. 2006).

4.3 Lipid Raft Microdomains and TCR Microclusters

The detergent-insoluble glycolipid-enriched membrane (GEM) fraction, referred to as lipid raft (Hancock 2006), has been extensively analyzed as a plasma-membrane microdomain for TCR signaling and often in the context of the immunological synapse (Shaw 2006). It has been shown that various signal components are localized in lipid raft. Those include Src family kinases, Ras, G proteins, adaptor proteins such as LAT, as well as various GPI-anchored proteins. Cross linking of ganglioside GM1 by the cholera toxin-B subunit (CT-B), induced lipid patches colocalized with Lck, LAT, and TCRs (Janes et al. 1999) and lead to T cell activation. The functional significance of lipid raft was shown by the observation that LAT mutant lacking palmitoylation site, which was not localized in lipid raft fraction, failed to induce T cell activation signals (Zhang et al. 1998). In addition, it has been shown that CD28 engagement led to the clustering of raft microdomains at

←——————————————————————————————

Fig. 3 (continued) MHC–peptide (MHCp) (*blue*) triggers the clustering of TCR and the transient association of CD4–Lck, which phosphorylates CD3ζ and zeta-chain associated protein kinase 70 kDa (ZAP-70). Activated ZAP-70 phosphorylates the downstream adaptors (*light blue*): linker for activation of T cells (LAT), Src homology 2 domain-containing leukocyte-specific phosphoprotein of 76 kDa (SLP-76), and Grb2-related adaptor protein (Gads). The phosphorylated adaptors assemble together and lead to main pathways for T cell activation: LAT–growth factor receptor-bound protein 2 (Grb2) for Ras–mitogen-activated protein kinase (MAPK) signaling and SLP-76–Vav–Wiskott–Aldrich syndrome protein (WASp) for actin polymerization. Phospholipase C (PLC) γ1 (*orange*), which is activated by interleukin-2 tyrosine kinase (Itk), cleavages phosphatidylinositol-4,5-bisphosphate (PIP$_2$) into diacylglycerol (DAG) and inositol-triphosphate (IP$_3$) responsible for NFAT–calcineurin pathway. Upon ligand binding, CD28 (*green*) translocates to TCR microclusters and recruits phosphatydilinositol-3 kinase (PI3K) and protein kinase C θ (PKCθ). PI3K produces phosphatidylinositol 3,4,5-trisphosphate (PIP$_3$), which ensures the connection to PI3K–Akt pathway. PKCθ leads to nuclear factor-κB pathway through the caspase recruitment domain-containing membrane-associated guanylate kinase protein-1 (CARMA1)–Bcl10–mucosa-associated-lymphoid-tissue lymphoma-translocation gene 1 (MALT1) complex

the immunological synapse (Viola et al. 1999), and PKCθ was recruited there (Bi et al. 2001). In spite of these initial studies for important roles of lipid raft as the platform for recruiting signaling molecules for T cell activation and the colocalization with immunological synapse (c-SMAC), there are accumulating data to demonstrate no critical role for activation. The raft-associated molecules including Lck, Fyn, GM1, and cholesterol were not highly concentrated at TCR microclusters (Bunnell et al. 2002), and fluorescence resonance energy transfer (FRET) among GPI-linked proteins was not detected even in the presence of focal condensation of GPI-linked proteins or CT-B (Glebov and Nichols 2004). We analyzed the relationship between the TCR microclusters and lipid raft. The lipid raft probes did not accumulate in the TCR microclusters (A. Hashimoto-Tane, T.Y., T.S.; unpublished observations). Furthermore, single-molecule imaging analyses illustrated the coclustering of CD2, LAT, and Lck microdomains, which required protein–protein interactions but not lipid rafts (Douglass and Vale 2005). In contrast, the FRET analysis using a lipid raft probe demonstrated the B cell receptor (BCR)–lipid raft association but this association was limited at the newly formed BCR microclusters and induced just transiently for a few seconds in B cells (Sohn et al. 2008). Collecting together, although lipid raft does not appear to support as the platform for TCR microclusters and protein interaction within TCR microclusters is critical for activation signals, the functional nanoscale association with TCR microclusters remained elusive. On the other hand, the new technology, transmission electron microscopy of plasma membrane sheets, suggests pre-existing protein clusters on plasma membrane in cholesterol-enriched domains despite raft or non-raft-associating domains (Lillemeier et al. 2006)

5   c-SMAC Function

5.1   Dual Functions in TCR Signaling

In the conventional immunological synapse, the c-SMAC, as the site for TCR clustering, was suggested to control TCR signaling. However, the finding of the TCR microcluster leads us to reconsider this issue. The pattern of the immunological synapse suggested a causal relationship between TCR radial position and its signaling activity. Prolonged signaling was generated at the trapped periphery of the c-SMACs but not in the center (Mossman et al. 2005). On the other hand, the patterning "TCRs inside and LFA-1 outside" was required for stable contact, normal PKCθ clustering, and interferon (IFN)-γ secretion (Doh and Irvine 2006). Shaw and colleagues first proposed that the c-SMAC was involved in TCR degradation by analyzing CD2AP-deficient T cells exhibiting no generation of c-SMACs but augmented responses (Lee et al. 2003). Further observations supporting this hypothesis followed; a lipid for multivesicular body for degradation, lysobisphosphatidic acid (LBPA), was localized at the c-SMAC after strong TCR stimulation (Varma

et al. 2006) and the enrichment of ubiquitin and Cbl-b recruitment at the immunological synapse (Wiedemann et al. 2005). CD45 required for the initial activation of
Lck is topologically excluded from the synapse (Shaw and Dustin 1997; Davis and
van der Merwe 2006), but later is recruited back to the c-SMAC to terminate TCR
signaling by dephosphorylation of phosphoproteins in the TCR microclusters
(Johnson et al. 2000; Varma et al. 2006). In contrast, there are some suggestions
of a possible function of the c-SMAC for the activation of signaling. ZAP-70 is
partially recruited to the c-SMAC under some restricted conditions (Yokosuka et al.
2005) and SLP-76 microclusters in Jurkat cells stimulated upon anti-CD3-antibody-
coated coverslips transmigrate to the perinuclear space (Bunnell et al. 2006). It is
suggested that stronger TCR stimulation causes earlier and stronger degradation at
the c-SMAC whereas weaker stimulation results in prolonged accumulation of
phospho-tyrosine and PIP3 (Cemerski et al. 2008), and further that fully phosphorylated CD3ζ is translocated into the c-SMAC upon stimulation with a low-dose
peptide. Recently, we showed that costimulation signal is sustained in cSMAC by
demonstrating that CD28 and PKCθ formed clusters at the c-SMAC in a manner
depending on the CD28–CD80 binding (Yokosuka et al. 2008). For this regulation,
it is noteworthy that the c-SMAC has two functionally different regions (see
Sect. 7.2). The clustering of PKCθ at the c-SMAC is a hallmark of the conventional
immunological synapse and leads to caspase recruitment domain-containing
membrane-associated guanylate kinase protein-1 (CARMA1) activation and
Bcl10 assembly for nuclear factor-κB (NF-κB) activation. It has been reported
that Bcl10 was placed at the cytoplasmic face of the c-SMAC and formed
"punctate and oligomeric killing or activating domains transducing signals"
(POLKADOTS) (Schaefer et al. 2004). Collectively, based on these reports,
there may be differential regulation of signaling pathways; TCR microclusters
induce a calcium response and actin polymerization through the ZAP-70–LAT–
SLP-76–PLCγ1 pathway, whereas the c-SMAC may be induce NF-κB activation
through the PKCθ–Bcl10 pathway.

5.2 Cell Polarity and the c-SMAC

The c-SMAC appears to regulate cell polarity. The MTOC was relocated to the
CTL–target cell interface (Kupfer and Dennert 1984) and lytic granules were
transported along microtubules toward the MTOC and secreted at a unique region
along the c-SMAC (Stinchcombe et al. 2001; Faroudi et al. 2003; Stinchcombe et al.
2006). The translocation was regulated by formin – but not Arp2/3-mediated actin
nucleation (Billadeau et al. 2007; Gomez et al. 2007). Russel and colleagues first
demonstrated that the cell polarity proteins: Scribble, Crumbs3, and Par3, which
were initially identified in epithelial cells, were also asymmetrically distributed in
T cells (Ludford-Menting et al. 2005). Cell polarity is crucial for the asymmetrical
division of the T cell developing to an effector or memory lineage (Chang et al.

2007). Kupfer et al. demonstrated directionality in cytokine secretion by T helper (Th) cells, similar to the MTOC (Kupfer et al. 1991). Pooling of effector cytokines at the immunological synapse effectively differentiates Th1/2 cells by the regulation of IFN-γ receptor 1 condensation and signal transducer and activator of transcription 1 (STAT1) recruitment (Maldonado et al. 2004, 2009). In contrast, tumor necrosis factor and the chemokine CCL3 are released in all directions, even from T–APC conjugates (Huse et al. 2006), suggesting that there are two types of spatial regulation of cytokine secretion: polarized secretion toward synapse and non-polarized secretion. Conversely, the chemokine receptor CCR5, but not CCR7, was sequestrated at the T cell–APC interface, making the cell insensitive to chemotactic gradients and to obtain costimulatory signaling through chemokine receptors (Molon et al. 2005).

6 Heterogeneity of the Immunological Synapse and the c-SMAC

The immunological synapse was originally characterized in T cells as the c-SMAC and p-SMAC. Although this structural concept is widely accepted to occur in other lymphoid cells, it is not necessarily associated with any segregation into the SMACs, and sometimes other characteristic structures are induced; e.g., the lytic synapse on CTLs (Stinchcombe et al. 2001) and the inhibitory synapse and the microclusters on NK cells (Davis and Dustin 2004; Orange 2008).

A variety of the immunological synapses are generated in different contexts. Some T cell lines are activated without forming any c-SMACs (Purtic et al. 2005). Immature thymocytes form multifocal CD3 and Lck clusters, but not a c-SMAC (Hailman et al. 2002; Richie et al. 2002). At the T cell–dendritic cell (DC) interface, TCR submicronic contact spots can be visualized by electron microscopy, and these multifocal TCR clusters can fully induce T cell activation without large-scale segregation of TCR and LFA-1 (Brossard et al. 2005). These examples lead us to conclude that T cells do not require c-SMAC formation in every situation. Upon stimulation with lower-dose antigen or a weaker stimulus, CTLs can kill their target cells without forming c-SMACs (Faroudi et al. 2003; Purbhoo et al. 2004). The requirement for c-SMAC formation to induce T cell activation depends on TCR characteristics. In the case of low-affinity/avidity TCR, c-SMAC formation is well correlated with T cell activation induction (Purtic et al. 2005). However, Davis and colleagues have shown that just ten MHCp can induce the typical immunological synapse, three MHCp can induce cytotoxicity (Purbhoo et al. 2004) and, further, only one MHCp can induce transient calcium responses (Irvine et al. 2002). Since these small numbers of antigen-peptide-bearing MHCs induce activation in collaboration with self-peptide-bearing MHCs, the relationship with TCR-microclusters has to be determined. Collectively, T cells can be activated even in the absence of c-SMAC formation, where TCR microclusters play central roles in transducing activation signals.

7 Costimulation Regulation by TCR Microclusters and the c-SMAC

7.1 Costimulation and TCR Microclusters

Most costimulatory receptors and their ligands are localized at the immunological synapse where they might modify T cell activation (Alegre et al. 2001; Acuto and Michel 2003) (Table 1). The discovery of the TCR microcluster led us to reevaluate the structural and functional features of T cell activation at the immunological synapse. Recently, we found a small clustering of CD28 at the T cell–bilayer or T cell–APC interface, which was named "CD28 microclusters" (Yokosuka et al. 2008). Their formation depends on binding to the ligands CD80/CD86. High-density ligands generate clear clustering of CD28. At the beginning of antigen stimulation, these microclusters are completely colocalized with TCR microclusters and are then translocated toward the center to form a c-SMAC. There are few molecules that translocate into c-SMAC after colocalization in TCR microclusters. The movement of CD28 suggests the existence of a molecule that translocates from microclusters to the c-SMAC together. Although CD28 signaling has been analyzed for years, critical molecules in this pathway and the relationship between CD28 and TCR signaling pathways have not been defined yet. For a decade, biochemical analyses have suggested some candidates such as PI3K, protein phosphatase 2A (PP2A), Grb2, Gads, interleukin-2 tyrosine kinase (Itk), Vav, and Akt (Alegre et al. 2001; Acuto and Michel 2003), but most of these molecules function downstream of TCR as well as CD28. PI3K, which has been thought to be the most critical molecule in this pathway, dissociates from the TCR–CD28 microclusters in the same way as other TCR signaling molecules such as SLP-76. In contrast, PKCθ translocates to the outer region of the c-SMAC and remains there for more than 1 h, suggesting its contribution for sustained T cell signaling. Indeed, blockade of CD28–CD80 interaction by CTLA-4-Ig resulted in the disappearance of the annular accumulation of not only CD28 but also PKCθ at the c-SMAC, indicating that CD28 recruits PKCθ to the c-SMAC. The functional importance of PKCθ for full T cell activation and maturation is consistent with previous functional and biological studies as well as with the phenotypes of PKCθ-deficient mice (Sun et al. 2000; Pfeifhofer et al. 2003) and PKCθ imaging (Monks et al. 1997; Monks et al. 1998).

7.2 Functional Subregions Within the c-SMAC

High-resolution images of T cells on antigen-presenting lipid bilayers revealed two distinct regions within the c-SMAC (Yokosuka et al. 2008) (Fig. 4). One is a TCR/CD3 high-density (CD3^{hi}) region, the traditional c-SMAC, and another is a TCR/CD3 low- (CD3^{lo}) and CD28 high-density region. The CD3^{hi} c-SMAC is a rigid

Table 1 Costimulation at the immunological synapse

Receptor on T cell	Ligand on APC	Location in immunological synapse	Functions at immunological synapse	References
CD28	CD80 (B7-1), CD86 (B7-2)	Whole synapse, c-SMAC	Lipid raft recruitment, actin rearrangement, enlarge conjugation area, PKCθ segregation, Filamin-A association, TCR segregation, Lck autophosphorylation, CD28 phosphorylation	(Kaga et al. 1998; Viola et al. 1999; Bromley et al. 2001; Holdorf et al. 2002; Huang et al. 2002; Wetzel et al. 2002; Salazar-Fontana et al. 2003; Tskvitaria-Fuller et al. 2003; Tavano et al. 2004; Tseng et al. 2005; Hayashi and Altman 2006; Tavano et al. 2006)
CTLA4	CD80 (B7-1), CD86 (B7-2)	Whole synapse, c-SMAC	Reduction ZAP-70 microcluster, reduction lipid raft expression, enhancement adhesion	(Linsley et al. 1996; Martin et al. 2001; Darlington et al. 2002; Egen and Allison 2002; Pentcheva-Hoang et al. 2004; Schneider et al. 2005; Schneider et al. 2008)
ICOS	ICOSL (B7-H2,CD275)	Whole synapse	PI3K recruitment	(Fos et al. 2008)
PD-1	PD-L1 (B7-H1), PD-L2 (B7-DC)	Whole synapse	Reduction PKCθ concentration	(Lazar-Molnar et al. 2008)
CD40	CD40L (CD152)	Whole synapse, c-SAMC, various patterning	Fascin accumulation, maybe T cell help signal	(Boisvert et al. 2004; Rothoeft et al. 2006; Barcia et al. 2008)
4-1BB	4-1BBL	Whole synapse	Granzyme B recruitment, bystander T cell activation	(Stephan et al. 2007)
CD38	CD31	Whole synapse	Lipid raft recruitment, PKCθ recruitment, calcium response enhancement	(Zubiaur et al. 2002; Munoz et al. 2008)
CD26	ADA–ADA receptor coupling	Whole synapse	Reduction antigen dose, cytokine secretion enhancement	(Pacheco et al. 2005)
CD6	CD116 (ALCAM)	c-SMAC	T–APC conjugation enhancement, immunological synapse maturation, syntenin-1 binding, cytoskeletal molecule association	(Gimferrer et al. 2004; Gimferrer et al. 2005; Ibanez et al. 2006)
VLA4	VCAM1	ND	Blockade of SLP-76 microcluster centripetal translocation, retain phosphorylation	(Nguyen et al. 2008)

ADA adenosine deaminase; *ALCAM* activaed leukocyte cell adhesion molecule; *VLA4* very late antigen-4; *VCAM1* vascular adhesion molecule-1; *ND* not determined

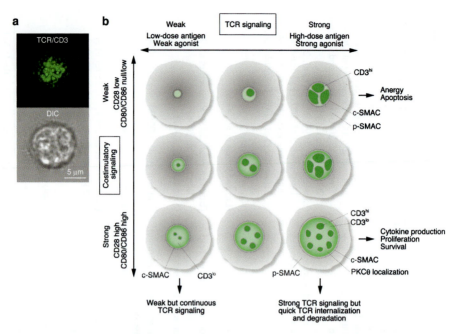

Fig. 4 The c-SMAC composition characterized by the strength of TCR and costimulatory signaling. (**a**) The two regions with the different density of CD3, CD3-high (CD3^{hi}) and CD3-low (CD3^{lo}), were identified within the central-supramolecular activation cluster (c-SMAC) in a T cell expressing EGFP-tagged CD3ζ settled on a antigen-presenting lipid bilayer (*top*) (Yokosuka et al. 2008). The figure at the bottom is a differential interference contrast (DIC) image of the one at the top. (**b**) The scheme presents our hypothesis in the relationship between the T cell response and the TCR/CD3 composition within the c-SMAC. The c-SMAC size correlates with the TCR signal strength. Without costimulation, stronger TCR signaling induces more intensive internalization and degradation of TCRs forming the CD3^{hi} regions, which may result in T cell anergy or apoptosis. CD28-mediated costimulation increases the area of the CD3^{lo} region that is constructed by CD28, lower level of TCR/CD3, and protein kinase C θ (PKCθ), which results in the cytokine production and T cell survival. PKCθ is dynamically reorganized at the relatively outer region of the CD3^{lo} region in an annular form

structure that had lost the ability of lateral movement of receptors and does not contain any tyrosine phosphorylated proteins. In contrast, the CD3^{lo} c-SMAC maintains rapid lateral movement and demonstrates colocalization of both CD28 and PKCθ. Structurally, it is located at the outer region of the entire c-SMAC in an annular form. Formation of the CD3^{hi} c-SMAC is limited to strong TCR stimulation, whereas the CD3^{lo} c-SMAC is formed and continuously colocalized with PKCθ following weak stimulation, even if the CD3^{hi} c-SMAC is not detected. PKCθ recruitment to the c-SMAC is dependent on TCR-mediated signaling from the initially and sequentially formed TCR microclusters; furthermore, the amount of PKCθ in the c-SMAC and the area occupied by PKCθ within the c-SMAC are dependent on the density of the costimulatory receptor and its ligand. Taken together, these features of CD3^{hi} and CD3^{lo} c-SMAC imply that the CD3^{hi} c-SMAC might be the result of TCR internalization and degradation and that the CD3^{lo} c-SMAC might function in continuous costimulatory signaling for sustained T cell activation (Saito and Yokosuka 2006; Dustin 2009; Yokosuka and Saito 2009).

8   T cell Activation Models and the TCR Microcluster Model

Several models for the initiation of TCR signaling have been discussed over the years (Box 1). We propose here the "TCR microcluster model" (Saito and Yokosuka 2006; Seminario and Bunnell 2008; Yokosuka and Saito 2009). Based on the finding that the TCR microcluster is the signalosome and the minimal unit for T cell activation, we propose that a single microcluster induces transient signals in the limited time span but that the continuous generation of TCR microclusters in a spatially and temporally regulated manner provides the sustained signals required for full T cell activation. The formation of both TCR microclusters and the c-SMAC is dependent on the avidity of TCR, which influences the activation/degradation balance. Furthermore, several different modes of costimulation can modulate activation status.

The "multimerization model" is the fundamental basis of the TCR microcluster model (Davis et al. 2007; Seminario and Bunnell 2008). Because dimerized TCRs can induce the initial and transient calcium response, the minimal unit for signal transduction could be a dimer. However, there is a correlation between the stimulation strength and microcluster formation, and thus a microcluster might be at the limit of what can be imaged by current technologies. Whereas a dimer provides a digital signal, a microcluster may convert this into an analog signal as the sum of the initial inputs. There is supportive evidence for the functional importance of receptor multimerization, such as the conformational change of CD3ζ (Aivazian and Stern 2000) and multimodal clustering of adaptors (Houtman et al. 2006). Endogenous peptides could have a synergistic function with dimeric MHC, but this function is still controversial from the view of the microcluster model, since endogenous MHCp failed to enhance TCR triggering on lipid bilayers (Ma et al. 2008).

The "kinetic segregation model" (Davis and van der Merwe 2006) is featured by the grossly segregated c-SMAC and p-SMAC, but the microcluster model seems to be the opposite. The initial small-sized microclusters of TCR–MHCp are scattered over the entire interface, which is filled with tall molecules LFA-1–ICAM-1 (Yokosuka et al. 2005; Varma et al. 2006; Kaizuka et al. 2007). These molecules are clearly excluded from the TCR microclusters, whereas smaller molecules CD28–CD80 are colocalized there (Yokosuka et al. 2008). Consequently, the TCR and CD28 move to the c-SMAC, whereas the LFA-1 and CD45 enclose the TCR–CD28 as a p-SMAC and c-SMAC, respectively. Therefore, the kinetic segregation model is tightly connected with the microcluster model at the microscale.

The microcluster model is also reminiscent of the "serial triggering model" (Valitutti et al. 1995). Each microcluster is generated transiently and induces short-term signals, but TCR microclusters continue to be generated from the initiation of cell–cell contact to SMAC formation. This system represents serial triggering at the large scale.

Box 1: T cell activation models

Kinetic proofreading model

As a quantitative model, McKeithan (McKeithan 1995) and McConnell (Rabinowitz et al. 1996) hypothesized that T cell activation was governed by the half-life ($t_{1/2}$) of the TCR–MHCp interaction. The temporal lag between ligand binding and receptor signaling may elicit qualitatively different signals. Longer $t_{1/2}$ determines a strong response induced by agonists or strong agonists, and shorter $t_{1/2}$ determines a weaker response by weak agonists, null peptides, or antagonists (Davis et al. 1998).

Serial triggering model

T cell activation requires sustained activation for several hours. TCR affinity to MHCp is low, and TCR activation induces only a brief spike of intracellular signals. To solve this paradoxical requirement for T cell activation, Lanzavecchia and his colleagues set up this model to explain how a small number of agonist MHCp governed the activation and down-modulation of a large number of TCRs. They suspected that a single complex could serially engage and trigger up to approximately 200 TCRs (Valitutti et al. 1995). The dissociation rate calculated from kinetics of TCR–MHCp is likely to this model. For T cell activation, approximately 8,000 TCRs are required to be triggered (Viola and Lanzavecchia 1996).

Kinetic segregation model

van der Merwe first proposed this model by the topological view of the cell surface molecules at the T cell–APC interface (Davis and van der Merwe 1996; Shaw and Dustin 1997). The tight intercellular contact causes the segregation of the molecules by sizes of their ectodomain. This model is supported by the structural features and kinetics of the immunological synapse proved by segregation patterning (Monks et al. 1998; Grakoui et al. 1999): the smaller receptors in the center whose distance is 15 nm and the taller adhesion molecules in the periphery whose distance is 42 nm (Davis and van der Merwe 2006).

Multimerization model

This model shows that the minimum unit of T cell activation is known to be a dimer on the basis of antibody-induced dimerization (Imboden and Stobo

1985) and crystal structure of dimeric MHC (Brown et al. 1993). Initial but transient calcium response is induced by a single MHCp, but monomeric MHCp in solution fails to stimulate most T cells (Boniface et al. 1998; Cochran et al. 2000), with one exception (Delon et al. 1998). More multi-oligomeric ligands induce more substantial TCR clods and more intensive T cell activation (Boniface et al. 1998). This model is supported by other evidences: clustering-induced conformational change of CD3ζ being more accessible for Lck (Aivazian and Stern 2000) and multimodal cluster formation of multimeric and multipoint binding of receptors and adaptors (Houtman et al. 2006).

Conformational change model
The crystal structures of TCR–MHCp (Garcia et al. 1996; Reinherz et al. 1999) were solved in late 1990s and the subtle differences of TCR–MHCp characterized. Although structural change has not obtained upon antigen binding by the ectodomain of TCR, biochemical data revealed that the TCR–MHCp ligation induces the structural change TCR–CD3 complex, particularly in CD3ε, which exposes the proline-rich sequence and recruits Nck to induce downstream signaling (Gil et al. 2002; Mingueneau et al. 2008). This model is also hinted by the conformational change in Igα upon BCR engagements by membrane-binding antigens (Tolar et al. 2005).

Pseudo-dimer model
Quite a few MHCs carry cognate antigen peptides for the responsible TCRs, whereas a great majority of MHCs carry endogenous self-peptides. Davis and colleagues modified the "dimer of dimers model" on the basis of this phenomenon, and the crystallographic study which showed CD4 tail associating with Lck was far from their own TCR/CD3 complex than expected (Davis et al. 2007). Upon the stimulation by artificial MHC dimers carrying an agonist peptide on one MHC and a self-peptide on another, T cells respond to the particular repertoires of self-peptides (Krogsgaard et al. 2005). In this model, the fast off rate of TCR–self-MHCp would engage hundreds or thousands of different TCRs that could drive signaling up to the required threshold for T cell activation.

TCR microcluster model
For the present proposed model, see the text.

9 Concluding Remarks

In this review, we have reconsidered the bona fide functions of the immunological synapse and discussed the features of the TCR microcluster, a novel cluster of TCRs dynamically assembling the downstream signaling molecules. Compared to the classical idea of the immunological synapse, the microcluster model is able to explain better the mechanisms of T cell activation from the most critical point of view of spatial-temporal regulation of the "signalosome." TCR microclusters dynamically change during the course of T cell recognition and activation within the immunological synapse. After the initial binding of a TCR with an MHC/ peptide, TCR assembles to form clusters at the initial contact area. Thereafter, the TCR microclusters exhibit spatial translocation from the peripheral edge to the center and, chronologically, association and dissociation with kinases and adaptors during their movement toward the center, and accumulation and internalization at the c-SMAC. Individual signaling molecules may behave differentially along with the movement of the TCR microcluster: ZAP-70 only transiently associates with the TCR microcluster at the periphery; accumulated PKCθ remains for hours at the midpoint; and TCRs are internalized and degraded at the center.

The analysis of TCR microclusters provides novel insights into the dynamic regulation of T cell signaling not only at the immunological synapse but also within the entire cell. Further analysis by spatio-temporal imaging of TCR signaling will unveil the complex network of the regulatory systems for T cell activation and function.

Acknowledgments We thank the former and current members of the laboratory for discussions and M. Dustin, R. Varma, A. Shaw, M. Tokunaga, K. Sogawa, and A. Tane for collaborations. T. Y. and T. S. are supported by a Grant-in-Aid for Priority Area Research from the Ministry of Education, Culture, Sports, Science and Technology of Japan.

References

Acuto O, Michel F (2003) CD28-mediated co-stimulation: a quantitative support for TCR signalling. Nat Rev Immunol 3:939–951

Aivazian D, Stern LJ (2000) Phosphorylation of T cell receptor zeta is regulated by a lipid dependent folding transition. Nat Struct Biol 7:1023–1026

Alegre ML, Frauwirth KA, Thompson CB (2001) T-cell regulation by CD28 and CTLA-4. Nat Rev Immunol 1:220–228

Allenspach EJ, Cullinan P, Tong J, Tang Q, Tesciuba AG, Cannon JL, Takahashi SM, Morgan R, Burkhardt JK, Sperling AI (2001) ERM-dependent movement of CD43 defines a novel protein complex distal to the immunological synapse. Immunity 15:739–750

Balagopalan L, Barr VA, Sommers CL, Barda-Saad M, Goyal A, Isakowitz MS, Samelson LE (2007) c-Cbl-mediated regulation of LAT-nucleated signaling complexes. Mol Cell Biol 27:8622–8636

Barcia C, Gomez A, de Pablos V, Fernandez-Villalba E, Liu C, Kroeger KM, Martin J, Barreiro AF, Castro MG, Lowenstein PR, Herrero MT (2008) CD20, CD3, and CD40 ligand microclusters segregate three-dimensionally in vivo at B-cell-T-cell immunological synapses after viral immunity in primate brain. J Virol 82:9978–9993

Barda-Saad M, Braiman A, Titerence R, Bunnell SC, Barr VA, Samelson LE (2004) Dynamic molecular interactions linking the T cell antigen receptor to the actin cytoskeleton. Nat Immunol 6:80–89

Bi K, Tanaka Y, Coudronniere N, Sugie K, Hong S, van Stipdonk MJ, Altman A (2001) Antigen-induced translocation of PKC-theta to membrane rafts is required for T cell activation. Nat Immunol 2:556–563

Billadeau DD, Nolz JC, Gomez TS (2007) Regulation of T-cell activation by the cytoskeleton. Nat Rev Immunol 7:131–143

Boisvert J, Edmondson S, Krummel MF (2004) Immunological synapse formation licenses CD40-CD40L accumulations at T-APC contact sites. J Immunol 173:3647–3652

Boniface JJ, Rabinowitz JD, Wulfing C, Hampl J, Reich Z, Altman JD, Kantor RM, Beeson C, McConnell HM, Davis MM (1998) Initiation of signal transduction through the T cell receptor requires the multivalent engagement of peptide/MHC ligands [corrected]. Immunity 9:459–466

Braiman A, Barda-Saad M, Sommers CL, Samelson LE (2006) Recruitment and activation of PLCgamma1 in T cells: a new insight into old domains. EMBO J 25:774–784

Bromley SK, Iaboni A, Davis SJ, Whitty A, Green JM, Shaw AS, Weiss A, Dustin ML (2001) The immunological synapse and CD28-CD80 interactions. Nat Immunol 2:1159–1166

Brossard C, Feuillet V, Schmitt A, Randriamampita C, Romao M, Raposo G, Trautmann A (2005) Multifocal structure of the T cell – dendritic cell synapse. Eur J Immunol 35:1741–1753

Brown JH, Jardetzky TS, Gorga JC, Stern LJ, Urban RG, Strominger JL, Wiley DC (1993) Three-dimensional structure of the human class II histocompatibility antigen HLA-DR1. Nature 364:33–39

Bunnell SC, Kapoor V, Trible RP, Zhang W, Samelson LE (2001) Dynamic actin polymerization drives T cell receptor-induced spreading: a role for the signal transduction adaptor LAT. Immunity 14:315–329

Bunnell SC, Hong DI, Kardon JR, Yamazaki T, McGlade CJ, Barr VA, Samelson LE (2002) T cell receptor ligation induces the formation of dynamically regulated signaling assemblies. J Cell Biol 158:1263–1275

Bunnell SC, Singer AL, Hong DI, Jacque BH, Jordan MS, Seminario MC, Barr VA, Koretzky GA, Samelson LE (2006) Persistence of cooperatively stabilized signaling clusters drives T-cell activation. Mol Cell Biol 26:7155–7166

Campi G, Varma R, Dustin ML (2005) Actin and agonist MHC-peptide complex-dependent T cell receptor microclusters as scaffolds for signaling. J Exp Med 202:1031–1036

Cemerski S, Das J, Giurisato E, Markiewicz MA, Allen PM, Chakraborty AK, Shaw AS (2008) The balance between T cell receptor signaling and degradation at the center of the immunological synapse is determined by antigen quality. Immunity 29:414–422

Chang JT, Palanivel VR, Kinjyo I, Schambach F, Intlekofer AM, Banerjee A, Longworth SA, Vinup KE, Mrass P, Oliaro J, Killeen N, Orange JS, Russell SM, Weninger W, Reiner SL (2007) Asymmetric T lymphocyte division in the initiation of adaptive immune responses. Science 315:1687–1691

Cochran JR, Cameron TO, Stern LJ (2000) The relationship of MHC-peptide binding and T cell activation probed using chemically defined MHC class II oligomers. Immunity 12:241–250

Costello PS, Gallagher M, Cantrell DA (2002) Sustained and dynamic inositol lipid metabolism inside and outside the immunological synapse. Nat Immunol 3:1082–1089

Darlington PJ, Baroja ML, Chau TA, Siu E, Ling V, Carreno BM, Madrenas J (2002) Surface cytotoxic T lymphocyte-associated antigen 4 partitions within lipid rafts and relocates to the immunological synapse under conditions of inhibition of T cell activation. J Exp Med 195:1337–1347

Davis DM, Dustin ML (2004) What is the importance of the immunological synapse? Trends Immunol 25:323–327

Davis SJ, van der Merwe PA (1996) The structure and ligand interactions of CD2: implications for T-cell function. Immunol Today 17:177–187

Davis SJ, van der Merwe PA (2006) The kinetic-segregation model: TCR triggering and beyond. Nat Immunol 7:803–809

Davis MM, Boniface JJ, Reich Z, Lyons D, Hampl J, Arden B, Chien Y (1998) Ligand recognition by alpha beta T cell receptors. Annu Rev Immunol 16:523–544

Davis MM, Krogsgaard M, Huse M, Huppa J, Lillemeier BF, Li QJ (2007) T cells as a self-referential, sensory organ. Annu Rev Immunol 25:681–695

Delon J, Gregoire C, Malissen B, Darche S, Lemaitre F, Kourilsky P, Abastado JP, Trautmann A (1998) CD8 expression allows T cell signaling by monomeric peptide-MHC complexes. Immunity 9:467–473

Delon J, Kaibuchi K, Germain RN (2001) Exclusion of CD43 from the immunological synapse is mediated by phosphorylation-regulated relocation of the cytoskeletal adaptor moesin. Immunity 15:691–701

Depoil D, Fleire S, Treanor BL, Weber M, Harwood NE, Marchbank KL, Tybulewicz VL, Batista FD (2008) CD19 is essential for B cell activation by promoting B cell receptor-antigen microcluster formation in response to membrane-bound ligand. Nat Immunol 9:63–72

Doh J, Irvine DJ (2006) Immunological synapse arrays: patterned protein surfaces that modulate immunological synapse structure formation in T cells. Proc Natl Acad Sci USA 103:5700–5705

Douglass AD, Vale RD (2005) Single-molecule microscopy reveals plasma membrane micro-domains created by protein-protein networks that exclude or trap signaling molecules in T Cells. Cell 121:937–950

Dustin ML (2009) The cellular context of T cell signaling. Immunity 30:482–492

Egen JG, Allison JP (2002) Cytotoxic T lymphocyte antigen-4 accumulation in the immunological synapse is regulated by TCR signal strength. Immunity 16:23–35

Faroudi M, Utzny C, Salio M, Cerundolo V, Guiraud M, Muller S, Valitutti S (2003) Lytic versus stimulatory synapse in cytotoxic T lymphocyte/target cell interaction: manifestation of a dual activation threshold. Proc Natl Acad Sci USA 100:14145–14150

Fleire SJ, Goldman JP, Carrasco YR, Weber M, Bray D, Batista FD (2006) B cell ligand discrimination through a spreading and contraction response. Science 312:738–741

Fos C, Salles A, Lang V, Carrette F, Audebert S, Pastor S, Ghiotto M, Olive D, Bismuth G, Nunes JA (2008) ICOS ligation recruits the p50alpha PI3K regulatory subunit to the immunological synapse. J Immunol 181:1969–1977

Freiberg BA, Kupfer H, Maslanik W, Delli J, Kappler J, Zaller DM, Kupfer A (2002) Staging and resetting T cell activation in SMACs. Nat Immunol 3:911–917

Garcia KC, Degano M, Stanfield RL, Brunmark A, Jackson MR, Peterson PA, Teyton L, Wilson IA (1996) An alphabeta T cell receptor structure at 2.5 A and its orientation in the TCR-MHC complex. Science 274:209–219

Gil D, Schamel WW, Montoya M, Sanchez-Madrid F, Alarcon B (2002) Recruitment of Nck by CD3 epsilon reveals a ligand-induced conformational change essential for T cell receptor signaling and synapse formation. Cell 109:901–912

Gimferrer I, Calvo M, Mittelbrunn M, Farnos M, Sarrias MR, Enrich C, Vives J, Sanchez-Madrid F, Lozano F (2004) Relevance of CD6-mediated interactions in T cell activation and proliferation. J Immunol 173:2262–2270

Gimferrer I, Ibanez A, Farnos M, Sarrias MR, Fenutria R, Rosello S, Zimmermann P, David G, Vives J, Serra-Pages C, Lozano F (2005) The lymphocyte receptor CD6 interacts with syntenin-1, a scaffolding protein containing PDZ domains. J Immunol 175:1406–1414

Glebov OO, Nichols BJ (2004) Lipid raft proteins have a random distribution during localized activation of the T-cell receptor. Nat Cell Biol 6:238–243

Gomez TS, McCarney SD, Carrizosa E, Labno CM, Comiskey EO, Nolz JC, Zhu P, Freedman BD, Clark MR, Rawlings DJ, Billadeau DD, Burkhardt JK (2006) HS1 functions as an essential actin-regulatory adaptor protein at the immune synapse. Immunity 24:741–752

Gomez TS, Kumar K, Medeiros RB, Shimizu Y, Leibson PJ, Billadeau DD (2007) Formins regulate the actin-related protein 2/3 complex-independent polarization of the centrosome to the immunological synapse. Immunity 26:177–190

Grakoui A, Bromley SK, Sumen C, Davis MM, Shaw AS, Allen PM, Dustin ML (1999) The immunological synapse: a molecular machine controlling T cell activation. Science 285:221–227

Hailman E, Burack WR, Shaw AS, Dustin ML, Allen PM (2002) Immature CD4(+)CD8(+) thymocytes form a multifocal immunological synapse with sustained tyrosine phosphorylation. Immunity 16:839–848

Hancock JF (2006) Lipid rafts: contentious only from simplistic standpoints. Nat Rev Mol Cell Biol 7:456–462

Hayashi K, Altman A (2006) Filamin A is required for T cell activation mediated by protein kinase C-theta. J Immunol 177:1721–1728

Holdorf AD, Lee KH, Burack WR, Allen PM, Shaw AS (2002) Regulation of Lck activity by CD4 and CD28 in the immunological synapse. Nat Immunol 3:259–264

Houtman JC, Yamaguchi H, Barda-Saad M, Braiman A, Bowden B, Appella E, Schuck P, Samelson LE (2006) Oligomerization of signaling complexes by the multipoint binding of GRB2 to both LAT and SOS1. Nat Struct Mol Biol 13:798–805

Huang J, Lo PF, Zal T, Gascoigne NR, Smith BA, Levin SD, Grey HM (2002) CD28 plays a critical role in the segregation of PKC theta within the immunologic synapse. Proc Natl Acad Sci USA 99:9369–9373

Huang Y, Comiskey EO, Dupree RS, Li S, Koleske AJ, Burkhardt JK (2008) The c-Abl tyrosine kinase regulates actin remodeling at the immune synapse. Blood 112:111–119

Huppa JB, Davis MM (2003) T-cell-antigen recognition and the immunological synapse. Nat Rev Immunol 3:973–983

Huse M, Lillemeier BF, Kuhns MS, Chen DS, Davis MM (2006) T cells use two directionally distinct pathways for cytokine secretion. Nat Immunol 7:247–255

Ibanez A, Sarrias MR, Farnos M, Gimferrer I, Serra-Pages C, Vives J, Lozano F (2006) Mitogen-activated protein kinase pathway activation by the CD6 lymphocyte surface receptor. J Immunol 177:1152–1159

Ilani T, Vasiliver-Shamis G, Vardhana S, Bretscher A, Dustin ML (2009) T cell antigen receptor signaling and immunological synapse stability require myosin IIA. Nat Immunol 10:531–539

Imboden JB, Stobo JD (1985) Transmembrane signalling by the T cell antigen receptor. Perturbation of the T3-antigen receptor complex generates inositol phosphates and releases calcium ions from intracellular stores. J Exp Med 161:446–456

Irvine DJ, Purbhoo MA, Krogsgaard M, Davis MM (2002) Direct observation of ligand recognition by T cells. Nature 419:845–849

Itoh K, Sakakibara M, Yamasaki S, Takeuchi A, Arase H, Miyazaki M, Nakajima N, Okada M, Saito T (2002) Cutting edge: negative regulation of immune synapse formation by anchoring lipid raft to cytoskeleton through Cbp-EBP50-ERM assembly. J Immunol 168:541–544

Janes PW, Ley SC, Magee AI (1999) Aggregation of lipid rafts accompanies signaling via the T cell antigen receptor. J Cell Biol 147:447–461

Johnson KG, Bromley SK, Dustin ML, Thomas ML (2000) A supramolecular basis for CD45 tyrosine phosphatase regulation in sustained T cell activation. Proc Natl Acad Sci USA 97:10138–10143

Kaga S, Ragg S, Rogers KA, Ochi A (1998) Stimulation of CD28 with B7-2 promotes focal adhesion-like cell contacts where Rho family small G proteins accumulate in T cells. J Immunol 160:24–27

Kaizuka Y, Douglass AD, Varma R, Dustin ML, Vale RD (2007) Mechanisms for segregating T cell receptor and adhesion molecules during immunological synapse formation in Jurkat T cells. Proc Natl Acad Sci USA 104:20296–20301

Krogsgaard M, Li QJ, Sumen C, Huppa JB, Huse M, Davis MM (2005) Agonist/endogenous peptide-MHC heterodimers drive T cell activation and sensitivity. Nature 434:238–243

Krummel MF, Davis MM (2002) Dynamics of the immunological synapse: finding, establishing and solidifying a connection. Curr Opin Immunol 14:66–74

Krummel MF, Sjaastad MD, Wulfing C, Davis MM (2000) Differential clustering of CD4 and CD3zeta during T cell recognition. Science 289:1349–1352

Kupfer A, Dennert G (1984) Reorientation of the microtubule-organizing center and the Golgi apparatus in cloned cytotoxic lymphocytes triggered by binding to lysable target cells. J Immunol 133:2762–2766

Kupfer A, Mosmann TR, Kupfer H (1991) Polarized expression of cytokines in cell conjugates of helper T cells and splenic B cells. Proc Natl Acad Sci USA 88:775–779

Lazar-Molnar E, Yan Q, Cao E, Ramagopal U, Nathenson SG, Almo SC (2008) Crystal structure of the complex between programmed death-1 (PD-1) and its ligand PD-L2. Proc Natl Acad Sci USA 105:10483–10488

Lee KH, Dinner AR, Tu C, Campi G, Raychaudhuri S, Varma R, Sims TN, Burack WR, Wu H, Wang J, Kanagawa O, Markiewicz M, Allen PM, Dustin ML, Chakraborty AK, Shaw AS (2003) The immunological synapse balances T cell receptor signaling and degradation. Science 302:1218–1222

Lillemeier BF, Pfeiffer JR, Surviladze Z, Wilson BS, Davis MM (2006) Plasma membrane-associated proteins are clustered into islands attached to the cytoskeleton. Proc Natl Acad Sci USA 103:18992–18997

Linsley PS, Bradshaw J, Greene J, Peach R, Bennett KL, Mittler RS (1996) Intracellular trafficking of CTLA-4 and focal localization towards sites of TCR engagement. Immunity 4:535–543

Ludford-Menting MJ, Oliaro J, Sacirbegovic F, Cheah ET, Pedersen N, Thomas SJ, Pasam A, Iazzolino R, Dow LE, Waterhouse NJ, Murphy A, Ellis S, Smyth MJ, Kershaw MH, Darcy PK, Humbert PO, Russell SM (2005) A network of PDZ-containing proteins regulates T cell polarity and morphology during migration and immunological synapse formation. Immunity 22:737–748

Ma Z, Sharp KA, Janmey PA, Finkel TH (2008) Surface-anchored monomeric agonist pMHCs alone trigger TCR with high sensitivity. PLoS Biol 6:e43

Maldonado RA, Irvine DJ, Schreiber R, Glimcher LH (2004) A role for the immunological synapse in lineage commitment of CD4 lymphocytes. Nature 431:527–532

Maldonado RA, Soriano MA, Perdomo LC, Sigrist K, Irvine DJ, Decker T, Glimcher LH (2009) Control of T helper cell differentiation through cytokine receptor inclusion in the immunological synapse. J Exp Med 206:877–892

Martin M, Schneider H, Azouz A, Rudd CE (2001) Cytotoxic T lymphocyte antigen 4 and CD28 modulate cell surface raft expression in their regulation of T cell function. J Exp Med 194:1675–1681

McCarthy C, Shepherd D, Fleire S, Stronge VS, Koch M, Illarionov PA, Bossi G, Salio M, Denkberg G, Reddington F, Tarlton A, Reddy BG, Schmidt RR, Reiter Y, Griffiths GM, van der Merwe PA, Besra GS, Jones EY, Batista FD, Cerundolo V (2007) The length of lipids bound to human CD1d molecules modulates the affinity of NKT cell TCR and the threshold of NKT cell activation. J Exp Med 204:1131–1144

McConnell HM, Watts TH, Weis RM, Brian AA (1986) Supported planar membranes in studies of cell-cell recognition in the immune system. Biochim Biophys Acta 864:95–106

McKeithan TW (1995) Kinetic proofreading in T-cell receptor signal transduction. Proc Natl Acad Sci USA 92:5042–5046

Mingueneau M, Sansoni A, Gregoire C, Roncagalli R, Aguado E, Weiss A, Malissen M, Malissen B (2008) The proline-rich sequence of CD3epsilon controls T cell antigen receptor expression on and signaling potency in preselection CD4+CD8+ thymocytes. Nat Immunol 9:522–532

Molon B, Gri G, Bettella M, Gomez-Mouton C, Lanzavecchia A, Martinez AC, Manes S, Viola A (2005) T cell costimulation by chemokine receptors. Nat Immunol 6:465–471

Monks CR, Kupfer H, Tamir I, Barlow A, Kupfer A (1997) Selective modulation of protein kinase C-theta during T-cell activation. Nature 385:83–86

Monks CR, Freiberg BA, Kupfer H, Sciaky N, Kupfer A (1998) Three-dimensional segregation of supramolecular activation clusters in T cells. Nature 395:82–86

Mor A, Philips MR (2006) Compartmentalized Ras/MAPK signaling. Annu Rev Immunol 24:771–800

Mossman KD, Campi G, Groves JT, Dustin ML (2005) Altered TCR signaling from geometrically repatterned immunological synapses. Science 310:1191–1193

Mugnier B, Nal B, Verthuy C, Boyer C, Lam D, Chasson L, Nieoullon V, Chazal G, Guo XJ, He HT, Rueff-Juy D, Alcover A, Ferrier P (2008) Coronin-1A links cytoskeleton dynamics to TCR alpha beta-induced cell signaling. PLoS ONE 3:e3467

Munoz P, Mittelbrunn M, de la Fuente H, Perez-Martinez M, Garcia-Perez A, Ariza-Veguillas A, Malavasi F, Zubiaur M, Sanchez-Madrid F, Sancho J (2008) Antigen-induced clustering of surface CD38 and recruitment of intracellular CD38 to the immunologic synapse. Blood 111:3653–3664

Nguyen K, Sylvain NR, Bunnell SC (2008) T cell costimulation via the integrin VLA-4 inhibits the actin-dependent centralization of signaling microclusters containing the adaptor SLP-76. Immunity 28:810–821

Nolz JC, Gomez TS, Zhu P, Li S, Medeiros RB, Shimizu Y, Burkhardt JK, Freedman BD, Billadeau DD (2006) The WAVE2 complex regulates actin cytoskeletal reorganization and CRAC-mediated calcium entry during T cell activation. Curr Biol 16:24–34

Norcross MA (1984) A synaptic basis for T-lymphocyte activation. Ann Immunol (Paris) 135D:113–134

Orange JS (2008) Formation and function of the lytic NK-cell immunological synapse. Nat Rev Immunol 8:713–725

Pacheco R, Martinez-Navio JM, Lejeune M, Climent N, Oliva H, Gatell JM, Gallart T, Mallol J, Lluis C, Franco R (2005) CD26, adenosine deaminase, and adenosine receptors mediate costimulatory signals in the immunological synapse. Proc Natl Acad Sci USA 102:9583–9588

Paul WE, Seder RA (1994) Lymphocyte responses and cytokines. Cell 76:241–251

Paul WE, Brown M, Hornbeck P, Mizuguchi J, Ohara J, Rabin E, Snapper C, Tsang W (1987) Regulation of B-lymphocyte activation, proliferation, and differentiation. Ann NY Acad Sci 505:82–89

Pentcheva-Hoang T, Egen JG, Wojnoonski K, Allison JP (2004) B7–1 and B7–2 selectively recruit CTLA-4 and CD28 to the immunological synapse. Immunity 21:401–413

Pfeifhofer C, Kofler K, Gruber T, Tabrizi NG, Lutz C, Maly K, Leitges M, Baier G (2003) Protein kinase C theta affects Ca2+ mobilization and NFAT cell activation in primary mouse T cells. J Exp Med 197:1525–1535

Purbhoo MA, Irvine DJ, Huppa JB, Davis MM (2004) T cell killing does not require the formation of a stable mature immunological synapse. Nat Immunol 5:524–530

Purtic B, Pitcher LA, van Oers NS, Wulfing C (2005) T cell receptor (TCR) clustering in the immunological synapse integrates TCR and costimulatory signaling in selected T cells. Proc Natl Acad Sci USA 102:2904–2909

Rabinowitz JD, Beeson C, Lyons DS, Davis MM, McConnell HM (1996) Kinetic discrimination in T-cell activation. Proc Natl Acad Sci USA 93:1401–1405

Reinherz EL, Tan K, Tang L, Kern P, Liu J, Xiong Y, Hussey RE, Smolyar A, Hare B, Zhang R, Joachimiak A, Chang HC, Wagner G, Wang J (1999) The crystal structure of a T cell receptor in complex with peptide and MHC class II. Science 286:1913–1921

Revy P, Sospedra M, Barbour B, Trautmann A (2001) Functional antigen-independent synapses formed between T cells and dendritic cells. Nat Immunol 2:925–931

Richie LI, Ebert PJ, Wu LC, Krummel MF, Owen JJ, Davis MM (2002) Imaging synapse formation during thymocyte selection: inability of CD3zeta to form a stable central accumulation during negative selection. Immunity 16:595–606

Rothoeft T, Balkow S, Krummen M, Beissert S, Varga G, Loser K, Oberbanscheidt P, van den Boom F, Grabbe S (2006) Structure and duration of contact between dendritic cells and T cells are controlled by T cell activation state. Eur J Immunol 36:3105–3117

Roumier A, Olivo-Marin JC, Arpin M, Michel F, Martin M, Mangeat P, Acuto O, Dautry-Varsat A, Alcover A (2001) The membrane-microfilament linker ezrin is involved in the formation of the immunological synapse and in T cell activation. Immunity 15:715–728

Rozdzial MM, Malissen B, Finkel TH (1995) Tyrosine-phosphorylated T cell receptor zeta chain associates with the actin cytoskeleton upon activation of mature T lymphocytes. Immunity 3:623–633

Saito T, Yokosuka T (2006) Immunological synapse and microclusters: the site for recognition and activation of T cells. Curr Opin Immunol 18:305–313

Salazar-Fontana LI, Barr V, Samelson LE, Bierer BE (2003) CD28 engagement promotes actin polymerization through the activation of the small Rho GTPase Cdc42 in human T cells. J Immunol 171:2225–2232

Sasahara Y, Rachid R, Byrne MJ, de la Fuente MA, Abraham RT, Ramesh N, Geha RS (2002) Mechanism of recruitment of WASP to the immunological synapse and of its activation following TCR ligation. Mol Cell 10:1269–1281

Schaefer BC, Kappler JW, Kupfer A, Marrack P (2004) Complex and dynamic redistribution of NF-kappaB signaling intermediates in response to T cell receptor stimulation. Proc Natl Acad Sci USA 101:1004–1009

Schneider H, Valk E, da Rocha Dias S, Wei B, Rudd CE (2005) CTLA-4 up-regulation of lymphocyte function-associated antigen 1 adhesion and clustering as an alternate basis for coreceptor function. Proc Natl Acad Sci USA 102:12861–12866

Schneider H, Smith X, Liu H, Bismuth G, Rudd CE (2008) CTLA-4 disrupts ZAP70 microcluster formation with reduced T cell/APC dwell times and calcium mobilization. Eur J Immunol 38:40–47

Seminario MC, Bunnell SC (2008) Signal initiation in T-cell receptor microclusters. Immunol Rev 221:90–106

Shaw AS (2006) Lipid rafts: now you see them, now you don't. Nat Immunol 7:1139–1142

Shaw AS, Dustin ML (1997) Making the T cell receptor go the distance: a topological view of T cell activation. Immunity 6:361–369

Singer AL, Bunnell SC, Obstfeld AE, Jordan MS, Wu JN, Myung PS, Samelson LE, Koretzky GA (2004) Roles of the proline-rich domain in SLP-76 subcellular localization and T cell function. J Biol Chem 279:15481–15490

Sloan-Lancaster J, Presley J, Ellenberg J, Yamazaki T, Lippincott-Schwartz J, Samelson LE (1998) ZAP-70 association with T cell receptor zeta (TCRzeta): fluorescence imaging of dynamic changes upon cellular stimulation. J Cell Biol 143:613–624

Sohn HW, Tolar P, Pierce SK (2008) Membrane heterogeneities in the formation of B cell receptor-Lyn kinase microclusters and the immune synapse. J Cell Biol 182:367–379

Spitaler M, Emslie E, Wood CD, Cantrell D (2006) Diacylglycerol and protein kinase D localization during T lymphocyte activation. Immunity 24:535–546

Stauffer TP, Meyer T (1997) Compartmentalized IgE receptor-mediated signal transduction in living cells. J Cell Biol 139:1447–1454

Stephan MT, Ponomarev V, Brentjens RJ, Chang AH, Dobrenkov KV, Heller G, Sadelain M (2007) T cell-encoded CD80 and 4–1BBL induce auto- and transcostimulation, resulting in potent tumor rejection. Nat Med 13:1440–1449

Stinchcombe JC, Bossi G, Booth S, Griffiths GM (2001) The immunological synapse of CTL contains a secretory domain and membrane bridges. Immunity 15:751–761

Stinchcombe JC, Majorovits E, Bossi G, Fuller S, Griffiths GM (2006) Centrosome polarization delivers secretory granules to the immunological synapse. Nature 443:462–465

Stoll S, Delon J, Brotz TM, Germain RN (2002) Dynamic imaging of T cell-dendritic cell interactions in lymph nodes. Science 296:1873–1876

Sun Z, Arendt CW, Ellmeier W, Schaeffer EM, Sunshine MJ, Gandhi L, Annes J, Petrzilka D, Kupfer A, Schwartzberg PL, Littman DR (2000) PKC-theta is required for TCR-induced NF-kappaB activation in mature but not immature T lymphocytes. Nature 404:402–407

Tavano R, Gri G, Molon B, Marinari B, Rudd CE, Tuosto L, Viola A (2004) CD28 and lipid rafts coordinate recruitment of Lck to the immunological synapse of human T lymphocytes. J Immunol 173:5392–5397

Tavano R, Contento RL, Baranda SJ, Soligo M, Tuosto L, Manes S, Viola A (2006) CD28 interaction with filamin-A controls lipid raft accumulation at the T-cell immunological synapse. Nat Cell Biol 8:1270–1276

Tolar P, Sohn HW, Pierce SK (2005) The initiation of antigen-induced B cell antigen receptor signaling viewed in living cells by fluorescence resonance energy transfer. Nat Immunol 6:1168–1176

Tseng SY, Liu M, Dustin ML (2005) CD80 cytoplasmic domain controls localization of CD28, CTLA-4, and protein kinase Ctheta in the immunological synapse. J Immunol 175:7829–7836

Tskvitaria-Fuller I, Rozelle AL, Yin HL, Wulfing C (2003) Regulation of sustained actin dynamics by the TCR and costimulation as a mechanism of receptor localization. J Immunol 171:2287–2295

Valitutti S, Muller S, Cella M, Padovan E, Lanzavecchia A (1995) Serial triggering of many T-cell receptors by a few peptide-MHC complexes. Nature 375:148–151

Varma R, Campi G, Yokosuka T, Saito T, Dustin ML (2006) T cell receptor-proximal signals are sustained in peripheral microclusters and terminated in the central supramolecular activation cluster. Immunity 25:117–127

Vicente-Manzanares M, Sanchez-Madrid F (2004) Role of the cytoskeleton during leukocyte responses. Nat Rev Immunol 4:110–122

Viola A, Lanzavecchia A (1996) T cell activation determined by T cell receptor number and tunable thresholds. Science 273:104–106

Viola A, Schroeder S, Sakakibara Y, Lanzavecchia A (1999) T lymphocyte costimulation mediated by reorganization of membrane microdomains. Science 283:680–682

Wetzel SA, McKeithan TW, Parker DC (2002) Live-cell dynamics and the role of costimulation in immunological synapse formation. J Immunol 169:6092–6101

Wiedemann A, Muller S, Favier B, Penna D, Guiraud M, Delmas C, Champagne E, Valitutti S (2005) T-cell activation is accompanied by an ubiquitination process occurring at the immunological synapse. Immunol Lett 98:57–61

Yokosuka T, Saito T (2009) Dynamic regulation of T-cell costimulation through TCR–CD28 microclusters. Immunol Rev 229:27–40

Yokosuka T, Sakata-Sogawa K, Kobayashi W, Hiroshima M, Hashimoto-Tane A, Tokunaga M, Dustin ML, Saito T (2005) Newly generated T cell receptor microclusters initiate and sustain T cell activation by recruitment of Zap70 and SLP-76. Nat Immunol 6:1253–1262

Yokosuka T, Kobayashi W, Sakata-Sogawa K, Takamatsu M, Hashimoto-Tane A, Dustin ML, Tokunaga M, Saito T (2008) Spatiotemporal regulation of T cell costimulation by TCR-CD28 microclusters and protein kinase C theta translocation. Immunity 29:589–601

Zhang W, Trible RP, Samelson LE (1998) LAT palmitoylation: its essential role in membrane microdomain targeting and tyrosine phosphorylation during T cell activation. Immunity 9:239–246

Zipfel PA, Bunnell SC, Witherow DS, Gu JJ, Chislock EM, Ring C, Pendergast AM (2006) Role for the Abi/wave protein complex in T cell receptor-mediated proliferation and cytoskeletal remodeling. Curr Biol 16:35–46

Zubiaur M, Fernandez O, Ferrero E, Salmeron J, Malissen B, Malavasi F, Sancho J (2002) CD38 is associated with lipid rafts and upon receptor stimulation leads to Akt/protein kinase B and Erk activation in the absence of the CD3-zeta immune receptor tyrosine-based activation motifs. J Biol Chem 277:13–22

Signaling Amplification at the Immunological Synapse

Antonella Viola, Rita Lucia Contento, and Barbara Molon

Contents

Abstract The immunological synapse is a dynamic structure, formed between a T cell and one or more antigen presenting cells, characterized by lipid and protein segregation, signaling compartmentalization, and bidirectional information exchange through soluble and membrane-bound transmitters. In addition, the immunological synapse is the site where signals delivered by the T cell receptors, adhesion molecules, as well as costimulatory and coinhibitory receptors are decoded and integrated. Signaling modulation and tunable activation thresholds allow T cells to interpret the context in which the antigen is presented, recognize infectious stimuli, and finally decide between activation and tolerance. In this review, we discuss some strategies used by membrane receptors to tune activation signals in T cells.

A. Viola (✉)
Laboratory of Adaptive Immunity, Department of Translational Medicine, University of Milan, I.R.C.C.S. Istituto Clinico Humanitas, Via Manzoni 113, 20089, Rozzano, Milan, Italy
e-mail: antonella.viola@humanitas.it

R.L. Contento
Laboratory of Adaptive Immunity, I.R.C.C.S. Istituto Clinico Humanitas, Via Manzoni 113, 20089, Rozzano, Milan, Italy

B. Molon
Istituto Oncologico Veneto I.R.C.C.S., Via Gattamelata 64, 35128, Padua, Italy

T. Saito and F.D. Batista (eds.), *Immunological Synapse*,
Current Topics in Microbiology and Immunology 340,
DOI 10.1007/978-3-642-03858-7_6, © Springer-Verlag Berlin Heidelberg 2010

1 Introduction

The adaptive immune response is initiated by activation of T and B lymphocytes in secondary lymphoid tissues, where dendritic cells (DCs) carry antigens collected in the periphery. In the case of T lymphocytes, T cell receptors (TCRs) recognize and interact with specific antigenic complexes formed by antigen-derived peptides bound to membrane proteins encoded by the class I or class II genes of the major histocompatibility complex (MHC) and expressed on the DC surface. Since a single DC presents on its membrane many different combinations of peptide–MHC (pMHC) molecules, the number of specific antigenic complexes for a T cell can be very low (10–100) (Harding and Unanue 1990; Christinck et al. 1991; Sykulev et al. 1996). For example, while a single antigenic complex elicits a transient calcium influx, at least ten pMHC complexes are required to induce the formation of the immunological synapse (Irvine et al. 2002). T cell priming is therefore a very sensitive process because it induces a variety of cellular responses including proliferation, secretion of cytokines, and cytotoxic mediators, but it is initiated by very few ligands.

Another key feature of the immune response is its specificity: T cells must be able to discriminate precisely between an infectious stimulus and a noninfectious one and tune their response in accordance with the molecular context in which the antigen is presented. Establishing checkpoints for signaling is therefore a very important aspect in T cell activation (Acuto et al. 2008).

As discussed in this review, T cell sensitivity and specificity are extremely interconnected and both depend on T cell costimulatory molecules, which integrate and amplify TCR signaling at the immunological synapse. While the activating and inhibitory molecular interactions have half-lives in the order of seconds (Davis et al. 1998), the duration of signaling that is required to achieve T cell priming ranges from a few to several hours (Iezzi et al. 1998; Lanzavecchia et al. 1999). During the prolonged interaction with the DC, the T lymphocyte integrates all signals delivered by its TCRs as well as stimulatory and inhibitory receptors. This signaling integration ensures the amplification required for sensitivity, as well as the checkpoints required for specificity.

2 CD28 and Lipid Rafts

T cell priming is strongly influenced by signals delivered through the costimulatory molecule CD28. In contrast to adhesion molecules, such as the leukocyte function-associated antigen 1 (LFA-1), which exert their costimulatory action by facilitating and prolonging the contact between the antigen presenting cell (APC) and the T cell (Bachmann et al. 1997), CD28 lowers the T cell activation threshold and allows T cell priming by few antigenic complexes (Viola and Lanzavecchia 1996). Several reports have demonstrated that CD28 can enhance several signaling pathways leading to gene transcription (Pages et al. 1994; Su et al. 1994; Tuosto and Acuto

1998; Viola et al. 1999; Viola 2001; Acuto and Michel 2003), suggesting that CD28 acts as a general amplifier of early TCR signaling. Indeed, T cells from CD28-deficient mice can be activated using higher doses of antigen, demonstrating that the signals delivered by CD28 can be easily replaced by stronger TCR signaling (Shahinian et al. 1993; Kundig et al. 1996). Thus, CD28 represents a signaling amplifier for naive T cells and therefore determines the sensitivity of the adaptive immune response. CD28 ligands, namely B7-1 and B7-2, are expressed at high levels by pathogen-activated professional APC, such as mature DCs, as well as activated B cells and macrophages. On most APC populations, B7-2 is expressed constitutively at low levels and is rapidly upregulated upon activation, whereas B7-1 is inducibly expressed later after activation (Freeman et al. 1993; Hathcock et al. 1994; van Vliet et al. 2007). In DCs, the switch from an immature to an inflammatory phenotype expressing CD28 ligands and capable of inducing T cell priming depends on the interaction between pattern recognition receptors (PRRs) and pathogen-associated molecular patterns. For example, Toll-like receptor (TLR) signaling pathways regulate the activation of different transcription factors leading to expression of costimulatory molecules and chemokine receptors and to the production of inflammatory cytokines (Janeway et al. 1989; Medzhitov and Janeway 2002; Akira et al. 2006). In addition, inflammatory cytokines may themselves trigger DC maturation in the absence of microbial stimulation (Blanco et al. 2008).

CD28 costimulation is therefore possible when APCs present antigens in the context of infection and/or inflammation. This system allows the use of T cell sensitivity in favor of specificity: TCR signaling will be amplified and T cells will be primed only if "danger" signals are present in our body. In other words, a qualitative signal, such as presence or absence of inflammation, can be interpreted through quantitative and tunable events, such as phosphorylation of signaling mediators, and calcium influxes.

Although several laboratories have investigated CD28 downstream signals, the precise mechanism of CD28-mediated costimulation is not clearly understood. Several molecules, such as phosphoinositide 3-kinase (PI3K) (Pages et al. 1994; Harada et al. 2003), lymphocyte specific protein tyrosine kinase (Lck) (Holdorf et al. 1999; Liu et al. 2000), growth factor receptor-bound protein 2 (Grb2) (Raab et al. 1995), Grb2-related adaptor protein (Gads) (Watanabe et al. 2006), IL2-inducible T cell kinase (Itk), the guaninenucleotide exchange factor Vav (Villalba et al. 2000), protein kinase B (PKB) (also known as Akt) (Kane et al. 2001), protein phosphatase 2A (PP2A) (Chuang et al. 2000; Alegre et al. 2001), and protein kinase C θ(PKCθ) (Villalba et al. 2000), have been implicated in the CD28-mediated pathway. In the case of PKCθ, it has been recently shown that CD28 is responsible for recruitment of the kinase into TCR–CD28 microclusters and for its retaining at a spatially unique and dynamic subregion of central supramolecular activation cluster (Yokosuka et al. 2008).

While searching for a mechanism responsible for CD28-induced amplification of the TCR signaling cascade, we hypothesized that costimulation might promote membrane lipid rearrangement at the immunological synapse and thus generate an environment in which signals are protected from phosphatases and amplified. Indeed, we had shown that in the absence of CD28 costimulation, tyrosine phosphorylation of TCR signaling mediators is very transient since they are dephosphorylated in a few seconds by the action of phosphatases. By contrast, when CD28 costimulation is provided, the stability of TCR-induced phosphorylation is long-lasting and persists for minutes (Viola et al. 1999). Interestingly, we found that stimulation of resting T cells with anti-CD3 plus anti-CD28 antibody-coated beads induces recruitment of the ganglioside GM1, a membrane raft marker, to the TCR triggering site (Viola et al. 1999). Several studies confirmed and expanded this initial observation (Dupre et al. 2002; Paccani et al. 2005; Round et al. 2005) and suggested that raft recruitment into the immunological synapse occurs only in T cells with high activation stringency (Ebert et al. 2000; Balamuth et al. 2001; Kovacs et al. 2002) and requires CD28 signaling (Viola et al. 1999; Tavano et al. 2004; Tavano et al. 2006).

Membrane rafts are small (10–200 nm in diameter), heterogeneous, highly dynamic, sterol- and sphingolipid-enriched domains that compartmentalize cellular processes. They have been implicated in protein sorting in several cell types (Schuck and Simons 2004), but the precise role of membrane rafts in organizing receptor assembly at the immunological synapse is not fully understood. However, the correlation between the capacity of a molecule (either a signaling molecule or a fluorescent probe) to be recruited into the immune synapse and its preference for a "raft environment" is quite strong. At the T cell synapse, membrane rafts may function as platforms for the formation of multicomponent transduction complexes. Indeed, these microdomains are constitutively enriched in proteins involved in the early phases of TCR signaling, such as the Src family kinases Lck and Fyn, the adapter protein LAT, phosphoprotein associated with glycosphingolipid-enriched domains (PAG) or Csk-activating protein (Cbp), and Lck-interacting molecule (LIME) (Pizzo and Viola 2004). Furthermore, the composition of raft-associated proteins changes after T cell stimulation, suggesting that rafts are dynamic platforms for T cell signaling. Thus, upon TCR stimulation many signaling proteins become concentrated in rafts, including the zeta-associated protein 70, the phospholipase Cγ, Vav, PKB, and PKCθ (Pizzo and Viola 2004).

As already mentioned, T cell stimulation by APCs results in a dramatic redistribution of membrane rafts toward the immunological synapse, and this process requires CD28 signaling (Tavano et al. 2004; Tavano et al. 2006). On the other hand, CD28 has been long recognized as an important organizer of the actin cytoskeleton. The TCR–CD28-triggered polymerization of actin at the immune synapse is regulated by the action of the guanine nucleotide-exchange factor VAV, the small Rho GTPase CDC42, the Wiscott–Aldrich Syndrome protein (WASP), and the ARP2/3 complex. However, the mechanism of membrane raft mobilization into the immunological synapse was unclear until recently.

The ARP2/3 complex cooperates with filamins, which are actin cross-linking proteins, to generate and maintain the cortical actin cytoskeleton (Stossel et al. 2001). It has been suggested that the linkages between actin filaments formed by the ARP2/3 complex are metastable and dissociate, whereas interactions between the actin-binding protein filamin A (FLNa) and actin filaments are stable for long periods of time (Flanagan et al. 2001). Interestingly, FLNa, which is expressed in T cells, was recently shown to interact with CD28 in a stimulation-dependent manner (Tavano et al. 2006). After physiological stimulation, CD28 recruits FLNa into the immunological synapse (Tavano et al. 2006), where FLNa organizes TCR (Hayashi and Altman 2006) and CD28 signaling (Tavano et al. 2006). RNA interference (RNAi)-mediated knockdown of FLNa expression resulted in loss of accumulation of membrane rafts at the immunological synapse, as well as impairment of CD28-dependent costimulation (Tavano et al. 2006). In addition, mutations in the CD28 cytoplasmic tail that led to abrogation of the CD28–FLNa interaction also resulted in impaired mobilization of membrane rafts to the immunological synapse (Tavano et al. 2004; Tavano et al. 2006). These data strongly indicate a role for FLNa in the recruitment of membrane rafts into the immunological synapse and suggest that CD28 signaling provides for a membrane-raft-based compartmentalization of key signaling intermediates at the immunological synapse for amplification of TCR-derived signals.

3 Chemokines and Their Receptors

Chemokines are small cytokines with selective chemoattractant properties coordinating the homeostatic circulation of leukocytes as well as their migration towards sites of inflammation or injury. Homeostatic chemokines are constitutively produced and involved in maintaining leukocyte trafficking, as well as the architecture of secondary lymphoid organs, whereas inflammatory chemokines are produced by activated cells and recruit leukocytes to inflamed tissues. Similar to cytokines and costimulatory molecules, chemokine and chemokine receptor synthesis is regulated by infectious and inflammatory stimuli, such as TLR and nuclear oligomerization domain (NOD)-like family ligands (Park et al. 2007; Werts et al. 2007; Serbina et al. 2008). Although their major role is to direct leukocyte trafficking, chemokines can be useful in helping T cells to interpret the context in which an antigen is presented. We have demonstrated that the T cell chemokine receptors CCR5 and CXCR4 are recruited into the immunological synapse during T cell–APC interaction (Molon et al. 2005). When approaching an APC, T cells emit CCR5 (or CXCR4)-enriched protrusions that indent the APC surface; this situation resembles the concentration of chemokine receptors at the leading edge of chemoattractant-stimulated T cells (Gomez-Mouton et al. 2004). These interactions culminate in the formation of a stable synapse, where CCR5 and CXCR4 are stably concentrated. Chemokine receptor accumulation at the T cell synapse requires secretion of chemokines by the APC, substantiating an important role for the activation state of the APC in this process. The consequence of chemokine release at the immunological synapse and of chemokine receptor recruitment into this region is T cell costimulation. Indeed, during T cell activation, CCL5 and CXCL12 chemokines enhance T cell proliferation and cytokine production (Taub 1996; Karpus et al.

1997; Molon et al. 2005), suggesting that at the immunological synapse chemokines function as soluble immunotransmitters and are potent T cell activators.

At the T cell synapse, chemokine receptor triggering modifies, and is modified by, other receptor pathways in a complex signaling cross-talk. For example, both TCR and chemokine receptors activate adhesion molecules through inside-out signaling (Dustin and Springer 1989; Constantin et al. 2000), whereas CD28 and chemokine receptors participate in TCR signaling amplification. Interestingly, TCR triggering modifies chemokine receptor signaling properties (Molon et al. 2005), too. Chemokines receptors are seven transmembrane spanning proteins coupled to heterotrimeric G protein – i.e., G protein-coupled receptors (GPCRs). Chemokine binding to chemokine receptors dissociates $G\alpha_i$, the $G\alpha$ most commonly associated with those receptors, and $G\beta\gamma$ subunits of the heterotrimeric G proteins, leading to calcium flux and activation of the PI3K, and the small Rho GTPases signaling pathways, among others (Thelen and Stein 2008). Consistent with G_i association, the majority of chemokine responses are inhibited by treatment with pertussis toxin (PTx) (Goldman et al. 1985). Nevertheless, in some circumstances, PTx cannot completely block chemokine-induced responses owing to chemokine receptor association to G proteins other than G_i, such as $G_{q/11}$ or G_{16} (Thelen and Stein 2008). Interestingly, chemokine receptor accumulation at the immunological synapse is insensitive to PTx treatment, indicating that the process does not involve G_i-mediated signaling (Molon et al. 2005). Compatible with this, we found that chemokine recognition in the context of the immunological synapse induces a $G_{q/11}$-mediated CCR5 signaling, suggesting that chemokine receptor signaling pathways are modified by TCR triggering (Molon et al. 2005). Notably, coupling of G_q to the chemokine receptors delays their internalization, explaining the accumulation of CCR5 and CXCR4 at the T cell immunological synapse. In this scenario, chemokine receptors prolong the duration of T cell–APC interaction and facilitate T cell activation by increasing LFA-1 affinity (Tybulewicz 2002; Shamri et al. 2005), reinforcing T cell–APC pair attraction and avoiding premature splitting due to other chemoattractant sources. In addition to stabilization of the immune synapse, chemokine receptors may induce costimulation through specific signaling pathways cooperating with the TCR. For example, G_q-mediated signaling triggers the translocation of nuclear factor of activated T cells (NFAT) to the nucleus (Boss et al. 1996); moreover, chemokine receptors bind FLNa (Jimenez-Baranda et al. 2007), suggesting that actin reorganization is a common strategy used by CD28 and chemokine receptors to amplify TCR signaling (Fig. 1).

Although CD28 and chemokine receptor may share some signaling intermediates in delivering TCR costimulatory signals, they may operate in very different physiological contexts. Indeed, while CD28 is expressed on naïve T cells, the expression of chemokine receptors is finely tuned during all stages of T cell activation. We have demonstrated that the costimulatory properties of CCR5 and CXCR4 chemokine receptors depend on their ability to form heterodimers (Contento et al. 2008). CXCR4 and CCR5 homodimers are not recruited into the immunological synapse and do not costimulate T cell activation, although they are perfectly functional in inducing chemotactic responses (Contento et al. 2008),

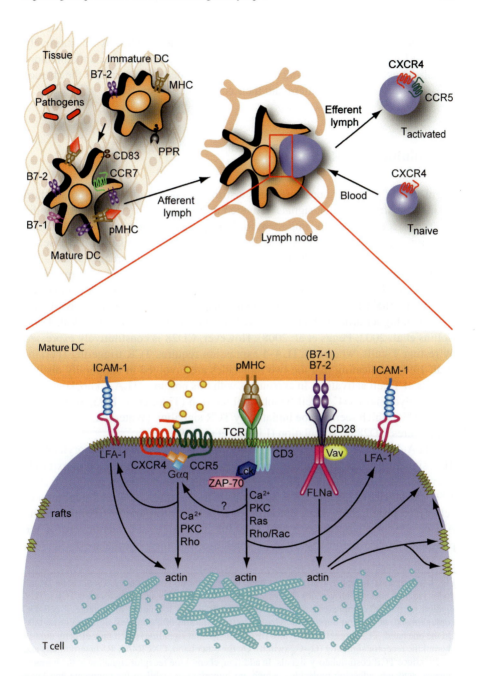

Fig. 1 Costimulation at the immunological synapse. In peripheral tissues, resting DCs recognize pathogens through pattern recognition receptors (PPRs). Signals delivered by PPRs allow DCs to switch from an immature to a mature, inflammatory phenotype. Mature DCs upregulate the expression of costimulatory molecules, such as B7-1 and B7-2, and of the CCR7 chemokine

indicating that chemokine receptor homo- and heterodimers have distinctive signaling and biological properties. Interestingly, while CXCR4 is constitutively expressed in T cells, CCR5 expression is induced by antigenic or inflammatory stimuli. Thus, the context in which T cells are activated will determine the chemokine receptor expression pattern and their costimulatory functions.

4 Coinhibitory Receptors

Regulation of T cell responses requires a stringent control of the turn-on and turn off mechanisms. Negative signals delivered at the immunological synapse by the inhibitory receptors may be important for limiting the size and duration of immune responses and, thus, for maintaining the equilibrium between health and disease. Interestingly, the two CD28 ligands, B7-1 and B7-2, which are crucial for initiating T cell responses, are required to deliver negative signals to T cells and turn them off. The CTLA-4 (cytotoxic T lymphocyte antigen-4) coinhibitory molecule belongs to the CD28:B7 immunoglobulin superfamily and binds to B7-1 and B7-2 with higher affinity than does CD28 (Brunet et al. 1987; Linsley et al. 1991; Collins et al. 2002; Peggs et al. 2008). However, CD28 is constitutively expressed by resting T cells, whereas CTLA-4 expression requires TCR triggering (Perkins et al. 1996), indicating that the two molecules are involved in temporally distinct process of T cell activation. In agreement with this notion, CTLA-4 knockout mice die of polyclonal CD4$^+$ T cell lymphoproliferation (Tivol et al. 1995; Waterhouse et al. 1995), which seems to be initiated by TCR signaling (Waterhouse et al. 1997) and requires CD28 co stimulation (Linsley et al. 1991).

CTLA-4 coligation with the TCR results in reduced tyrosine phosphorylation of TCR signaling effectors (Guntermann and Alexander 2002), inhibition of extracellular signal-regulated kinase (ERK)/c-Jun N-terminal kinase pathways (Calvo et al. 1997), reduced NF-kB and AP-1 activation (Olsson et al. 1999) and inhibition of cell cycle progression, IL-2 secretion, and T cell proliferation (Krummel and Allison 1996). Competition with CD28 for its ligands and recruitment of the phosphatases Src homology 2 (SH2) domain-containing phosphatase-1 (SHP-1),

---

Fig. 1 (continued) receptor, which allows them to migrate into lymph nodes. T cells enter lymph nodes via high endothelial venules (HEVs) and actively scan DC's surface with their TCRs. TCR ligation by pMHC complexes expressed on DC leads to the formation of a stable T cell–DC conjugate and, at the immunological synapse, to the initiation of a complex signaling cross-talk. On the one hand, TCR triggering activates LFA-1 (inside-out signaling) and it may directly modify chemokine receptor signaling (G_i–G_q switch). On the other hand, CXCR4/CCR5 heterodimers and CD28 induce TCR costimulatory signals. In addition, chemokine receptor signaling at the immune synapse activates adhesion molecules, which are important to stabilize the conjugate and favor TCR ligation. All receptors induce massive rearrangements of the actin cytoskeleton at the immunological synapse, an event required to stabilize the T cell–DC pair. In addition, CD28. interaction with the actin-binding protein FLNa induces accumulation of membrane rafts at the synapse, a process that may be crucial to amplify TCR-induced signal transduction

SHP-2, and PP2A into the immune synapse are among the possible mechanisms responsible for CTLA-4 coinhibition (Teft et al. 2006). In addition, CTLA-4 may counteract TCR-induced stop signals and increase T cell motility (Schneider et al. 2006), thus reducing the stability of the T cell–APC conjugate.

Another negative regulator of the TCR signaling, belonging to the CD28:B7 immunoglobulin superfamily, is the PD-1 (programmed death-1) receptor, which is expressed on activated T cells, as well as B cells, monocytes, and natural killer T (NKT) cells (Peggs et al. 2008). PD-1 knockout mice develop antibody-mediated autoimmune diseases (Nishimura et al. 1999; Nishimura et al. 2001) and, accordingly, in T cells, PD-1 interaction with its ligands – PD-L1 and PD-L2 – results in recruitment of SHP-1 and SHP-2 and inhibition of proliferation and cytokine production (Keir et al. 2008). Interestingly, PD-L1, which is not only expressed on APCs but also on resting and activated T cells, can bind B7-1 (Butte et al. 2007) and act as a coinhibitory receptor in T cells in vitro and in vivo (Latchman et al. 2004).

5 Conclusions

The immunological synapse is an exquisite site for cross-talk among several signaling pathways. Adhesion molecules, chemokines, as well as costimulatory and coinhibitory receptors are all involved in the complex process of tuning TCR signaling and T cell activation thresholds. This is achieved through two major strategies: the control of the stability of the T cell–APC conjugate, and/or the generation around the TCR of a molecular environment that either amplifies or inhibits protein tyrosine phosphorylation (Fig. 2).

Although we can describe detailed signaling pathways for most of the single receptors acting at the immune synapse, we still do not know how these pathways are integrated during the various phases of T cell activation. An integrated view of

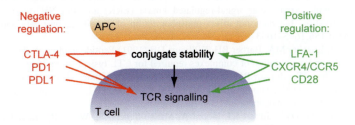

Fig. 2 Two strategies to tune T cell activation. Costimolatory and coinhibitory receptors may tune T cell activation acting at two different levels: conjugate stability or signal transduction. Adhesion molecules facilitate T cell activation by stabilizing T cell–APC interaction, whereas CD28 and PD1/PD1L tune the amplitude of TCR signaling. Interestingly, CTLA-4 and the CXCR4/CCR5 heterodimer operate at both levels, delivering signals that modify conjugate stability and T cell activation

the immunological synapse signaling would allow us to understand the contribution of each ligand–receptor pair to T cell dysfunctions in pathology and to design novel immunotherapeutic strategies.

Acknowledgments A.V. is supported by the Italian Association for Cancer Research (AIRC); Telethon; Ministero dell'Università e della Ricerca (MIUR); Istituto Superiore di Sanità; Alleanza Contro il Cancro; the DoD Army Medical Research, USA; the Cancer Research Institute of New York; the EMBO Young Investigator Program; E-rare 2007; EC FP7 HEALTH-F4-2008-201106.

References

Acuto O, Michel F (2003) CD28-mediated co-stimulation: a quantitative support for TCR signalling. Nat Rev Immunol 3:939–951

Acuto O, Bartolo VD, Michel F (2008) Tailoring T-cell receptor signals by proximal negative feedback mechanisms. Nat Rev Immunol 8:699–712

Akira S, Uematsu S, Takeuchi O (2006) Pathogen recognition and innate immunity. Cell 124:783–801

Alegre ML, Frauwirth KA, Thompson CB (2001) T-cell regulation by CD28 and CTLA-4. Nat Rev Immunol 1:220–228

Bachmann MF, McKall-Faienza K, Schmits R, Bouchard D, Beach J, Speiser DE, Mak TW, Ohashi PS (1997) Distinct roles for LFA-1 and CD28 during activation of naive T cells: adhesion versus costimulation. Immunity 7:549–557

Balamuth F, Leitenberg D, Unternaehrer J, Mellman I, Bottomly K (2001) Distinct patterns of membrane microdomain partitioning in Th1 and th2 cells. Immunity 15:729–738

Blanco P, Palucka AK, Pascual V, Banchereau J (2008) Dendritic cells and cytokines in human inflammatory and autoimmune diseases. Cytokine Growth Factor Rev 19:41–52

Boss V, Talpade DJ, Murphy TJ (1996) Induction of NFAT-mediated transcription by Gq-coupled receptors in lymphoid and non-lymphoid cells. J Biol Chem 271:10429–10432

Brunet JF, Denizot F, Luciani MF, Roux-Dosseto M, Suzan M, Mattei MG, Golstein P (1987) A new member of the immunoglobulin superfamily – CTLA-4. Nature 328:267–270

Butte MJ, Keir ME, Phamduy TB, Sharpe AH, Freeman GJ (2007) Programmed death-1 ligand 1 interacts specifically with the B7-1 costimulatory molecule to inhibit T cell responses. Immunity 27:111–122

Calvo CR, Amsen D, Kruisbeek AM (1997) Cytotoxic T lymphocyte antigen 4 (CTLA-4) interferes with extracellular signal-regulated kinase (ERK) and Jun NH2-terminal kinase (JNK) activation, but does not affect phosphorylation of T cell receptor zeta and ZAP70. J Exp Med 186:1645–1653

Christinck ER, Luscher MA, Barber BH, Williams DB (1991) Peptide binding to class I MHC on living cells and quantitation of complexes required for CTL lysis. Nature 352:67–70

Chuang E, Fisher TS, Morgan RW, Robbins MD, Duerr JM, Vander Heiden MG, Gardner JP, Hambor JE, Neveu MJ, Thompson CB (2000) The CD28 and CTLA-4 receptors associate with the serine/threonine phosphatase PP2A. Immunity 13:313–322

Collins AV, Brodie DW, Gilbert RJ, Iaboni A, Manso-Sancho R, Walse B, Stuart DI, van der Merwe PA, Davis SJ (2002) The interaction properties of costimulatory molecules revisited. Immunity 17:201–210

Constantin G, Majeed M, Giagulli C, Piccio L, Kim JY, Butcher EC, Laudanna C (2000) Chemokines trigger immediate beta2 integrin affinity and mobility changes: differential regulation and roles in lymphocyte arrest under flow. Immunity 13:759–769

Contento RL, Molon B, Boularan C, Pozzan T, Manes S, Marullo S, Viola A (2008) CXCR4-CCR5: a couple modulating T cell functions. Proc Natl Acad Sci USA 105:10101–10106

Davis MM, Boniface JJ, Reich Z, Lyons D, Hampl J, Arden B, Chien Y (1998) Ligand recognition by alpha beta T cell receptors. Annu Rev Immunol 16:523–544

Dupre L, Aiuti A, Trifari S, Martino S, Saracco P, Bordignon C, Roncarolo MG (2002) Wiskott-Aldrich syndrome protein regulates lipid raft dynamics during immunological synapse formation. Immunity 17:157–166

Dustin ML, Springer TA (1989) T-cell receptor cross-linking transiently stimulates adhesiveness through LFA-1. Nature 341:619–624

Ebert PJ, Baker JF, Punt JA (2000) Immature CD4+CD8+ thymocytes do not polarize lipid rafts in response to TCR-mediated signals. J Immunol 165:5435–5442

Flanagan LA, Chou J, Falet H, Neujahr R, Hartwig JH, Stossel TP (2001) Filamin A, the Arp2/3 complex, and the morphology and function of cortical actin filaments in human melanoma cells. J Cell Biol 155:511–517

Freeman GJ, Gribben JG, Boussiotis VA, Ng JW, Restivo VA Jr, Lombard LA, Gray GS, Nadler LM (1993) Cloning of B7-2: a CTLA-4 counter-receptor that costimulates human T cell proliferation. Science 262:909–911

Goldman DW, Chang FH, Gifford LA, Goetzl EJ, Bourne HR (1985) Pertussis toxin inhibition of chemotactic factor-induced calcium mobilization and function in human polymorphonuclear leukocytes. J Exp Med 162:145–156

Gomez-Mouton C, Lacalle RA, Mira E, Jimenez-Baranda S, Barber DF, Carrera AC, Martinez AC, Manes S (2004) Dynamic redistribution of raft domains as an organizing platform for signaling during cell chemotaxis. J Cell Biol 164:759–768

Guntermann C, Alexander DR (2002) CTLA-4 suppresses proximal TCR signaling in resting human CD4(+) T cells by inhibiting ZAP-70 Tyr(319) phosphorylation: a potential role for tyrosine phosphatases. J Immunol 168:4420–4429

Harada Y, Ohgai D, Watanabe R, Okano K, Koiwai O, Tanabe K, Toma H, Altman A, Abe R (2003) A single amino acid alteration in cytoplasmic domain determines IL-2 promoter activation by ligation of CD28 but not inducible costimulator (ICOS). J Exp Med 197:257–262

Harding CV, Unanue ER (1990) Quantitation of antigen-presenting cell MHC class II/peptide complexes necessary for T-cell stimulation. Nature 346:574–576

Hathcock KS, Laszlo G, Pucillo C, Linsley P, Hodes RJ (1994) Comparative analysis of B7-1 and B7-2 costimulatory ligands: expression and function. J Exp Med 180:631–640

Hayashi K, Altman A (2006) Filamin A is required for T cell activation mediated by protein kinase C-theta. J Immunol 177:1721–1728

Holdorf AD, Green JM, Levin SD, Denny MF, Straus DB, Link V, Changelian PS, Allen PM, Shaw AS (1999) Proline residues in CD28 and the Src homology (SH)3 domain of Lck are required for T cell costimulation. J Exp Med 190:375–384

Iezzi G, Karjalainen K, Lanzavecchia A (1998) The duration of antigenic stimulation determines the fate of naive and effector T cells. Immunity 8:89–95

Irvine DJ, Purbhoo MA, Krogsgaard M, Davis MM (2002) Direct observation of ligand recognition by T cells. Nature 419:845–849

Janeway CA Jr, Yagi J, Conrad PJ, Katz ME, Jones B, Vroegop S, Buxser S (1989) T-cell responses to Mls and to bacterial proteins that mimic its behavior. Immunol Rev 107:61–88

Jimenez-Baranda S, Gomez-Mouton C, Rojas A, Martinez-Prats L, Mira E, Ana Lacalle R, Valencia A, Dimitrov DS, Viola A, Delgado R, Martinez AC, Manes S (2007) Filamin-A regulates actin-dependent clustering of HIV receptors. Nat Cell Biol 9:838–846

Kane LP, Andres PG, Howland KC, Abbas AK, Weiss A (2001) Akt provides the CD28 costimulatory signal for up-regulation of IL-2 and IFN-gamma but not TH2 cytokines. Nat Immunol 2:37–44

Karpus WJ, Lukacs NW, Kennedy KJ, Smith WS, Hurst SD, Barrett TA (1997) Differential CC chemokine-induced enhancement of T helper cell cytokine production. J Immunol 158:4129–4136

Keir ME, Butte MJ, Freeman GJ, Sharpe AH (2008) PD-1 and its ligands in tolerance and immunity. Annu Rev Immunol 26:677–704

Kovacs B, Maus MV, Riley JL, Derimanov GS, Koretzky GA, June CH, Finkel TH (2002) Human CD8+ T cells do not require the polarization of lipid rafts for activation and proliferation. Proc Natl Acad Sci USA 99:15006–15011

Krummel MF, Allison JP (1996) CTLA-4 engagement inhibits IL-2 accumulation and cell cycle progression upon activation of resting T cells. J Exp Med 183:2533–2540

Kundig TM, Shahinian A, Kawai K, Mittrucker HW, Sebzda E, Bachmann MF, Mak TW, Ohashi PS (1996) Duration of TCR stimulation determines costimulatory requirement of T cells. Immunity 5:41–52

Lanzavecchia A, Lezzi G, Viola A (1999) From TCR engagement to T cell activation: a kinetic view of T cell behavior. Cell 96:1–4

Latchman YE, Liang SC, Wu Y, Chernova T, Sobel RA, Klemm M, Kuchroo VK, Freeman GJ, Sharpe AH (2004) PD-L1-deficient mice show that PD-L1 on T cells, antigen-presenting cells, and host tissues negatively regulates T cells. Proc Natl Acad Sci USA 101:10691–10696

Linsley PS, Brady W, Urnes M, Grosmaire LS, Damle NK, Ledbetter JA (1991) CTLA-4 is a second receptor for the B cell activation antigen B7. J Exp Med 174:561–569

Liu Y, Witte S, Liu YC, Doyle M, Elly C, Altman A (2000) Regulation of protein kinase Ctheta function during T cell activation by Lck-mediated tyrosine phosphorylation. J Biol Chem 275:3603–3609

Medzhitov R, Janeway CA Jr (2002) Decoding the patterns of self and nonself by the innate immune system. Science 296:298–300

Molon B, Gri G, Bettella M, Gomez-Mouton C, Lanzavecchia A, Martinez AC, Manes S, Viola A (2005) T cell costimulation by chemokine receptors. Nat Immunol 6:465–471

Nishimura H, Nose M, Hiai H, Minato N, Honjo T (1999) Development of lupus-like autoimmune diseases by disruption of the PD-1 gene encoding an ITIM motif-carrying immunoreceptor. Immunity 11:141–151

Nishimura H, Okazaki T, Tanaka Y, Nakatani K, Hara M, Matsumori A, Sasayama S, Mizoguchi A, Hiai H, Minato N, Honjo T (2001) Autoimmune dilated cardiomyopathy in PD-1 receptor-deficient mice. Science 291:319–322

Olsson C, Riesbeck K, Dohlsten M, Michaelsson E (1999) CTLA-4 ligation suppresses CD28-induced NF-kappaB and AP-1 activity in mouse T cell blasts. J Biol Chem 274:14400–14405

Paccani SR, Boncristiano M, Patrussi L, Ulivieri C, Wack A, Valensin S, Hirst TR, Amedei A, Del Prete G, Telford JL, D'Elios MM, Baldari CT (2005) Defective Vav expression and impaired F-actin reorganization in a subset of patients with common variable immunodeficiency characterized by T-cell defects. Blood 106:626–634

Pages F, Ragueneau M, Rottapel R, Truneh A, Nunes J, Imbert J, Olive D (1994) Binding of phosphatidylinositol-3-OH kinase to CD28 is required for T-cell signalling. Nature 369:327–329

Park JH, Kim YG, Shaw M, Kanneganti TD, Fujimoto Y, Fukase K, Inohara N, Nunez G (2007) Nod1/RICK and TLR signaling regulate chemokine and antimicrobial innate immune responses in mesothelial cells. J Immunol 179:514–521

Peggs KS, Quezada SA, Allison JP (2008) Cell intrinsic mechanisms of T-cell inhibition and application to cancer therapy. Immunol Rev 224:141–165

Perkins D, Wang Z, Donovan C, He H, Mark D, Guan G, Wang Y, Walunas T, Bluestone J, Listman J, Finn PW (1996) Regulation of CTLA-4 expression during T cell activation. J Immunol 156:4154–4159

Pizzo P, Viola A (2004) Lipid rafts in lymphocyte activation. Microbes Infect 6:686–692

Raab M, Cai YC, Bunnell SC, Heyeck SD, Berg LJ, Rudd CE (1995) p56Lck and p59Fyn regulate CD28 binding to phosphatidylinositol 3-kinase, growth factor receptor-bound protein GRB-2, and T cell-specific protein-tyrosine kinase ITK: implications for T-cell costimulation. Proc Natl Acad Sci USA 92:8891–8895

Round JL, Tomassian T, Zhang M, Patel V, Schoenberger SP, Miceli MC (2005) Dlgh1 coordinates actin polymerization, synaptic T cell receptor and lipid raft aggregation, and effector function in T cells. J Exp Med 201:419–430

Schneider H, Downey J, Smith A, Zinselmeyer BH, Rush C, Brewer JM, Wei B, Hogg N, Garside P, Rudd CE (2006) Reversal of the TCR stop signal by CTLA-4. Science 313:1972–1975

Schuck S, Simons K (2004) Polarized sorting in epithelial cells: raft clustering and the biogenesis of the apical membrane. J Cell Sci 117:5955–5964

Serbina NV, Jia T, Hohl TM, Pamer EG (2008) Monocyte-mediated defense against microbial pathogens. Annu Rev Immunol 26:421–452

Shahinian A, Pfeffer K, Lee KP, Kundig TM, Kishihara K, Wakeham A, Kawai K, Ohashi PS, Thompson CB, Mak TW (1993) Differential T cell costimulatory requirements in CD28-deficient mice. Science 261:609–612

Shamri R, Grabovsky V, Gauguet JM, Feigelson S, Manevich E, Kolanus W, Robinson MK, Staunton DE, von Andrian UH, Alon R (2005) Lymphocyte arrest requires instantaneous induction of an extended LFA-1 conformation mediated by endothelium-bound chemokines. Nat Immunol 6:497–506

Stossel TP, Condeelis J, Cooley L, Hartwig JH, Noegel A, Schleicher M, Shapiro SS (2001) Filamins as integrators of cell mechanics and signalling. Nat Rev Mol Cell Biol 2:138–145

Su B, Jacinto E, Hibi M, Kallunki T, Karin M, Ben-Neriah Y (1994) JNK is involved in signal integration during costimulation of T lymphocytes. Cell 77:727–736

Sykulev Y, Joo M, Vturina I, Tsomides TJ, Eisen HN (1996) Evidence that a single peptide-MHC complex on a target cell can elicit a cytolytic T cell response. Immunity 4:565–571

Taub DD (1996) Chemokine-leukocyte interactions. The voodoo that they do so well. Cytokine Growth Factor Rev 7:355–376

Tavano R, Gri G, Molon B, Marinari B, Rudd CE, Tuosto L, Viola A (2004) CD28 and lipid rafts coordinate recruitment of Lck to the immunological synapse of human T lymphocytes. J Immunol 173:5392–5397

Tavano R, Contento RL, Baranda SJ, Soligo M, Tuosto L, Manes S, Viola A (2006) CD28 interaction with filamin-A controls lipid raft accumulation at the T-cell immunological synapse. Nat Cell Biol 8:1270–1276

Teft WA, Kirchhof MG, Madrenas J (2006) A molecular perspective of CTLA-4 function. Annu Rev Immunol 24:65–97

Thelen M, Stein JV (2008) How chemokines invite leukocytes to dance. Nat Immunol 9:953–959

Tivol EA, Borriello F, Schweitzer AN, Lynch WP, Bluestone JA, Sharpe AH (1995) Loss of CTLA-4 leads to massive lymphoproliferation and fatal multiorgan tissue destruction, revealing a critical negative regulatory role of CTLA-4. Immunity 3:541–547

Tuosto L, Acuto O (1998) CD28 affects the earliest signaling events generated by TCR engagement. Eur J Immunol 28:2131–2142

Tybulewicz VL (2002) Chemokines and the immunological synapse. Immunology 106:287–288

van Vliet SJ, den Dunnen J, Gringhuis SI, Geijtenbeek TB, van Kooyk Y (2007) Innate signaling and regulation of Dendritic cell immunity. Curr Opin Immunol 19:435–440

Villalba M, Coudronniere N, Deckert M, Teixeiro E, Mas P, Altman A (2000) A novel functional interaction between Vav and PKCtheta is required for TCR-induced T cell activation. Immunity 12:151–160

Viola A (2001) The amplification of TCR signaling by dynamic membrane microdomains. Trends Immunol 22:322–327

Viola A, Lanzavecchia A (1996) T cell activation determined by T cell receptor number and tunable thresholds. Science 273:104–106

Viola A, Schroeder S, Sakakibara Y, Lanzavecchia A (1999) T lymphocyte costimulation mediated by reorganization of membrane microdomains. Science 283:680–682

Watanabe R, Harada Y, Takeda K, Takahashi J, Ohnuki K, Ogawa S, Ohgai D, Kaibara N, Koiwai O, Tanabe K, Toma H, Sugamura K, Abe R (2006) Grb2 and Gads exhibit different interactions with CD28 and play distinct roles in CD28-mediated costimulation. J Immunol 177:1085–1091

Waterhouse P, Penninger JM, Timms E, Wakeham A, Shahinian A, Lee KP, Thompson CB, Griesser H, Mak TW (1995) Lymphoproliferative disorders with early lethality in mice deficient in Ctla-4. Science 270:985–988

Waterhouse P, Bachmann MF, Penninger JM, Ohashi PS, Mak TW (1997) Normal thymic
    selection, normal viability and decreased lymphoproliferation in T cell receptor-transgenic
    CTLA-4-deficient mice. Eur J Immunol 27:1887–1892
Werts C, le Bourhis L, Liu J, Magalhaes JG, Carneiro LA, Fritz JH, Stockinger S, Balloy V,
    Chignard M, Decker T, Philpott DJ, Ma X, Girardin SE (2007) Nod1 and Nod2 induce CCL5/
    RANTES through the NF-kappaB pathway. Eur J Immunol 37:2499–2508
Yokosuka T, Kobayashi W, Sakata-Sogawa K, Takamatsu M, Hashimoto-Tane A, Dustin ML,
    Tokunaga M, Saito T (2008) Spatiotemporal regulation of T cell costimulation by TCR-CD28
    microclusters and protein kinase C theta translocation. Immunity 29:589–601

Multiple Microclusters: Diverse Compartments Within the Immune Synapse

Stephen C. Bunnell

Contents

S.C. Bunnell
Department of Pathology, Tufts University Medical School, Jaharis Bldg., Rm. 512, 150 Harrison
Ave., Boston, MA 02111, USA
e-mail: Stephen.Bunnell@tufts.edu

T. Saito and F.D. Batista (eds.), *Immunological Synapse*,   123
Current Topics in Microbiology and Immunology 340,
DOI 10.1007/978-3-642-03858-7_7, © Springer-Verlag Berlin Heidelberg 2010

Abstract The activation of classical αβ T cells is initiated when the T cell receptor (TCR) recognizes peptide antigens presented by major histocompatibility complex (pMHC) molecules. This recognition always occurs at the junction of a T cell and antigen-presenting cell (APC). Existing models of T cell activation accurately explain the sensitivity and selectivity of antigen recognition within the immunological synapse. However, these models have not fully incorporated the diverse microcluster types revealed by current imaging technologies. It is increasingly clear that a better understanding of T cell activation will require an appreciation of the diverse signaling assemblies arising within the immune synapse, the interrelationships between these structures, and the mechanisms by which underlying cytoskeletal systems govern their assembly and fate. Here, we will provide a brief framework for understanding these issues, review our contributions to current knowledge, and provide perspectives on the future of this rapidly advancing field.

1 Challenges in Antigen Recognition

The adaptive immune system plays an essential role in the defense against pathogenic microorganisms. Randomly assembled clonotypic receptors allow lymphocytes to recognize a nearly unlimited repertoire of antigens. In most vertebrates, T lymphocytes recognize foreign and self-derived antigens that are presented by endogenous major histocompatibility complex (MHC) proteins. This ability, coupled with developmental pruning of the initial T cell receptor (TCR) repertoire, enables T cells to distinguish self from non-self. This capacity allows T cells to play a crucial role in the orchestration of effective immune responses.

The properties of the TCR are constrained by the need to meet two conflicting imperatives. On the one hand, T cells must rapidly identify and respond to pathogenic organisms in order to prevent life-threatening infections. On the other hand, T cells must be finely tuned to prevent spontaneous self-recognition and the initiation of autoimmune responses. These pressures have resulted in the development of systems that ensure encounters between rare T cells and antigen-bearing antigen-presenting cells (APCs) and enable the recognition of low doses of antigens with exquisite fidelity. The recognition of antigens by the rare T cells bearing cognate TCRs is facilitated by the coordinated recruitment of T cells and APCs to secondary lymphoid organs. Once present in these organs, T cells migrate rapidly across stromal cell networks (Bajenoff et al. 2006). Current estimates suggest that this rapid scanning allows a single antigen-bearing APC to be tested by 500–5,000 T cells/h (Breart and Bousso 2006). Recent estimates suggest that the frequency of T cells capable of recognizing a given antigen is approximately 1 in 300,000 (Moon et al. 2007). Given these parameters, T cells of the appropriate specificity will come into contact with antigen-bearing APCs within the first hours to days of an infection. To effectively initiate successful immune responses, these potential recognition events must be efficiently converted into productive signals, while hundreds of thousands of irrelevant interactions must fail. This sensitivity and specificity is achieved through the formation of a specialized junction linking the T cell and APC, known as an immunological synapse. Both systems require the dynamic modulation of the T cell cytoskeleton. In the first case, these changes enable circulating T cells to be recruited into lymphoid organs and to be converted into polarized T cells capable of rapid migration. In the second case, these changes enable T cells that engage antigen to stop migrating and to form the synaptic structures that support optimal antigen recognition.

2   T Cell Migration and Synapsis

Circulating T cells are roughly spherical and are densely coated with microvilli. These narrow membrane extensions contain bundled actin filaments and possess a distinct tip structure. Microvilli contribute to the entry of circulating T cells into secondary lymphoid organs by facilitating T cell rolling on high endothelial venules (HEVs). Rolling is initiated when proteins enriched at the tips of microvilli engage ligands expressed on the vascular endothelial cells that comprise the HEV wall (Springer 1994). These interactions, coupled with the shear forces exerted by fluid flow within the HEV, cause T cells to roll along the surface of the HEV. Leukocyte rolling is an active process in which microvilli function as springs and tethers to resist the intense shear forces encountered at the vascular wall (Park et al. 2002; Snapp et al. 2002). This requires the coupling of the integrins and selectin ligands of the microvillus tip to underlying actin filaments and the capacity of underlying actin filaments to lengthen and develop tension in response to mechanical strain. These processes slow the rolling T cells, facilitating encounters with chemokines immobilized on the vessel wall. Chemokine receptors then trigger cytoplasmic signaling cascades which upregulate integrin affinity and avidity and promote T cell spreading on the vascular wall. This response requires the modification of rigid intermediate filament networks composed of vimentin and the remodeling of cortical actin networks stabilized by the ezrin/radixin/moesin (ERM) family of cytoskeletal adaptors (Brown et al. 2001; Shaw 2001; Nijhara et al. 2004). Subsequently, T cells exit the vascular space and enter the surrounding tissue. This process is initiated with the formation of integrin-dependent adhesive structures known as podosomes. Recent studies have demonstrated that T cells can pass directly through endothelial cells in a process known as transcellular diapedesis (Petri and Bixel 2006; Carman et al. 2007). This process is associated with the maturation of the pro-adhesive podosomes into invasive structures resembling the lamina-penetrating invadopodia of cancer cells.

T cells that have escaped circulation and entered secondary lymphoid organs are exposed to chemokines, which direct T cell polarization and the initiation of rapid amoeboid movement. These processes require the formation of domains with distinct cytoskeletal properties (Dustin 2008). The leading edge of the cell is composed of exploratory actin-rich structures that are driven forward by the dynamic polymerization of actin. At least two distinct structures are observed in this region: thin filopodia, which contain bundled actin filaments, and sheet-like lamellipodia, which contain branched actin filaments. At the base of the leading edge is the lamellum, which generates integrin-dependent adhesive contacts required for efficient locomotion (Ponti et al. 2004). The rear of the cell contains the microtubule-organizing center (MTOC) and is drawn into a tail-like structure referred to as a uropod (Sanchez-Madrid and Serrador 2009). This trailing structure is assembled through the action of myosin II and is the primary site of membrane internalization in crawling cells (Jacobelli et al. 2004; Samaniego et al. 2007). The uropod is also enriched in moesin, the ERM-interacting membrane glycoproteins CD43 and CD44, and the polarity-regulating proteins Dlg and Scribble (del Pozo et al. 1998; Ludford-Menting et al. 2005). Collectively, these systems define an axis of polarity compatible with directed migration. Movement is accomplished through the generation of adhesive contact at the leading edge, the application of myosin II-dependent forces, and the detachment of adhesive structures at the rear of the cell (Morin et al. 2008).

In response to antigen, T cells stop crawling and form an immunological synapse. Stopping is accompanied by the reorientation of the protrusive and adhesive systems of crawling T cells, so that movements parallel to the migration substrate are redirected toward the stimulatory surface (Krummel and Macara 2006; Dustin 2008). Since the APC presents a barrier to movement, these systems are redirected outward, along the surface of the APC. In this manner, the front-to-rear axis characteristic of migrating T cells is converted into the symmetric edge-to-center axis characteristic of the immune synapse. Thus, actin-rich regions at the boundary of the synapse correspond to the leading edge and lamellum found in migratory T cells. Similarly, the center of the synapse, which excludes integrins and recruits the MTOC, corresponds to the rear of a crawling T cell. In addition, myosin II-dependent cytoskeletal flows are reoriented so as to transport material from the rear of the cell toward the synapse, and from the edge of the synapse toward the center of the synapse (Wulfing and Davis 1998; Ilani et al. 2009). However, other components of the uropod, including moesin, CD43, CD44, Dlg, and Scribble, are retained at the rear of the cell, within a "distal pole complex" (DPC) opposite the contact interface (Cullinan et al. 2002; Ludford-Menting et al. 2005). Thus, T cells participating in immune synapses retain a front-to-back axis defined by ERM-interacting proteins and polarity proteins, but extensively modify a distinct axis orchestrating MTOC positioning, myosin II-dependent membrane flows, and integrin-dependent locomotion.

The stopping behavior associated with the formation of an immune synapse allows T cells to ignore the abundant extraneous stimuli provided by the majority of the APC present in secondary lymphoid organs. In addition, T cell stopping facilitates the identification of additional cognate pMHC, which may be diluted several thousandfold among irrelevant pMHC (Valitutti et al. 1995). Although the sustained delivery of antigen-dependent signals is essential for optimal T cell proliferation, the signals transmitted during this period do not require sustained monogamous interactions between T cells and APCs (Huppa et al. 2003; Friedl et al. 2005; Henrickson et al. 2008). In fact, T cells activated and observed in vivo, within intact lymphoid organs, initially alternate between periods of mobility and conjugate formation. These interactions result in the upregulation of numerous activation markers, demonstrating that T cells are capable of integrating signals that are distributed in space and time. During this migratory phase, signals initiated by the TCR suppress the dissolution of synapses; nevertheless, the boundaries of the immune synapse remain dynamic and permit T cell reorientation toward APCs bearing higher doses of antigen (Negulescu et al. 1996; Depoil et al. 2005). These properties are well suited for the recognition of rare and widely dispersed antigens, and for the identification of the most potent APC within the local microenvironment.

3   Models of Antigen Recognition

T cell activation is associated with the downmodulation of several thousand TCR molecules by much smaller numbers of cognate pMHC (Valitutti et al. 1995). The *serial triggering* hypothesis proposes that this is achieved through the serial recognition of an individual pMHC by tens to hundreds of TCR molecules. In this model, the immune synapse anchors the responding T cell to an APC, facilitating efficient serial recognition of pMHC. However, the demand for efficient serial recognition is at odds with the *kinetic proofreading* hypothesis (McKeithan 1995). This model predicts that the correlation between pMHC half-life and antigenicity is a direct result of the time required to assemble a potent signaling complex at the TCR. The opposing demands of these hypotheses explain the observation that efficient T cell activation occurs only within a narrow range of pMHC half-lives (Davis et al. 1998).

The relatively short half-lives of agonist pMHC inevitably impact the affinity of interaction with the TCR. In addition, the unusual nature of the TCR–pMHC interaction limits the surface available for the selective recognition of distinct antigenic peptides. Given these constraints, how is selective antigen recognition achieved? *Topological* models of T-cell activation posit that the immune synapse generates domains of membrane apposition that are dominated by a distinct parameter, known as the two-dimensional affinity (Shaw and Dustin 1997). This parameter becomes progressively more important as the separation of the membranes decreases and as the rigidity of the confining membranes increases. The TCR and pMHC are ideally suited to this mode of interaction in that they are short, jointly spanning only 13 nm, their interacting surfaces face directly outwards, and their interaction is not thought to involve major structural rearrangements in the direction of confinement (Kuhns et al. 2006). Although the TCR–pMHC pair is dwarfed by the abundant glycoproteins CD43 and CD45, the repulsive interactions mediated by these proteins are expected to be overcome by the pro-adhesive functions of integrins, such as LFA-1 (Springer 1990). Because the distance spanned by LFA-1 and ICAM-1 is large, and because cognate pMHC are rare, abundant accessory molecules, such as CD2, are predicted to enforce rigid membrane separations compatible with TCR engagement (Dustin et al. 1996a). Junctions with these properties could reduce the steric barriers to pMHC recognition, facilitate encounters between the TCR and pMHC, and appropriately orient the TCR and pMHC with respect to one another. Furthermore, these tightly apposed membrane domains could exclude the large tyrosine phosphatases CD45 and CD148, thereby creating permissive domains for signal initiation by the TCR.

4 The Structure of the Immune Synapse

In the late 1990s, the Kupfer laboratory revealed the first detailed views of the immune synapses formed between CD4+ T cells and antigen-presenting B cells (Monks et al. 1997). *En face* views of these synapses, generated using optical deconvolution and digital reconstruction techniques, revealed distinct concentric domains (Monks et al. 1998; Freiberg et al. 2002). These domains are commonly referred to as supramolecular activation complexes (SMACs). The formation of a compact cluster rich in the TCR was predictive of T-cell activation, and could be induced only by agonist peptides (Monks et al. 1998). This central SMAC (cSMAC) was also enriched in PKCθ and marked the site of MTOC recruitment (Monks et al. 1997). A pro-adhesive domain enriched in LFA-1 and Talin was observed in response to either antagonist or agonist peptides; this domain typically surrounded the cSMAC, and was therefore denoted the peripheral SMAC (pSMAC). The distal SMAC (dSMAC), found at the boundary of the synapse, was initially defined as a domain containing CD45, which was largely absent from the cSMAC and pSMAC. However, CD45 is not significantly enriched in the dSMAC, and is found at comparable levels on all surfaces outside of the immune synapse (Johnson et al. 2000; Leupin et al. 2000; Freiberg et al. 2002). More recently, the dSMAC has been redefined as an actin-rich region containing circumferential lamellipodia (Varma et al. 2006; Dustin 2008). As discussed above, a fourth domain, known as the DPC, is found outside of the contact, at the opposite pole of the T cell (Cullinan et al. 2002; Ludford-Menting et al. 2005).

Within 1 year of the initial description of the cSMAC, the Dustin laboratory provided the first insights into the dynamic evolution of the immune synapse (Grakoui et al. 1999). In these studies, the APC was replaced by supported lipid bilayers bearing laterally mobile and fluorescently tagged ligands. In this manner, Dustin's group was able to dynamically visualize changes in the distributions of the TCR and the LFA-1 during the maturation of an immune synapse. The TCR was initially enriched in a thin ring at the boundary of the contact, outside of a central domain containing LFA-1. This pattern gradually inverted as the TCR was drawn into the center of the contact, creating patterns analogous to the cSMAC and pSMAC observed in conjugates. Consistent with these previous studies, the ability to form a central TCR cluster was strictly dependent on ligand quality. These studies also established that the assembly of a cSMAC was rigorously correlated with the half-life of the pMHC and was predictive of T-cell proliferation. Collectively, these discoveries provided direct support for the topological and kinetic proofreading models of T-cell activation. Perhaps more profoundly, these studies emphasized the crucial roles played by dynamic spatial rearrangements within the immune synapse and spurred the application of dynamic imaging techniques to the study of immune signaling.

Although these observations suggested that the cSMAC played a fundamental role in T cell activation, this hypothesis was dealt a blow by the discovery of multifocal immune synapses. These immune synapses exhibit multiple TCR clusters, which are small, are distributed throughout the contact, and persist without being consolidated into a central structure (Krummel and Davis 2002). In part, this distinction appears to be determined by intrinsic qualities of the T cell and APC. Compact central clusters analogous to those observed in the synapses formed by naive CD4$^+$ T cells and B cells were also reported in the synapses formed by Th1-polarized CD4$^+$ T cells and the cytotoxic synapses generated by naive CD8$^+$ T cells (Balamuth et al. 2001; Potter et al. 2001; Stinchcombe et al. 2001; Thauland et al. 2008). In contrast, multifocal synapses were identified in the synapses formed by thymocytes and Th2 polarized CD4$^+$ T cells, and in the synapses formed by naive T cells and dendritic cells (Balamuth et al. 2001; Hailman et al. 2002; Brossard et al. 2005; Dustin et al. 2006; Thauland et al. 2008). These cell types are all activated normally, indicating that the dispersed TCR clusters typical of multifocal synapses are competent to induce T cell activation.

5 Cytoskeletal Rearrangements Associated with Contact Formation

Although early descriptions of the immune synapse focused attention on the role of the cSMAC in T cell activation, this domain is not assembled quickly enough to participate in the rapid calcium responses triggered upon pMHC recognition. To clarify the topological context in which TCR engagement occurs, T cells were imaged using interference reflection microscopy (IRM), a technique that enables the visualization of cellular membranes apposed to the underlying substrate. These studies revealed that T cells migrating on lipid bilayers generate a striking arc of tight contact with the substrate at the tip of the leading edge (Dustin et al. 1996b). These leading contacts were separated from the cell body by a distinct gap, and were consistent with the extension of lamellipodia from the cell body toward the substrate. Since crawling T cells preferentially respond to APCs presented at the leading edge, TCR engagement was likely to be initiated within these small contacts (Negulescu et al. 1996). Calcium signals were subsequently observed following *de novo* TCR engagement in the periphery of a newly formed, expanding contact. However, these studies did not provide the temporal resolution required to separate contact initiation from its sequelae (Grakoui et al. 1999).

To understand the behavior of these early contact structures in greater detail, the Samelson laboratory dynamically visualized the synapses formed between Jurkat

T cells and coverslips bearing immobilized stimulatory antibodies specific for CD3ε (Bunnell et al. 2001). Using confocal IRM (cIRM), which is capable of resolving exceedingly small differences in membrane–substrate spacing, we were able to visualize the earliest contacts generated by protrusive structures (Bunnell et al. 2003). In the absence of a stimulatory ligand, this structure remained constant in size and drifted slowly across the substrate. In contrast, stimulatory surfaces triggered the expansion of the initial structure and the development of thin, arc-shaped contacts distal to the previous boundary of the synapse. This rapid change in morphology was completed within seconds, producing a poorly sealed synapse, characterized by dispersed contact points and large gaps. Thereafter, the expanding synapse exhibited increasing radial symmetry, which resulted from the cyclical formation of arc-shaped contacts at sites distal to the outermost existing contacts. This phase of synapse expansion was marked by the progressive sealing of the gaps between contact points, and culminated in 3–5 min with the formation of a tightly sealed contact bounded by a circumferential adhesive ring. This arrangement persisted for an additional 10–15 min, during which the adhesive ring thinned and then broke down. Thereafter, the T cells gradually rounded, yielding a smaller contact surrounded by retraction fibers extending to the previous boundary of the synapse. These studies clarified the topological details of synapse formation and established that dramatic changes in T-cell morphology could be initiated by TCRs engaged within individual contacts no larger than 400 nm in diameter.

Using a variety of fluorescent imaging techniques, we established that the rapid morphological changes observed in the early synapse involve the extensive remodeling of the actin cytoskeleton (Bunnell et al. 2001; Bunnell et al. 2002). By imaging T cells expressing a chimera of actin and enhanced green fluorescent protein (EGFP), we established that the first points of contact were generated by filopodia and lamellipodia. The initial contact triggered the extension of larger, sheet-like lamellipodia from the T cell body, confirming that the initial triggering of the TCR occurs within contact domains rich in filamentous actin. The tips of these newly generated lamellipodia formed new contacts distal to the initial point of contact, producing the gaps observed by IRM. These gaps were not evident by standard confocal microscopy, but typically spanned ~120 nm, a distance too great to support receptor–ligand interactions (Bunnell et al. 2003). As they extended, these early lamellipodia merged, generating a symmetric circumferential lamellipodium. Actin also accumulated at the base of these pioneering lamellipodia, in dense fibers that extended vertically from the substrate. Both structures advanced in lockstep, and were continuously remodeled as polymerized actin was cleared from the center of the contact. As with our IRM studies, these observations suggested that the growth of the synapse is sustained by self-reinforcing cycles of contact formation and lamellipodial extension at the boundary of the synapse. Within 3–5 min, the circumferential lamellipodium was reduced in size as the dense actin-rich region reached the advancing boundary of the synapse. This dense circumferential ring corresponded to the adhesive ring observed by IRM and persisted in place for an additional 10–15 min. During this period, small, transient lamellipodia extended from the perimeter of the synapse. These structures clearly displayed retrograde actin flows, which were directed toward the center of the synapse (Bunnell et al. 2001; Nguyen et al. 2008). These flows supported the hypothesis that the movement of actin could be harnessed to drive the centralization of activated TCRs (Grakoui et al. 1999).

The program of cyclical contact expansion described above proceeds similarly with little regard for the T cell type, the mechanism of TCR ligation, or the mobility of the TCR ligand. In all model systems, the earliest TCR engagement occurs in an exploratory actin-rich structure. Resting cells plated on coverslips contact the substrate via pre-existing protrusive structures resembling filopodia (Bunnell et al. 2001, 2002; Barda-Saad et al. 2005). In contrast, migrating T cells preferentially recognize antigen within the tight contacts generated by the leading edge (Grakoui et al. 1999). The first productive contact triggers a rapid burst of expansion that is similar in extent and duration whether the T cells are stimulated on coverslips, lipid bilayers, or antigen-bearing APC (Tskvitaria-Fuller et al. 2003; Varma et al. 2006; Kaizuka et al. 2007). This expansion involves the cyclical extension of symmetric lamellipodia and the formation of a lagging ring of actin-dense structures. The primary difference between these models only becomes apparent once the immune synapse reaches its maximum extent. During this phase, the synapses elicited by immobile ligands maintain peak spreading, whereas the synapses induced by laterally mobile ligands gradually contract, permitting a partial rounding of the responding T cell. This difference is likely to result from the tethering of the TCR to the actin cytoskeleton (Rozdzial et al. 1995, 1998). The resulting linkage may permit immobilized TCR to resist the centripetal forces generated by retrograde actin flows and by myosin-dependent motors (Bunnell et al. 2001; Kaizuka et al. 2007; Nguyen et al. 2008; Ilani et al. 2009).

6   The Regulation of Contact Formation and Persistence

The role of cytoplasmic calcium in the initiation and maintenance of the immune synapse remains controversial. Based on the properties of its effectors, calcium elevations are likely to antagonize cell migration by disrupting the cortical actin cytoskeleton and by downregulating integrin-dependent adhesive contacts (Gremm and Wegner 2000; Franco and Huttenlocher 2005). This hypothesis is consistent with the observation that cytoplasmic calcium elevations arrest the movements of migratory T cells (Negulescu et al. 1996). Calcium elevations also contribute to the maintenance of monogamous conjugates, perhaps by suppressing integrin-dependent movements away from the APC (Negulescu et al. 1996; Delon et al. 1998). However, in studies involving resting T cells plated on stimulatory coverslips, we observed that transient cytoplasmic calcium elevations are required for maximal T cell spreading (Bunnell et al. 2001). This observation can be reconciled with the more general role of calcium by considering the initial states of the responding T cells. In the first two cases, the T cells were polarized, and had already dedicated a large pool of actin to cell migration. In the latter case, the responding T cell was in a resting state. We propose that the transient calcium elevations initiated following contact contribute to the remodeling of static pools of actin, liberating the cytoskeletal components required for rapid contact expansion.

We demonstrated that lamellipodia formed at the boundary of the expanding contact function as exploratory structures that preferentially generate contacts via their tips (Bunnell et al. 2001). Recent studies have shown that the Arp2/3 complex, which governs actin branching, plays a major role in the extension of lamellipodia during contact expansion (Gomez et al. 2007). Several protein families position and activate Arp2/3 complexes, and each family gives rise to a distinct set of actin-rich structures (Billadeau et al. 2007). The Arp2/3-activating Abi/WAVE complexes are regulated by Rac-family GTPases and have been decisively implicated in the assembly of lamellipodia. In T cells, the disruption of these complexes abolishes the extension of lamellipodia in response to TCR ligation (Nolz et al. 2006; Zipfel et al. 2006). The consequences associated with this change are profound, and include reductions in the area of contact, the inhibition of integrin-mediated adhesion, and the suppression of signals initiated by the TCR. Intriguingly, the Abi/WAVE complex "surfs" along the tips of growing lamellipodia, maintaining the position required to sustain the expansion of these lamellipodia (Zipfel et al. 2006). This surfing behavior may explain the ability of the TCR to influence actin polymerization at distal sites. We propose that the defective extension of lamellipodia in LAT-deficient cells, which do not effectively activate Rac, is caused by defects in the activation of Abi/WAVE complexes (Bunnell et al. 2001; Ku et al. 2001).

During the expansion of the immune synapse, circumferential lamellipodia are continuously remodeled, giving rise to a dense ring of actin-rich structures that extend vertically from the contact surface (Bunnell et al. 2001). These structures are similar in appearance to the podosome belts observed in osteoclasts (Jurdic et al. 2006; Luxenburg et al. 2007). Podosomes, which are the primary constituents of these belts, are composed of bundled actin filaments that dynamically incorporate actin monomers near the plasma membrane, at the base of a vertical "pillar." Podosome formation requires a distinct Arp2/3 activator, the Wiskott–Aldrich Syndrome protein (WASP), which is preferentially activated by Cdc42 (Tomasevic et al. 2007; Calle et al. 2008). Both WASP and Cdc42 are recruited to the immune synapse and contribute to its stabilization (Cannon et al. 2001; Labno et al. 2003; Tskvitaria-Fuller et al. 2006). This stabilization is likely to be mediated by the formation of a circumferential belt of podosomes. Therefore, we propose that the instability of the immune synapses formed by LAT-deficient T cells is due, at least in part, to the inability of these cells to recruit and activate WASP (Bunnell et al. 2001; Barda-Saad et al. 2005).

Our studies also raised the possibility that LAT and PLCγ1 indirectly regulate the stability of the immune synapse by controlling the organization of the microtubule cytoskeleton. Consistent with this hypothesis, the recruitment of the MTOC to the center of the contact is dependent on ZAP-70 and the downstream adaptors LAT and SLP-76 (Kuhne et al. 2003). Subsequent studies have shown that the MTOC is dynamically repositioned toward sites of active TCR signaling (Depoil et al. 2005;

Huse et al. 2007). In fact, local increases in the abundance of diacylglycerol are sufficient to reposition the MTOC within existing synapses (Quann et al. 2009). Given the role of LAT in the activation of diacylglycerol production by PLCγ1, the failure to appropriately polarize the MTOC could also contribute to the early dissociation of the contacts formed by LAT-mutant cells (Bunnell et al. 2001).

7 Signal Initiation within the Earliest Contact

In our 2001 study, we established that synapse expansion was dependent on the transient elevation of intracellular calcium. This indicated that biochemical events downstream of the TCR must progress to the point of initiating a calcium flux before the dynamic expansion of the immune synapse could begin. Because a single sub-micrometer contact point was sufficient to initiate these dramatic morphological rearrangements, we reasoned that the entire TCR-proximal signaling apparatus must be recruited into the initial contact within the relatively short period of time between contact initiation and expansion. At the time, a series of dynamic studies employing either bilayers or conjugates had provided precedents for this view. These studies revealed that calcium elevations preceded the consolidation of the cSMAC, and occurred within 30–60 s of the formation of peripheral TCR clusters less than 1 μm in diameter (Grakoui et al. 1999; Johnson et al. 2000; Krummel et al. 2000).

8 The TCR Microcluster

In 2002, we demonstrated that immobilized antibodies trigger the recruitment of the TCR into well-defined "microclusters" ~500 nm in diameter (Bunnell et al. 2002). Notably, these structures were comparable in size to the filopodial contacts observed in our previous studies. Consistent with their predicted role in signal initiation, these TCR microclusters colocalized with ZAP-70 and were the primary sites of phosphotyrosine accumulation in the synapse. Using an EGFP chimera, we established that ZAP-70 microclusters were preferentially assembled at the expanding boundary of the synapse, in regions of tight contact with the substrate. However, the resulting ZAP-70 microclusters remained stationary, reflecting their interaction with the immobilized TCR. Crucially, the assembly of the TCR into microclusters was independent of Src-family tyrosine kinases; this property indicated that microclusters could precede the initiation of downstream signals by the TCR. In conjunction with concurrent studies employing T cell–APC conjugates, our observations provided the first direct evidence for the recruitment of downstream signaling molecules into the small, peripheral TCR microclusters formed prior to the consolidation of the cSMAC (Freiberg et al. 2002; Lee et al. 2002). In addition, our studies established the competence of individual TCR microclusters by revealing that peak calcium elevations often occur when the synapse consists of a single point contact comparable in size to one TCR microcluster. In landmark studies employing total internal reflection fluorescent microscopy, the Dustin and Saito laboratories observed analogous TCR microclusters on pMHC-bearing lipid bilayers (Campi et al. 2005; Yokosuka et al. 2005). These structures also recruited ZAP-70, and were remarkably similar to the structures observed on immobilized antibodies with respect to their size, tyrosine phosphorylation, peripheral nucleation, insensitivity to Src-family kinase inhibition, and capacity to elicit calcium responses. However, in contrast to our model, the fluid bilayer preserved the centripetal movements responsible for the consolidation of the TCR into a cSMAC. In an elegant extension of these studies, Varma et al. demonstrated that the sustained calcium signals associated with persistent synapses are entirely driven by newly formed TCR microclusters arising in the periphery of the contact (Varma et al. 2006). Collectively, these observations emphasized the roles played by peripheral TCR microclusters in the initiation and maintenance of downstream signals, and de-emphasized the contribution of the cSMAC to these processes.

8.1   Rapid Signal Initiation in TCR Microclusters

The *kinetic proofreading* model of T-cell activation posits that the pMHC half-lives associated with productive T-cell activation are dictated by the speeds of the biochemical processes that drive the formation of competent signaling complexes following TCR ligation (McKeithan 1995; Davis et al. 1998). Our ability to observe the recruitment of downstream signaling molecules to the TCR in intact cells enabled us to test this hypothesis directly (Bunnell et al. 2002). Using cIRM in conjunction with confocal fluorescence microscopy, we were able to show that ZAP-70 is recruited to the TCR within 15 s of contact formation. Building on previous photobleaching studies, we established that the recruitment of ZAP-70 to the TCR is extremely rapid, with half-maximal recoveries occurring within 7–10 s. Our studies also indicated that downstream signaling complexes must be assembled with similar speed, as calcium responses could be initiated within 12 s of the formation of a single 'point' contact. Comparable speeds of signal initiation were observed in studies employing pMHC-bearing lipid bilayers, demonstrating that our results were not artifacts arising from differences in ligand affinity and mobility (Campi et al. 2005; Yokosuka et al. 2005). The precision of these measurements was not superseded until 2007, in studies employing primary T cells plated on immobilized and photoactivatable pMHC (Huse et al. 2007). These studies indicated that LAT phosphorylation could be observed within 4 s. Diacylglycerol production and calcium flux lagged slightly, and were observed within 6–7 s. These measurements were all compatible with the half-lives of agonist pMHC, and therefore demonstrated that T cells can generate fully competent signaling complexes within the window of time dictated by individual pMHC recognition events.

8.2   TCR Microclusters as Topological Confinement Domains

Topological models of T-cell activation predict that antigen recognition occurs within tight contact domains that provide membrane separations compatible with TCR engagement and provide a permissive signaling environment by excluding large tyrosine phosphatases. In our 2002 study, we demonstrated that TCR is selectively engaged and activated within distinct membrane domains that are closely apposed to the substrate (Bunnell et al. 2002). This observation supported topological models of T cell activation, and suggested that the relevant domains of tight membrane apposition would be similar in size to the observed TCR microclusters. Subsequently, transmission electron microscopy (TEM) studies of antigen-induced T cell–dendritic cell synapses validated this prediction (Brossard et al. 2005). These synapses contained tightly apposed membrane domains that excluded LFA-1 and were comparable in size to TCR microclusters, averaging 220–300 nm in diameter. In the same 2002 study, we established that TCR/ZAP-70 microclusters exclude CD45, which was otherwise distributed uniformly throughout the synapse. Similarly, CD45 was excluded from TCR microclusters elicited on pMHC-bearing lipid bilayers (Varma et al. 2006). Collectively, these studies confirmed the existence of membrane microdomains with the topological properties required to facilitate TCR engagement and to exclude large phosphatases, such as CD45 and CD148.

8.3   TCR Microclusters and the Kinetic Segregation Hypothesis

The *kinetic segregation* model incorporates aspects of the *topological* and *kinetic proofreading* models; however, this model was the first to explicitly incorporate the small sizes of the topological confinement domains associated with TCR microclusters (Davis and van der Merwe 2006). In fact, this model requires that the topological confinement domains that generate permissive signaling environments remain small, so as to permit TCRs ligated by non-agonist pMHC to escape before becoming fully phosphorylated. This model, which was profoundly influenced by the discovery of TCR microclusters, has proven highly effective. For example, subsequent studies have confirmed that the size-dependent exclusion of tyrosine phosphatases from tight contacts contributes to the establishment of a permissive microenvironment for TCR signaling (Irles et al. 2003; Lin and Weiss 2003). Conversely, chimeric receptors that increase the length of the TCR–pMHC complex, or that loosen the rigid membrane spacing enforced by accessory molecules, inhibit T cell activation (Choudhuri et al. 2005; Milstein et al. 2008). Signal Initiation within the Earliest Contact

9   The SLP-76 Microcluster

The rapid initiation of calcium fluxes following the formation of a TCR microcluster indicated that competent signaling complexes must be assembled within a comparable time frame. In addition, the restricted distribution of phosphotyrosine indicated that these signaling complexes would be assembled in close proximity to the TCR. Using a series of fluorescent chimeras, we confirmed that LAT, Grb2, Gads, and SLP-76 are rapidly and continuously recruited into peripheral microclusters that are similar in size to TCR microclusters (Bunnell et al. 2002). Pair-wise immunofluorescent studies, performed in cells fixed after 2 min of stimulation, revealed that these molecules extensively colocalize with one another and with ZAP-70 in TCR microclusters. Subsequent analyses have extended the list of signaling molecules dynamically recruited into microclusters to include Lck, SOS1, Vav1, Nck, WASP, and PLCγ1 (Bunnell et al. 2002; Barda-Saad et al. 2005; Douglass and Vale 2005; Braiman et al. 2006; Bunnell et al. 2006; Houtman et al. 2006). These adaptors and effectors are sufficient to mediate critical TCR-proximal biochemical events, including tyrosine phosphorylation; the activation of the small GTPases Ras, Rac, and Cdc42; actin polymerization; and the production of second messengers, which include diacylglycerol and inositol 1,4,5-trisphosphate. In addition, we established that a pivotal negative regulator of T cell activation, the ubiquitin ligase c-Cbl, is recruited into these microclusters (Bunnell et al. 2002; Balagopalan et al. 2007). Of these signaling molecules, only SLP-76 has been visualized on lipid bilayers, where it is also recruited into microclusters that contain the TCR and ZAP-70.

9.1   The Stabilization and Movement of SLP-76 Microclusters

Although SLP-76 initially colocalized with ZAP-70 in TCR microclusters, SLP-76 rapidly segregated into distinct structures that were transported toward the center of the immune synapse (Bunnell et al. 2002). Comparable structures formed on lipid bilayers and underwent analogous centripetal movements. In both systems, SLP-76 microclusters were transported at speeds ranging from 0 to 100 nm/s, depending on the time post stimulation and the position of the microcluster within the synapse (Yokosuka et al. 2005; Nguyen et al. 2008). In contrast, LAT, Grb2, and Gads did not undergo centripetal transport when overexpressed alone, and were rapidly cleared from the synapse (Bunnell et al. 2002). Subsequent analyses revealed that the persistence of SLP-76 microclusters is sensitive to the level of SLP-76 expression, and that the coexpression of SLP-76 with either LAT or Gads enhances the recruitment of these adaptors into persistent SLP-76 microclusters (Barr et al. 2006; Bunnell et al. 2006). In the absence of SLP-76, LAT was recruited into microclusters; however, these structures were labile and immobile (Bunnell et al. 2006). In contrast, mutations eliminating the membrane-distal Grb2-binding tyrosine phosphorylation sites in LAT completely eliminated its ability to enter microclusters (Houtman et al. 2006). Conversely, the recruitment of SLP-76 into persistent, centripetally transported microclusters required the integrity of the TCR-proximal signal apparatus, and was severely curtailed in the absence of Lck, ZAP-70, or LAT, or in the presence of dominant-negative forms of Gads or SLP-76

(Singer et al. 2004; Bunnell et al. 2006). These observations are consistent with a model in which Lck and ZAP-70 collaborate to phosphorylate LAT, which is assembled into Grb2-dependent oligomeric complexes that are stabilized and transported following the recruitment of Gads and SLP-76. Additional effector-binding motifs within SLP-76 contribute to the stability of this core complex, implicating Nck, Vav1, and Itk in the persistence and movement of SLP-76 micro-clusters (Bunnell et al. 2006). In contrast, persistence and movement were unaffected by the loss of PLCγ1; thus, this effector protein does not contribute to the overall stability of the SLP-76 microcluster (Bunnell et al. 2006).

9.2 The SLP-76 Microcluster as an Analog-to-Digital Converter

In modern variants of the *kinetic proofreading* model, the engaged TCR first gives rise to an anatgonistic signal mediated by SHP-1 and then, only after sufficient time has elapsed, triggers the formation of a complex capable of activating the serine-threonine kinase Erk (Stefanova et al. 2003; Altan-Bonnet and Germain 2005). Once Erk is activated, it phosphorylates Lck, which is thereby protected from inactivation by SHP-1. The removal of the inhibitory pressure exerted by SHP-1 drives a feed-forward loop that rapidly maximizes the activity of Erk, producing a binary all-or-nothing response. However, it is not intuitively obvious how Erk activation, which typically requires several minutes, influences the extremely rapid events that "encode" the quality of the pMHC ligand within seconds. We have proposed that this transfer of information requires the formation of SLP-76 microclusters (Seminario and Bunnell 2008). As discussed above, these structures contain adaptors and effectors that are known to activate Ras and trigger cascades resulting in the activation of Erk. Multiple perturbations impacting the components of SLP-76 microclusters lead to their dissociation within ~90 s of their formation (Bunnell et al. 2006). The uniform kinetics of microcluster disassembly, despite the diverse nature of these perturbations, could be explained by the involvement of an antagonistic pathway capable of disassembling these microclusters and by the existence of a feed-forward loop capable of promoting microcluster stabilization. These observations are compatible with models in which the quality of the pMHC interaction is rapidly encoded at the TCR and is subsequently decoded within SLP-76 microclusters. Thus, the ability of SLP-76 to enhance microcluster persis-tence may provide the primary mechanistic basis for its crucial roles in signaling pathways downstream of the TCR (Koretzky et al. 2006).

9.3 The Segregation of SLP-76 Microclusters from the TCR

Our 2002 and 2006 studies established that SLP-76 microclusters elicited by the TCR contain a "core" complex consisting of LAT, Gads, and SLP-76. These

SLP-76 microclusters persisted for several minutes as they moved toward the center of the contact, despite the fact that the TCR and ZAP-70 microclusters that gave rise to these structures were immobile (Bunnell et al. 2002, 2006). Photobleaching studies revealed that the pool of SLP-76 present in these microclusters is in dynamic equilibrium with the cytoplasmic pool of SLP-76; therefore, these microclusters remain competent to recruit SLP-76 long after departing their TCR-dependent sites of nucleation (Barr et al. 2006). These studies suggested that TCR/ZAP-70 microclusters and LAT/Gads/SLP-76 microclusters are distinct entities. This hypothesis was consistent with elegant TEM studies from the Oliver laboratory, which revealed that the mast cell receptor (FcεRI) and LAT are recruited into distinct, but adjacent, membrane domains ranging from 200 to 500 nm in size (Wilson et al. 2000, 2001). To clarify the kinetics with which SLP-76 segregates from the TCR, we directly observed peripheral TCR microclusters as they gave rise to SLP-76 microclusters (Nguyen et al. 2008). In contrast to our studies with LAT and SLP-76, we found that the TCR and SLP-76 microclusters colocalized only at the moment of SLP-76 microcluster nucleation. Subsequently, SLP-76 microclusters "stuck" to the boundaries of distinct TCR microclusters as they migrated toward the center of the synapse, behaving as if the TCR microclusters presented barriers to their movement. To date, it is unclear whether SLP-76 microclusters segregate from the TCR in bilayer-based systems, as the TCR is also translocated towards the center of the synapse in these models (Yokosuka et al. 2005). However, the Davis laboratory has reported the segregation of microcluster components from the TCR in primary T cells stimulated on immobilized pMHC (Lillemeier et al. 2006). Therefore, this discrepancy is unlikely to result from the quality of the stimulatory ligand, and is more likely to involve the resistance of immobilized ligands to translocation and internalization. Additional studies will be required to clarify whether SLP-76 microclusters segregate from the TCR under more physiological stimulation conditions, in which the available TCR ligands display intermediate lateral mobilities.

9.4   SLP-76 Microclusters Are Primarily Organized by Protein–Protein Scaffolds

The role of lipid rafts in the initiation of signals by antigen receptors remains an extremely contentious issue (Hancock 2006; Shaw 2006). For some time now, it has been clear that models involving large preassembled signaling platforms, which we facetiously refer to as "battleship" models, are not viable. In support of this assertion, the distributions of raft-resident GPI-anchored proteins were not appreciably impacted under conditions in which a raft-resident adaptor, LAT, was recruited into microclusters (Bunnell et al. 2002). Similarly, Src-family tyrosine kinase inhibitors abolished the recruitment of LAT into signaling microclusters, even though the TCR continued to be recruited into well-defined microclusters under these conditions (Bunnell et al. 2002). We also established that raft-resident mutants of LAT lacking their distal tyrosine phosphorylation sites were incapable of being recruited into SLP-76 microclusters (Bunnell et al. 2006). Douglass et al. came to similar conclusions after imaging single molecules of raft and non-raft probes (Douglass and Vale 2005). In these studies, raft probes diffused more freely through the plasma membrane, and were almost completely unaffected by activating stimuli. In contrast, the mobility of raft-resident proteins was almost entirely dictated by their ability to participate in protein–protein interactions. Nevertheless, it would be premature to dismiss the involvement of distinct lipid microenvironments in the activation of antigen receptors. For example, the TEM studies discussed immediately above have reported the segregation of the membrane into domains with distinct properties (Lillemeier et al. 2006). Similarly, dynamic studies employing dyes sensitive to the ordering of the plasma membrane have confirmed that raft-like domains arise during T-cell activation (Gaus et al. 2005). Elegant studies employing fluorescence resonance energy transfer (FRET) have identified similar changes accompanying B-cell activation (Sohn et al. 2008). Although these changes are likely to be driven by the assembly of protein-dependent scaffolds, it is certainly possible that the protein-driven packing of raft-resident proteins, such as LAT, into small microclusters will influence the local membrane composition. Thus, protein scaffolds may influence the local organization of the membrane, which may in turn influence the functions of proteins present within these microdomains.

10 Integrin Microclusters

Although integrins play critical roles in the formation of the immune synapse, relatively few studies have examined whether integrin signaling proceeds through the formation of microclusters. As early as 2003, the Koretzky laboratory demonstrated that LFA-1 was capable of driving SLP-76 into microclusters in neutrophils (Newbrough et al. 2003). However, integrins were not shown to elicit SLP-76 microclusters in T cells until this year (Baker et al. 2009). To date, only one study has directly addressed whether integrins themselves are recruited into microclusters in T cells. In this study, which employed antibody-bearing stimulatory bilayers, the TCR and LFA-1 were immediately assembled into distinct microclusters in the periphery of the synapse (Kaizuka et al. 2007). This differs from the situation observed with TCR and SLP-76 microclusters, which initially colocalize at their sites of origin in the cell periphery. As lamellipodial actin flowed toward the center of the contact, the TCR and integrin microclusters were swept inwards at comparable speeds. Single molecule studies revealed that the fates of these microclusters diverged as they approached the boundary of the cSMAC. Whereas individual TCR molecules proceeded through this boundary without hindrance, integrins were incapable of penetrating this barrier. Thus, that the cSMAC may act as a topological filter capable of excluding the taller integrin complexes.

10.1 Integrins Impact the Movement of SLP-76 Microclusters

Given the pivotal role of SLP-76 in T cell activation, we wished to determine whether the potent costimulatory signals transmitted by integrins impacted SLP-76 microclusters. Because previous studies had shown that VLA-4 could elicit the phosphorylation of SLP-76, we chose to evaluate the effects of VLA-4 on SLP-76 microclusters (Hunter et al. 2000). Costimulation through VLA-4 was highly effective, and enhanced TCR-dependent increases in cytoplasmic calcium levels and transcription factor activation. Although VLA-4 ligation increased the number of SLP-76 microclusters observed in response to low-dose stimulation of the TCR, comparable effects were observed using non-costimulatory pro-adhesive ligands, such as CD43 (Nguyen et al. 2008). However, the ligation of VLA-4 selectively inhibited the movement of SLP-76 microclusters toward the center of the immune synapse. This effect was associated with the retention of SLP-76 microclusters at their peripheral nucleation sites, and resulted in an overall increase in the colocalization of SLP-76 with phosphotyrosine in the cell periphery. This observation paralleled the work of Mossman et al. who demonstrated that tyrosine phosphorylation and T cell activation were both enhanced when the responding cells were stimulated on "gridded" lipid bilayers incapable of supporting long-range movements of TCR microclusters (Mossman et al. 2005). This led us to predict that VLA-4 was preventing the movement of SLP-76 microclusters through its impact on the actin cytoskeleton, rather than by inhibiting the molecular motors responsible for microcluster movement. In accordance with this hypothesis, VLA-4 ligation coordinately slowed the movement of SLP-76 and the underlying actin network. Furthermore, acute perturbations that arrested ongoing actin flows immediately halted the centripetal movement of SLP-76 microclusters. This observation was consistent with previous studies showing that comparable treatments halt the inward flow of TCR microclusters formed on lipid bilayers (Varma et al. 2006). Although we were not able to examine these movements in physiological conjugates, several precedents indicated that the lateral mobility of an integrin ligand within an APC influences the ultimate position of the corresponding integrin on the responding lymphocyte (Mittelbrunn et al. 2004; Carrasco and Batista 2006).

10.2 Adaptors Linking Integrins to SLP-76 Microclusters

Over the last several years, a series of publications has identified a pathway that has the potential to couple integrins to SLP-76 microclusters. Initially, the Koretzky laboratory established that the Gads-binding site within SLP-76 was dispensable for the transmission of integrin-dependent signals through SLP-76 (Judd et al. 2002; Abtahian et al. 2006). Our own studies indicated that the Src homology 2 (SH2) domain of SLP-76 plays a crucial role in the assembly of SLP-76 microclusters (Bunnell et al. 2006). This domain of SLP-76 binds to the adaptor protein ADAP, which is phosphorylated in response to VLA-4 ligation (Hunter et al. 2000). Subsequent studies confirmed that ADAP is the crucial intermediate that enables integrins to recruit SLP-76 into Gads-independent microclusters (Baker et al. 2009). The mechanisms coupling ADAP and SLP-76 to integrins are likely to involve a complex of proteins including SKAP55, Rap1, RIAM, and Talin (Han et al. 2006; Kliche et al. 2006; Menasche et al. 2007). ADAP interacts with SKAP55, and these proteins jointly regulate the recruitment of Rap1 to the plasma membrane. RIAM binds to ADAP and SKAP55, and facilitates the interaction of Rap1 with Talin. The presentation of Rap1 to Talin promotes the interaction of Talin with critical motifs in the tails of β-integrins (Lee et al. 2009). At present, it is unclear whether the interactions linking SLP-76, ADAP, and SKAP55 to Rap1, RIAM, and Talin are sufficient to limit the mobility of SLP-76 microclusters. Further, it is not clear whether the stimulatory integrins will reside within SLP-76 microclusters, or in distinct, laterally interacting integrin microclusters, as is observed for the TCR.

11   Accessory Microclusters

Diverse receptors possess the common structural and topological properties required to generate domains of membrane apposition compatible with the engagement of the TCR. Dynamic imaging studies recently established that at least two of these receptor families participate in microclusters, providing significant new insights into the general properties of these accessory receptors. The first family includes CD2 and its ligands, which are discussed below. The closely related SLAM family members are likely to play similar and overlapping roles in T-cell activation, but will not be discussed as they have recently been reviewed elsewhere (Schwartzberg et al. 2009). The second family includes the classical costimulatory receptor CD28 and its inhibitory counterpart CTLA-4. Although CD28 has typically received more attention as a costimulatory receptor, the overlapping functions of CD2 and CD28 have been appreciated for nearly a decade (Green et al. 2000).

11.1   CD2 Microclusters and the Inner Adhesion Ring

Almost two decades ago, Springer proposed that CD2 could facilitate the formation of the tight membrane juxtapositions required for optimal TCR engagement (Springer 1990). Subsequent studies confirmed that CD2 and LFA-1 are assembled into distinct contact domains, and determined that the accumulation of CD2 within the center of the synapse is governed by the interaction of the CD2 tail with the adaptor protein CD2AP (Dustin et al. 1998). The first studies to describe the formation of cSMAC-like structures on lipid bilayers also established that CD2 was recruited into an inner adhesion ring, which occupied the space between the TCR-rich cSMAC and the LFA-1 containing pSMAC (Grakoui et al. 1999). This inner ring clearly contributed to cell adhesion, although this role was most evident in the absence of integrin ligation (van der Merwe et al. 2000; Bromley et al. 2001). However, the positive role of CD2 was thrown into doubt when the disordered synapses formed in the absence of CD2AP were shown to result in enhanced TCR-dependent signals (Lee et al. 2003). These doubts were supported by the discovery that CD2 contributes to the formation of a large, central membrane invagination, which appears to contribute to the downmodulation of activated receptors (Singleton et al. 2006).

The recruitment of CD2 into signaling microclusters was first observed in T cells stimulated by TCR-specific immobilized antibodies (Douglass and Vale 2005). In these studies, CD2 colocalized with the TCR, Lck, and LAT in microclusters that excluded CD45. In addition, CD2 recruitment required the phosphorylation of LAT. Photobleaching studies revealed that CD2 dynamically exchanges between micro-clusters. However, these CD2-containing structures are not translocated within the plane of the contact, in marked contrast to the mobile SLP-76 microclusters observed in the same model system (Bunnell et al. 2002). This is somewhat perplexing, as the recruitment of CD2 into microclusters requires LAT, which is an integral component of SLP-76 microclusters. Therefore, it will be interesting to determine whether CD2 and SLP-76 display distinct patterns of clustering and movement when coordinately expressed in the same cells. Subsequent studies employing lipid bilayers revealed that CD2 is capable of initiating similar micro-clusters, which recruit the TCR and LAT, and exclude CD45 (Kaizuka et al. 2009). The coengagement of the TCR and CD2 results in the coordinated redistribution of both receptors into signaling microclusters. Over time, the TCR and CD2 gradually segregate from one another, giving rise to a dephosphorylated central cluster containing the TCR, and a phosphotyrosine-rich ring that accumulates CD2. These data indicate that the TCR and CD2 communicate with overlapping sets of downstream effectors, but display differing susceptibilities to downmodulation. Furthermore, these properties suggest that the CD2-rich inner adhesion ring observed in immune synapses contributes to T cell activation.

11.2 CD28 Microclusters Promote Costimulation and Stable Adhesion

In the first bilayer-based studies of the immune synapse, CD28 behaved differently than CD2 and was recruited into the cSMAC (Grakoui et al. 1999). However, studies employing APCs indicated that CD28 is coordinately enriched with $PKC\theta$ in an annular ring that surrounds the cSMAC, but remains internal to the pSMAC (Tseng et al. 2005). By manipulating the tail of the CD28 ligand, Tseng et al. were able to show that the position of CD28 was ultimately determined by the APC, and that the retention of CD28 in the annular ring was correlated with optimal T cell activation. Subsequent studies, employing lipid bilayers, revealed that CD28 is recruited into the TCR-rich signaling microclusters that are assembled upon contact initiation (Yokosuka et al. 2008). As in the studies with CD2, CD28 gradually segregated from the TCR, and formed an inner ring that surrounds the TCR, but remains internal to the integrin-rich pSMAC. This inner ring retained a dynamic composition, provided a docking platform for PKCθ within the immune synapse, and contributed to optimal T cell proliferation.

CD28 can contribute directly to T cell adhesion; however, its ability to participate in adhesive interactions is controlled by its tail and by signaling through the TCR (Bromley et al. 2001). In fact, the signaling pathways initiated by CD28 may have a greater impact on the formation of stable conjugates. Recent studies have indicated that CD28 and its inhibitory counterpart CTLA-4 reciprocally regulate stable adhesion and that this aspect of their function is responsible for the profound hyper-responsiveness observed in CTLA-4 deficient animals. This hypothesis is outlined in the "reverse stop" model of CTLA-4 function, in which CTLA-4 is thought to promote the disruption of productive conjugates by preferentially activating pro-migratory pathways (Rudd 2008).

12   The Bi-Functional cSMAC

One of the most intriguing features of the immune synapse is its capacity to boost weak signals and to moderate super-optimal signals. The inhibitory potential of the cSMAC was first suggested by the observation that the cSMAC was relatively poor in tyrosine-phosphorylated species, and was confirmed using T cells that exhibited aberrant synapses lacking well-defined cSMACs (Lee et al. 2002; Lee et al. 2003). These cells accumulated abnormally high levels of tyrosine phosphorylation in the synapse and failed to appropriately terminate antigen-dependent signals. In response these observations, Lee et al. developed a computational model in which a bi-functional cSMAC enhances T cell activation by concentrating pMHC ligands in the center of the contact and terminates signaling by promoting the internalization and degradation of fully activated TCR complexes.

12.1   Microcluster Centralization and Termination

In our early imaging studies, we readily identified a positive correlation between the centralization of SLP-76 microclusters and the efficiency of T cell activation (Bunnell et al. 2002). However, this relationship was difficult to interpret because microcluster centralization was tightly associated with microcluster persistence (Bunnell et al. 2006). Nevertheless, the colocalization of the inhibitory ubiquitin ligase c-Cbl with TCR and SLP-76 microclusters suggested that this situation was clarified somewhat when studies performed on lipid bilayers revealed that TCR microclusters are readily accumulated in the center of the synapse, whereas signaling microclusters containing either ZAP-70 or SLP-76 dissociate prior to their arrival in the cSMAC (Campi et al. 2005; Yokosuka et al. 2005). Subsequent studies progressively clarified that inhibitory functions were associated with microcluster centralization and cSMAC formation. Using immobilized stimuli, we demonstrated that SLP-76 microclusters undergoing centralization are rapidly internalized and disassembled. In addition, we determined that lipid raft- and ubiquitin-dependent pathways contribute to the movement and termination of SLP-76 microclusters (Barr et al. 2006). In the same year, the cSMAC was shown to contain significant amounts of lysobisphosphatidic acid (LBPA). The presence of this lipid, which assists the targeting of ubiquitinated proteins into degradative compartments, further clarified how the cSMAC could terminate TCR-dependent signals (Varma et al. 2006). Finally, in a comprehensive study from the Samelson laboratory, the ubiquitin ligase c-Cbl was shown to enter TCR and SLP-76 microclusters, to directly ubiquitinate LAT, and to promote the termination of these microclusters (Balagopalan et al. 2007). Collectively, these studies proved that ubiquitin-dependent internalization and degradation pathways direct the termination of TCR-dependent signals in the cSMAC.

12.2 Signal Amplification in the cSMAC

The positive role of the cSMAC in signal amplification has proven harder to establish experimentally. Hints of this function were apparent in the first studies examining microcluster movement on lipid bilayers (Yokosuka et al. 2005). In these studies, the lowest doses of pMHC resulted in the persistent detection of phosphorylated species of ZAP-70 in the center of the immune synapse. In a more exhaustive and conclusive study of this phenomenon, Cemerski et al. confirmed that, under conditions of low antigen abundance, the cSMAC generates sustained signals that contribute to productive T cell activation (Cemerski et al. 2008). Mathematical models of synapse formation suggest that this sustained phosphorylation is driven by the concentration of pMHC within the cSMAC and is enabled by the inability of weaker ligands to promote efficient TCR downmodulation.

13 Concluding Thoughts

13.1 Revisiting the SMACs: Toward Terms with Functional Definitions

The initial subdivision of the immune synapse into distinct SMACs was devised more than a decade ago. Although these concepts have proven useful, the recent explosion of studies examining microclusters, in all of their various forms, has yielded complexities that were not anticipated at the inception of this terminology. For example, the original definition of the dSMAC as a domain enriched in CD45 did not prove useful, as CD45 is present at comparable levels on the lateral surfaces of the T cell (Freiberg et al. 2002). However, the recent redefinition of the dSMAC as a zone defined by the thin circumferential lamellipodia associated with the immune synapse has much greater explanatory power (Dustin 2008). One of the primary advantages of the newer definition is that it identifies underlying cell biological processes characteristic of the domain. This has facilitated further insights into how this domain operates through the identification of parallels with other models systems. In this case, the re-definition led to the hypothesis that the retrograde actin flows characteristic of lamellipodia could contribute to the centripetal microcluster flows within the immune synapse (Varma et al. 2006; Nguyen et al. 2008).

In this vein, it is worth considering the unique properties of the distal tips of the lamellipodia that comprise the dSMAC. As noted above, TCR engagement during the expansion of the contact is almost exclusively restricted to these tips. How is this accomplished? Our own studies have identified the Abi/WAVE complex as a molecular marker for an exceedingly narrow domain at the distal tips of the circumferential lamellipodia of the dSMAC (Zipfel et al. 2006). We propose that these proteins form the core of specialized distal tip complex (DTC) that is involved in lamellipodial growth, the pre-positioning of pro-adhesive molecules, and the generation of mechanical forces required to approximate the T cell and APC membranes during scanning interactions, and to extrude large phosphatases such as CD45 from nascent contacts (Nolz et al. 2006, 2007; Billadeau et al. 2007). The latter concept provides a viable explanation for the requirement for dynamic actin polymerization in T cell activation, and is discussed elsewhere as the *mechanical segregation* model (Seminario and Bunnell 2008).

The correspondence between the pSMAC and Talin-dependent and integrin-mediated adhesion has remained remarkably robust. In addition, the discovery that myosin contributes to centripetal microcluster flows within the pSMAC has confirmed the usefulness of the recent analogy between the pSMAC and the lamellum (Dustin 2008; Ilani et al. 2009). However, the discovery of the multi-focal synapse demonstrated that definitions referring to the pSMAC "surrounding" a central TCR cluster have outlived their usefulness. Importantly, this domain does not appear to possess a specific membrane topology, and instead tolerates a wide range of membrane separations (Brossard et al. 2005). The high affinity of the integrin–ligand bond and the flexibility of the integrin leg domains may facilitate this behavior. This feature may play a crucial role in the relatively unrestricted movement of TCR and accessory microclusters through this domain.

After years of confusion, recent studies addressing the behaviors of CD2 and CD28 within the immune synapse have begun to clarify the confusing properties of the central domain that was originally defined as the cSMAC. However, it is becoming increasingly clear that this confusion has arisen because the "classical" cSMAC is actually composed of two distinct domains. The most central domain contains inert, dephosphorylated TCR that comprise a distinct, immobile pool. This domain is also enriched in LBPA, which is a marker for multivesicular bodies and lysosomes (Varma et al. 2006). In recent reviews, this domain has been referred to as the cSMACa or as the CD3^{hi} cSMAC (Dustin 2009; Yokosuka and Saito 2009). We suggest that this downmodulatory domain should continue to be referred to as the cSMAC.

Previous studies indicated that CD2 is present in an inner adhesion ring (Grakoui et al. 1999; van der Merwe et al. 2000). This domain, which fills the gap between the TCR-rich central domain and the classical pSMAC, is also highly enriched in CD28, which remains in a dynamic equilibrium and represents the primary site to which PKCθ is recruited (Yokosuka et al. 2008). This domain has been referred to as the cSMACb or as the CD3^{dim} cSMAC, and has been suggested to function as a "costimulatory signalosome" (Dustin 2009; Yokosuka and Saito 2009). This domain possesses many of the properties of the active TCR microclusters that arise in the periphery of the immune synapse. For the sake of clarity and simplicity, we suggest that the active domain interposed between the cSMAC and pSMAC should be referred to as an "inner" or "intermediate" SMAC (iSMAC). Given the involvement of CD2, CD28, and their associated signaling molecules in pathways leading to the activation of WASP, we suggest that this domain may possess many properties commonly associated with podosomes (Badour et al. 2003, 2007; Calle et al. 2008).

13.2   A Cell Biological Basis for Model-Independent Microclusters?

To date, microclusters have most frequently been observed using distinct planar systems involving either coverglass-immobilized antibodies or lipid bilayers bearing pMHC and ICAM-1. More recently, hybrids models have emerged. Thus, TCR microclusters have been observed on lipid bilayers functionalized with anti-CD3ε and ICAM-1, whereas "protein islands" and Grb2-positive microclusters have been observed using surface-immobilized pMHC (Lillemeier et al. 2006; Huse et al. 2007; Kaizuka et al. 2007). Together, these planar systems possess several very significant advantages. First, they enable the visualization of the entire contact interface in a single frame, enormously enhancing dynamic analyses of contact architecture. Second, these systems exploit the intrinsically higher resolution of the xy-plane relative to the z-axis (~0.2 μm vs. ~1.0 μm), offering images of superior quality to those derived by digital reconstruction from z-stacks. Third, these systems are compatible with TIRF microscopy, which offers a substantial increase in resolution along the z-axis. Finally, these systems enable the precise control of the stimulatory and costimulatory ligands presented on the substrate.

Despite significant differences in the affinity and mobility of the TCR ligands employed in each case, these model systems have yielded striking similarities. These include (1) the formation of TCR and ZAP-70 containing microclusters (Bunnell et al. 2002; Campi et al. 2005); (2) the specific exclusion of the tyrosine phosphatase CD45 from TCR microclusters (Bunnell et al. 2002; Varma et al. 2006); (3) the formation of signaling microclusters containing CD2, LAT, and SLP-76 (Bunnell et al. 2002; Campi et al. 2005; Douglass and Vale 2005; Yokosuka et al. 2005; Kaizuka et al. 2007); (4) the speed with which downstream scaffolds and effectors are recruited (Bunnell et al. 2002; Huse et al. 2007); (5) the intimate relationship between microcluster formation and calcium signaling (Bunnell et al. 2002; Campi et al. 2005); (6) the ligand densities required to support microcluster formation (Yokosuka et al. 2005; Varma et al. 2006; Nguyen et al. 2008); (7) the consistent sizes of microclusters (Varma et al. 2006; Nguyen et al. 2008); (8) the segregation of microclusters containing CD2, LAT, and SLP-76 from microclusters containing the TCR and ZAP-70 (Douglass and Vale 2005; Yokosuka et al. 2005; Lillemeier et al. 2006; Nguyen et al. 2008; Kaizuka et al. 2009); (9) the speed and directionality of SLP-76 movement (Bunnell et al. 2002; Yokosuka et al. 2005; Nguyen et al. 2008); (10) the peripheral origin of newly formed microclusters (Bunnell et al. 2002; Yokosuka et al. 2005); (11) the observation that barriers to microcluster centralization favor T-cell activation (Mossman et al. 2005; Nguyen et al. 2008); (12) the involvement of the actin cytoskeleton in microcluster movement (Varma et al. 2006; Nguyen et al. 2008; Ilani et al. 2009); and (13) the development of concentric zones characterized by divergent levels of tyrosine phosphorylation (Barda-Saad et al. 2005; Campi et al. 2005; Mossman et al. 2005; Nguyen et al. 2008). Although current models of T-cell activation acknowledge the crucial roles of ligand half-life and ligand size in the initiation of signals by the TCR, these observations indicate that the affinity, mobility, and size of the TCR ligand play unexpectedly small roles at the level of the microcluster.

Despite the higher affinities and divergent sizes of the antigen receptors involved, microclusters with very similar properties have been observed in mast cells, NK cells, and B cells (Wilson et al. 2000, 2001; Newbrough et al. 2003; Fleire et al. 2006; Silverman et al. 2006; Treanor et al. 2006; Depoil et al. 2008; Weber et al. 2008; Tolar et al. 2009). Based on the extensive parallels between the distinct models of microcluster formation outlined above, and between the diverse cell types listed here, we suggest that the properties of microclusters are dictated by conserved cell biological processes that are set in motion following the recognition of surface-associated antigens. These processes need not depend on the precise biophysical parameters that govern specific receptor–ligand interactions. We currently favor a *mechanical segregation model* in which protrusive actin structures generate the privileged contact domains predicted by the kinetic segregation model (Davis and van der Merwe 2006; Seminario and Bunnell 2008). We expect these structures to facilitate ligand recognition, and anticipate that the dimensions of these contact domains are dictated by the sizes of the actin-rich processes that give rise to them. Modern kinetic proofreading models suggest that rare triggering events of high quality flip a digital "switch" that enables the rapid population of a contact domain with activated receptors. However, we propse that the limited sizes of these structures will restrict the number of docking sites available for downstream effectors. Thus, the response profiles of immune cells could be channeled toward specific productive outputs, despite enormous variations in ligand quality and abundance. These are precisely the properties associated with T cell activation (Ma et al. 2008).

Acknowledgments S.C.B. was supported by an American Heart Association Scientist Development Grant, by an award from the Dana Foundation for Brain and Immuno-Imaging, and by the NIH (R01 AI076575-01A1).

References

Abtahian F, Bezman N, Clemens R, Sebzda E, Cheng L, Shattil SJ, Kahn ML, Koretzky GA (2006) Evidence for the requirement of ITAM domains but not SLP-76/Gads interaction for integrin signaling in hematopoietic cells. Mol Cell Biol 26:6936–6949

Altan-Bonnet G, Germain RN (2005) Modeling T cell antigen discrimination based on feedback control of digital ERK responses. PLoS Biol 3:e356

Badour K, Zhang J, Shi F, McGavin MK, Rampersad V, Hardy LA, Field D, Siminovitch KA (2003) The Wiskott-Aldrich syndrome protein acts downstream of CD2 and the CD2AP and PSTPIP1 adaptors to promote formation of the immunological synapse. Immunity 18:141–154

Badour K, McGavin MK, Zhang J, Freeman S, Vieira C, Filipp D, Julius M, Mills GB, Siminovitch KA (2007) Interaction of the Wiskott-Aldrich syndrome protein with sorting nexin 9 is required for CD28 endocytosis and cosignaling in T cells. Proc Natl Acad Sci USA 104:1593–1598

Bajenoff M, Egen JG, Koo LY, Laugier JP, Brau F, Glaichenhaus N, Germain RN (2006) Stromal cell networks regulate lymphocyte entry, migration, and territoriality in lymph nodes. Immunity 25:989–1001

Baker RG, Hsu CJ, Lee D, Jordan MS, Maltzman JS, Hammer DA, Baumgart T, Koretzky GA (2009) The adapter protein SLP-76 mediates "outside-in" integrin signaling and function in T cells. Mol Cell Biol 20:5578–5589

Balagopalan L, Barr VA, Sommers CL, Barda-Saad M, Goyal A, Isakowitz MS, Samelson LE (2007) c-Cbl mediated regulation of LAT-nucleated signaling complexes. Mol Cell Biol 27:8622–8636

Balamuth F, Leitenberg D, Unternaehrer J, Mellman I, Bottomly K (2001) Distinct patterns of membrane microdomain partitioning in Th1 and Th2 cells. Immunity 15:729–738

Barda-Saad M, Braiman A, Titerence R, Bunnell SC, Barr VA, Samelson LE (2005) Dynamic molecular interactions linking the T cell antigen receptor to the actin cytoskeleton. Nat Immunol 6:80–89

Barr VA, Balagopalan L, Barda-Saad M, Polishchuk R, Boukari H, Bunnell SC, Bernot KM, Toda Y, Nossal R, Samelson LE (2006) T-cell antigen receptor-induced signaling complexes: internalization via a cholesterol-dependent endocytic pathway. Traffic 7:1143–1162

Billadeau DD, Nolz JC, Gomez TS (2007) Regulation of T-cell activation by the cytoskeleton. Nat Rev Immunol 7:131–143

Braiman A, Barda-Saad M, Sommers CL, Samelson LE (2006) Recruitment and activation of PLCgamma1 in T cells: a new insight into old domains. Embo J 25:774–784

Breart B, Bousso P (2006) Cellular orchestration of T cell priming in lymph nodes. Curr Opin Immunol 18:483–490

Bromley SK, Iaboni A, Davis SJ, Whitty A, Green JM, Shaw AS, Weiss A, Dustin ML (2001) The immunological synapse and CD28-CD80 interactions. Nat Immunol 2:1159–1166

Brossard C, Feuillet V, Schmitt A, Randriamampita C, Romao M, Raposo G, Trautmann A (2005) Multifocal structure of the T cell – dendritic cell synapse. Eur J Immunol 35:1741–1753

Brown MJ, Hallam JA, Colucci-Guyon E, Shaw S (2001) Rigidity of circulating lymphocytes is primarily conferred by vimentin intermediate filaments. J Immunol 166:6640–6646

Bunnell SC, Kapoor V, Trible RP, Zhang W, Samelson LE (2001) Dynamic actin polymerization drives T cell receptor-induced spreading: a role for the signal transduction adaptor LAT. Immunity 14:315–329

Bunnell SC, Hong DI, Kardon JR, Yamazaki T, McGlade CJ, Barr VA, Samelson LE (2002) T cell receptor ligation induces the formation of dynamically regulated signaling assemblies. J Cell Biol 158:1263–1275

Bunnell SC, Barr VA, Fuller CL, Samelson LE (2003) High-resolution multicolor imaging of dynamic signaling complexes in T cells stimulated by planar substrates. Sci STKE 2003:PL8

Bunnell SC, Singer AL, Hong DI, Jacque BH, Jordan MS, Seminario MC, Barr VA, Koretzky GA, Samelson LE (2006) Persistence of cooperatively stabilized signaling clusters drives T-cell activation. Mol Cell Biol 26:7155–7166

Calle Y, Anton IM, Thrasher AJ, Jones GE (2008) WASP and WIP regulate podosomes in migrating leukocytes. J Microsc 231:494–505

Campi G, Varma R, Dustin ML (2005) Actin and agonist MHC-peptide complex-dependent T cell receptor microclusters as scaffolds for signaling. J Exp Med 202:1031–1036

Cannon JL, Labno CM, Bosco G, Seth A, McGavin MH, Siminovitch KA, Rosen MK, Burkhardt JK (2001) Wasp recruitment to the T cell:APC contact site occurs independently of Cdc42 activation. Immunity 15:249–259

Carman CV, Sage PT, Sciuto TE, de la Fuente MA, Geha RS, Ochs HD, Dvorak HF, Dvorak AM, Springer TA (2007) Transcellular diapedesis is initiated by invasive podosomes. Immunity 26:784–797

Carrasco YR, Batista FD (2006) B-cell activation by membrane-bound antigens is facilitated by the interaction of VLA-4 with VCAM-1. EMBO J 25:889–899

Cemerski S, Das J, Giurisato E, Markiewicz MA, Allen PM, Chakraborty AK, Shaw AS (2008) The balance between T cell receptor signaling and degradation at the center of the immunological synapse is determined by antigen quality. Immunity 29:414–422

Choudhuri K, Wiseman D, Brown MH, Gould K, van der Merwe PA (2005) T-cell receptor triggering is critically dependent on the dimensions of its peptide-MHC ligand. Nature 436:578–582

Cullinan P, Sperling AI, Burkhardt JK (2002) The distal pole complex: a novel membrane domain distal to the immunological synapse. Immunol Rev 189:111–122

Davis SJ, van der Merwe PA (2006) The kinetic-segregation model: TCR triggering and beyond. Nat Immunol 7:803–809

Davis MM, Boniface JJ, Reich Z, Lyons D, Hampl J, Arden B, Chien Y (1998) Ligand recognition by alpha beta T cell receptors. Annu Rev Immunol 16:523–544

del Pozo MA, Nieto M, Serrador JM, Sancho D, Vicente-Manzanares M, Martinez C, Sanchez-Madrid F (1998) The two poles of the lymphocyte: specialized cell compartments for migration and recruitment. Cell Adhes Commun 6:125–133

Delon J, Bercovici N, Raposo G, Liblau R, Trautmann A (1998) Antigen-dependent and -independent Ca2+ responses triggered in T cells by dendritic cells compared with B cells. J Exp Med 188:1473–1484

Depoil D, Zaru R, Guiraud M, Chauveau A, Harriague J, Bismuth G, Utzny C, Muller S, Valitutti S (2005) Immunological synapses are versatile structures enabling selective T cell polarization. Immunity 22:185–194

Depoil D, Fleire S, Treanor BL, Weber M, Harwood NE, Marchbank KL, Tybulewicz VL, Batista FD (2008) CD19 is essential for B cell activation by promoting B cell receptor-antigen microcluster formation in response to membrane-bound ligand. Nat Immunol 9:63–72

Douglass AD, Vale RD (2005) Single-molecule microscopy reveals plasma membrane microdomains created by protein-protein networks that exclude or trap signaling molecules in T cells. Cell 121:937–950

Dustin ML (2008) Hunter to gatherer and back: immunological synapses and kinapses as variations on the theme of amoeboid locomotion. Annu Rev Cell Dev Biol 24:577–596

Dustin ML (2009) The cellular context of T cell signaling. Immunity 30:482–492

Dustin ML, Ferguson LM, Chan PY, Springer TA, Golan DE (1996a) Visualization of CD2
interaction with LFA-3 and determination of the two-dimensional dissociation constant for
adhesion receptors in a contact area. J Cell Biol 132:465–474

Dustin ML, Miller JM, Ranganath S, Vignali DA, Viner NJ, Nelson CA, Unanue ER (1996b)
TCR-mediated adhesion of T cell hybridomas to planar bilayers containing purified MHC class
II/peptide complexes and receptor shedding during detachment. J Immunol 157:2014–2021

Dustin ML, Olszowy MW, Holdorf AD, Li J, Bromley S, Desai N, Widder P, Rosenberger F, van
der Merwe PA, Allen PM, Shaw AS (1998) A novel adaptor protein orchestrates receptor
patterning and cytoskeletal polarity in T-cell contacts. Cell 94:667–677

Dustin ML, Tseng SY, Varma R, Campi G (2006) T cell-dendritic cell immunological synapses.
Curr Opin Immunol 18:512–516

Fleire SJ, Goldman JP, Carrasco YR, Weber M, Bray D, Batista FD (2006) B cell ligand
discrimination through a spreading and contraction response. Science 312:738–741

Franco SJ, Huttenlocher A (2005) Regulating cell migration: calpains make the cut. J Cell Sci
118:3829–3838

Freiberg BA, Kupfer H, Maslanik W, Delli J, Kappler J, Zaller DM, Kupfer A (2002) Staging and
resetting T cell activation in SMACs. Nat Immunol 3:911–917

Friedl P, den Boer AT, Gunzer M (2005) Tuning immune responses: diversity and adaptation of
the immunological synapse. Nat Rev Immunol 5:532–545

Gaus K, Chklovskaia E, de St F, Groth B, Jessup W, Harder T (2005) Condensation of the plasma
membrane at the site of T lymphocyte activation. J Cell Biol 171:121–131

Gomez TS, Kumar K, Medeiros RB, Shimizu Y, Leibson PJ, Billadeau DD (2007) Formins
regulate the actin-related protein 2/3 complex-independent polarization of the centrosome to
the immunological synapse. Immunity 26:177–190

Grakoui A, Bromley SK, Sumen C, Davis MM, Shaw AS, Allen PM, Dustin ML (1999) The
immunological synapse: a molecular machine controlling T cell activation. Science 285:221–227

Green JM, Karpitskiy V, Kimzey SL, Shaw AS (2000) Coordinate regulation of T cell activation
by CD2 and CD28. J Immunol 164:3591–3595

Gremm D, Wegner A (2000) Gelsolin as a calcium-regulated actin filament-capping protein. Eur
J Biochem 267:4339–4345

Hailman E, Burack WR, Shaw AS, Dustin ML, Allen PM (2002) Immature CD4(+)CD8(+)
thymocytes form a multifocal immunological synapse with sustained tyrosine phosphorylation.
Immunity 16:839–848

Han J, Lim CJ, Watanabe N, Soriani A, Ratnikov B, Calderwood DA, Puzon-McLaughlin W,
Lafuente EM, Boussiotis VA, Shattil SJ, Ginsberg MH (2006) Reconstructing and deconstructing agonist-induced activation of integrin alphaIIbbeta3. Curr Biol 16:1796–1806

Hancock JF (2006) Lipid rafts: contentious only from simplistic standpoints. Nat Rev Mol Cell
Biol 7:456–462

Henrickson SE, Mempel TR, Mazo IB, Liu B, Artyomov MN, Zheng H, Peixoto A, Flynn MP,
Senman B, Junt T, Wong HC, Chakraborty AK, von Andrian UH (2008) T cell sensing of
antigen dose governs interactive behavior with dendritic cells and sets a threshold for T cell
activation. Nat Immunol 9:282–291

Houtman JC, Yamaguchi H, Barda-Saad M, Braiman A, Bowden B, Appella E, Schuck P,
Samelson LE (2006) Oligomerization of signaling complexes by the multipoint binding of
GRB2 to both LAT and SOS1. Nat Struct Mol Biol 13:798–805

Hunter AJ, Ottoson N, Boerth N, Koretzky GA, Shimizu Y (2000) Cutting edge: a novel function
for the SLAP-130/FYB adapter protein in beta 1 integrin signaling and T lymphocyte migration. J Immunol 164:1143–1147

Huppa JB, Gleimer M, Sumen C, Davis MM (2003) Continuous T cell receptor signaling required
for synapse maintenance and full effector potential. Nat Immunol 4:749–755

Huse M, Klein LO, Girvin AT, Faraj JM, Li QJ, Kuhns MS, Davis MM (2007) Spatial and temporal dynamics of T cell receptor signaling with a photoactivatable agonist. Immunity 27:76–88

Ilani T, Vasiliver-Shamis G, Vardhana S, Bretscher A, Dustin ML (2009) T cell antigen receptor signaling and immunological synapse stability require myosin IIA. Nat Immunol 10:531–539

Irles C, Symons A, Michel F, Bakker TR, van der Merwe PA, Acuto O (2003) CD45 ectodomain controls interaction with GEMs and Lck activity for optimal TCR signaling. Nat Immunol 4:189–197

Jacobelli J, Chmura SA, Buxton DB, Davis MM, Krummel MF (2004) A single class II myosin modulates T cell motility and stopping, but not synapse formation. Nat Immunol 5:531–538

Johnson KG, Bromley SK, Dustin ML, Thomas ML (2000) A supramolecular basis for CD45 tyrosine phosphatase regulation in sustained T cell activation. Proc Natl Acad Sci USA 97:10138–10143

Judd BA, Myung PS, Obergfell A, Myers EE, Cheng AM, Watson SP, Pear WS, Allman D, Shattil SJ, Koretzky GA (2002) Differential requirement for LAT and SLP-76 in GPVI versus T cell receptor signaling. J Exp Med 195:705–717

Jurdic P, Saltel F, Chabadel A, Destaing O (2006) Podosome and sealing zone: specificity of the osteoclast model. Eur J Cell Biol 85:195–202

Kaizuka Y, Douglass AD, Varma R, Dustin ML, Vale RD (2007) Mechanisms for segregating T cell receptor and adhesion molecules during immunological synapse formation in Jurkat T cells. Proc Natl Acad Sci USA 104:20296–20301

Kaizuka Y, Douglass AD, Vardhana S, Dustin ML, Vale RD (2009) The coreceptor CD2 uses plasma membrane microdomains to transduce signals in T cells. J Cell Biol 185:521–534

Kliche S, Breitling D, Togni M, Pusch R, Heuer K, Wang X, Freund C, Kasirer-Friede A, Menasche G, Koretzky GA, Schraven B (2006) The ADAP/SKAP55 signaling module regulates T-cell receptor-mediated integrin activation through plasma membrane targeting of Rap1. Mol Cell Biol 26:7130–7144

Koretzky GA, Abtahian F, Silverman MA (2006) SLP76 and SLP65: complex regulation of signalling in lymphocytes and beyond. Nat Rev Immunol 6:67–78

Krummel MF, Davis MM (2002) Dynamics of the immunological synapse: finding, establishing and solidifying a connection. Curr Opin Immunol 14:66–74

Krummel MF, Macara I (2006) Maintenance and modulation of T cell polarity. Nat Immunol 7:1143–1149

Krummel MF, Sjaastad MD, Wulfing C, Davis MM (2000) Differential clustering of CD4 and CD3zeta during T cell recognition. Science 289:1349–1352

Ku GM, Yablonski D, Manser E, Lim L, Weiss A (2001) A PAK1-PIX-PKL complex is activated by the T-cell receptor independent of Nck, Slp-76 and LAT. EMBO J 20:457–465

Kuhne MR, Lin J, Yablonski D, Mollenauer MN, Ehrlich LI, Huppa J, Davis MM, Weiss A (2003) Linker for activation of T cells, zeta-associated protein-70, and Src homology 2 domain-containing leukocyte protein-76 are required for TCR-induced microtubule-organizing center polarization. J Immunol 171:860–866

Kuhns MS, Davis MM, Garcia KC (2006) Deconstructing the form and function of the TCR/CD3 complex. Immunity 24:133–139

Labno CM, Lewis CM, You D, Leung DW, Takesono A, Kamberos N, Seth A, Finkelstein LD, Rosen MK, Schwartzberg PL, Burkhardt JK (2003) Itk functions to control actin polymerization at the immune synapse through localized activation of Cdc42 and WASP. Curr Biol 13:1619–1624

Lee KH, Holdorf AD, Dustin ML, Chan AC, Allen PM, Shaw AS (2002) T cell receptor signaling precedes immunological synapse formation. Science 295:1539–1542

Lee KH, Dinner AR, Tu C, Campi G, Raychaudhuri S, Varma R, Sims TN, Burack WR, Wu H, Wang J, Kanagawa O, Markiewicz M, Allen PM, Dustin ML, Chakraborty AK, Shaw AS (2003) The immunological synapse balances T cell receptor signaling and degradation. Science 302:1218–1222

Lee HS, Lim CJ, Puzon-McLaughlin W, Shattil SJ, Ginsberg MH (2009) RIAM activates integrins by linking talin to ras GTPase membrane-targeting sequences. J Biol Chem 284:5119–5127

Leupin O, Zaru R, Laroche T, Muller S, Valitutti S (2000) Exclusion of CD45 from the T-cell receptor signaling area in antigen-stimulated T lymphocytes. Curr Biol 10:277–280

Lillemeier BF, Pfeiffer JR, Surviladze Z, Wilson BS, Davis MM (2006) Plasma membrane-associated proteins are clustered into islands attached to the cytoskeleton. Proc Natl Acad Sci USA 103:18992–18997

Lin J, Weiss A (2003) The tyrosine phosphatase CD148 is excluded from the immunologic synapse and down-regulates prolonged T cell signaling. J Cell Biol 162:673–682

Ludford-Menting MJ, Oliaro J, Sacirbegovic F, Cheah ET, Pedersen N, Thomas SJ, Pasam A, Iazzolino R, Dow LE, Waterhouse NJ, Murphy A, Ellis S, Smyth MJ, Kershaw MH, Darcy PK, Humbert PO, Russell SM (2005) A network of PDZ-containing proteins regulates T cell polarity and morphology during migration and immunological synapse formation. Immunity 22:737–748

Luxenburg C, Geblinger D, Klein E, Anderson K, Hanein D, Geiger B, Addadi L (2007) The architecture of the adhesive apparatus of cultured osteoclasts: from podosome formation to sealing zone assembly. PLoS ONE 2:e179

Ma Z, Sharp KA, Janmey PA, Finkel TH (2008) Surface-anchored monomeric agonist pMHCs alone trigger TCR with high sensitivity. PLoS Biol 6:e43

McKeithan TW (1995) Kinetic proofreading in T-cell receptor signal transduction. Proc Natl Acad Sci USA 92:5042–5046

Menasche G, Kliche S, Chen EJ, Stradal TE, Schraven B, Koretzky G (2007) RIAM links the ADAP/SKAP-55 signaling module to Rap1, facilitating T-cell-receptor-mediated integrin activation. Mol Cell Biol 27:4070–4081

Milstein O, Tseng SY, Starr T, Llodra J, Nans A, Liu M, Wild MK, van der Merwe PA, Stokes DL, Reisner Y, Dustin ML (2008) Nanoscale increases in CD2-CD48-mediated intermembrane spacing decrease adhesion and reorganize the immunological synapse. J Biol Chem 283: 34414–34422

Mittelbrunn M, Molina A, Escribese MM, Yanez-Mo M, Escudero E, Ursa A, Tejedor R, Mampaso F, Sanchez-Madrid F (2004) VLA-4 integrin concentrates at the peripheral supramolecular activation complex of the immune synapse and drives T helper 1 responses. Proc Natl Acad Sci USA 101:11058–11063

Monks CRF, Kupfer H, Tamir I, Barlow A, Kupfer A (1997) Selective activation of protein kinase C-θ during T cell activation. Nature 385:83–86

Monks CR, Freiberg BA, Kupfer H, Sciaky N, Kupfer A (1998) Three-dimensional segregation of supramolecular activation clusters in T cells. Nature 395:82–86

Moon JJ, Chu HH, Pepper M, McSorley SJ, Jameson SC, Kedl RM, Jenkins MK (2007) Naive CD4(+) T cell frequency varies for different epitopes and predicts repertoire diversity and response magnitude. Immunity 27:203–213

Morin NA, Oakes PW, Hyun YM, Lee D, Chin YE, King MR, Springer TA, Shimaoka M, Tang JX, Reichner JS, Kim M (2008) Nonmuscle myosin heavy chain IIA mediates integrin LFA-1 de-adhesion during T lymphocyte migration. J Exp Med 205:195–205

Mossman KD, Campi G, Groves JT, Dustin ML (2005) Altered TCR signaling from geometrically repatterned immunological synapses. Science 310:1191–1193

Negulescu PA, Krasieva TB, Khan A, Kerschbaum HH, Cahalan MD (1996) Polarity of T cell shape, motility, and sensitivity to antigen. Immunity 4:421–430

Newbrough SA, Mocsai A, Clemens RA, Wu JN, Silverman MA, Singer AL, Lowell CA, Koretzky GA (2003) SLP-76 regulates Fcgamma receptor and integrin signaling in neutrophils. Immunity 19:761–769

Nguyen K, Sylvain NR, Bunnell SC (2008) T cell costimulation via the integrin VLA-4 inhibits the actin-dependent centralization of signaling microclusters containing the adaptor SLP-76. Immunity 28:810–821

Nijhara R, van Hennik PB, Gignac ML, Kruhlak MJ, Hordijk PL, Delon J, Shaw S (2004) Rac1 mediates collapse of microvilli on chemokine-activated T lymphocytes. J Immunol 173:4985–4993

Nolz JC, Gomez TS, Zhu P, Li S, Medeiros RB, Shimizu Y, Burkhardt JK, Freedman BD, Billadeau DD (2006) The WAVE2 complex regulates actin cytoskeletal reorganization and CRAC-mediated calcium entry during T cell activation. Curr Biol 16:24–34

Nolz JC, Medeiros RB, Mitchell JS, Zhu P, Freedman BD, Shimizu Y, Billadeau DD (2007) WAVE2 regulates high-affinity integrin binding by recruiting vinculin and talin to the immunological synapse. Mol Cell Biol 27:5986–6000

Park EY, Smith MJ, Stropp ES, Snapp KR, DiVietro JA, Walker WF, Schmidtke DW, Diamond SL, Lawrence MB (2002) Comparison of PSGL-1 microbead and neutrophil rolling: microvillus elongation stabilizes P-selectin bond clusters. Biophys J 82:1835–1847

Petri B, Bixel MG (2006) Molecular events during leukocyte diapedesis. Febs J 273:4399–4407

Ponti A, Machacek M, Gupton SL, Waterman-Storer CM, Danuser G (2004) Two distinct actin networks drive the protrusion of migrating cells. Science 305:1782–1786

Potter TA, Grebe K, Freiberg B, Kupfer A (2001) Formation of supramolecular activation clusters on fresh ex vivo CD8+ T cells after engagement of the T cell antigen receptor and CD8 by antigen-presenting cells. Proc Natl Acad Sci USA 98:12624–12629

Quann EJ, Merino E, Furuta T, Huse M (2009) Localized diacylglycerol drives the polarization of the microtubule-organizing center in T cells. Nat Immunol 10:627–635

Rozdzial MM, Malissen B, Finkel TH (1995) Tyrosine-phosphorylated T cell receptor zeta chain associates with the actin cytoskeleton upon activation of mature T lymphocytes. Immunity 3:623–633

Rozdzial MM, Pleiman CM, Cambier JC, Finkel TH (1998) pp 56Lck mediates TCR zeta-chain binding to the microfilament cytoskeleton. J Immunol 161:5491–5499

Rudd CE (2008) The reverse stop-signal model for CTLA4 function. Nat Rev Immunol 8:153–160

Samaniego R, Sanchez-Martin L, Estecha A, Sanchez-Mateos P (2007) Rho/ROCK and myosin II control the polarized distribution of endocytic clathrin structures at the uropod of moving T lymphocytes. J Cell Sci 120:3534–3543

Sanchez-Madrid F, Serrador JM (2009) Bringing up the rear: defining the roles of the uropod. Nat Rev Mol Cell Biol 10:353–359

Schwartzberg PL, Mueller KL, Qi H, Cannons JL (2009) SLAM receptors and SAP influence lymphocyte interactions, development and function. Nat Rev Immunol 9:39–46

Seminario MC, Bunnell SC (2008) Signal initiation in T-cell receptor microclusters. Immunol Rev 221:90–106

Shaw AS (2001) FERMing up the synapse. Immunity 15:683–686

Shaw AS (2006) Lipid rafts: now you see them, now you don't. Nat Immunol 7:1139–1142

Shaw A, Dustin ML (1997) Making the T cell receptor go the distance: a topological view of T cell activation. Immunity 6:361–369

Silverman MA, Shoag J, Wu J, Koretzky GA (2006) Disruption of SLP-76 interaction with Gads inhibits dynamic clustering of SLP-76 and FcepsilonRI signaling in mast cells. Mol Cell Biol 26:1826–1838

Singer AL, Bunnell SC, Obstfeld AE, Jordan MS, Wu JN, Myung PS, Samelson LE, Koretzky GA (2004) Roles of the proline-rich domain in SLP-76 subcellular localization and T cell function. J Biol Chem 279:15481–15490

Singleton K, Parvaze N, Dama KR, Chen KS, Jennings P, Purtic B, Sjaastad MD, Gilpin C, Davis MM, Wulfing C (2006) A large T cell invagination with CD2 enrichment resets receptor engagement in the immunological synapse. J Immunol 177:4402–4413

Snapp KR, Heitzig CE, Kansas GS (2002) Attachment of the PSGL-1 cytoplasmic domain to the actin cytoskeleton is essential for leukocyte rolling on P-selectin. Blood 99:4494–4502

Sohn HW, Tolar P, Pierce SK (2008) Membrane heterogeneities in the formation of B cell receptor-Lyn kinase microclusters and the immune synapse. J Cell Biol 182:367–379

Springer TA (1990) Adhesion receptors of the immune system. Nature 346:425–434

Springer TA (1994) Traffic signals for lymphocyte recirculation and leukocyte emigration: the multistep paradigm. Cell 76:301–314

Stefanova I, Hemmer B, Vergelli M, Martin R, Biddison WE, Germain RN (2003) TCR ligand discrimination is enforced by competing ERK positive and SHP-1 negative feedback pathways. Nat Immunol 4:248–254

Stinchcombe JC, Bossi G, Booth S, Griffiths GM (2001) The immunological synapse of CTL contains a secretory domain and membrane bridges. Immunity 15:751–761

Thauland TJ, Koguchi Y, Wetzel SA, Dustin ML, Parker DC (2008) Th1 and Th2 cells form morphologically distinct immunological synapses. J Immunol 181:393–399

Tolar P, Hanna J, Krueger PD, Pierce SK (2009) The constant region of the membrane immunoglobulin mediates B cell-receptor clustering and signaling in response to membrane antigens. Immunity 30:44–55

Tomasevic N, Jia Z, Russell A, Fujii T, Hartman JJ, Clancy S, Wang M, Beraud C, Wood KW, Sakowicz R (2007) Differential regulation of WASP and N-WASP by Cdc42, Rac1, Nck, and PI(4, 5)P2. Biochemistry 46:3494–3502

Treanor B, Lanigan PM, Kumar S, Dunsby C, Munro I, Auksorius E, Culley FJ, Purbhoo MA, Phillips D, Neil MA, Burshtyn DN, French PM, Davis DM (2006) Microclusters of inhibitory killer immunoglobulin-like receptor signaling at natural killer cell immunological synapses. J Cell Biol 174:153–161

Tseng SY, Liu M, Dustin ML (2005) CD80 cytoplasmic domain controls localization of CD28, CTLA-4, and protein kinase Ctheta in the immunological synapse. J Immunol 175:7829–7836

Tskvitaria-Fuller I, Rozelle AL, Yin HL, Wulfing C (2003) Regulation of sustained actin dynamics by the TCR and costimulation as a mechanism of receptor localization. J Immunol 171:2287–2295

Tskvitaria-Fuller I, Seth A, Mistry N, Gu H, Rosen MK, Wulfing C (2006) Specific patterns of Cdc42 activity are related to distinct elements of T cell polarization. J Immunol 177:1708–1720

Valitutti S, Muller S, Cella M, Padovan E, Lanzavecchia A (1995) Serial triggering of many T-cell receptors by a few peptide-MHC complexes. Nature 375:148–151

van der Merwe PA, Davis SJ, Shaw AS, Dustin ML (2000) Cytoskeletal polarization and redistribution of cell-surface molecules during T cell antigen recognition. Semin Immunol 12:5–21

Varma R, Campi G, Yokosuka T, Saito T, Dustin ML (2006) T cell receptor-proximal signals are sustained in peripheral microclusters and terminated in the central supramolecular activation cluster. Immunity 25:117–127

Weber M, Treanor B, Depoil D, Shinohara H, Harwood NE, Hikida M, Kurosaki T, Batista FD (2008) Phospholipase C-gamma2 and Vav cooperate within signaling microclusters to propagate B cell spreading in response to membrane-bound antigen. J Exp Med 205:853–868

Wilson BS, Pfeiffer JR, Oliver JM (2000) Observing FcepsilonRI signaling from the inside of the mast cell membrane. J Cell Biol 149:1131–1142

Wilson BS, Pfeiffer JR, Surviladze Z, Gaudet EA, Oliver JM (2001) High resolution mapping of mast cell membranes reveals primary and secondary domains of Fc(epsilon)RI and LAT. J Cell Biol 154:645–658

Wulfing C, Davis MM (1998) A receptor/cytoskeletal movement triggered by costimulation during T cell activation. Science 282:2266–2269

Yokosuka T, Saito T (2009) Dynamic regulation of T-cell costimulation through TCR-CD28 microclusters. Immunol Rev 229:27–40

Yokosuka T, Sakata-Sogawa K, Kobayashi W, Hiroshima M, Hashimoto-Tane A, Tokunaga M, Dustin ML, Saito T (2005) Newly generated T cell receptor microclusters initiate and sustain T cell activation by recruitment of Zap70 and SLP-76. Nat Immunol 6:1253–1262

Yokosuka T, Kobayashi W, Sakata-Sogawa K, Takamatsu M, Hashimoto-Tane A, Dustin ML, Tokunaga M, Saito T (2008) Spatiotemporal regulation of T cell costimulation by TCR-CD28 microclusters and protein kinase C theta translocation. Immunity 29:589–601

Zipfel PA, Bunnell SC, Witherow DS, Gu JJ, Chislock EM, Ring C, Pendergast AM (2006) Role for the Abi/wave protein complex in T cell receptor-mediated proliferation and cytoskeletal remodeling. Curr Biol 16:35–46

A Conformation-Induced Oligomerization Model for B cell Receptor Microclustering and Signaling

Pavel Tolar and Susan K. Pierce

Contents

Abstract The B cell receptor (BCR) generates both antigen-independent and dependent intracellular signals that are essential for B cell development and antibody responses against pathogens. However, the molecular mechanisms underlying the initiation of BCR signaling are not understood completely yet. The advent of new imaging technologies is allowing the earliest events in B cell signaling to be viewed both in vivo in lymphoid tissues and in vitro in living cells, in real-time, down to the single molecule level. Here we review recent progress in the use of these technologies to decipher the earliest events that follow B cell antigen recognition. Based on recent data using these techniques, we propose a model for the initiation of BCR signaling in which the binding of antigen induces a conformational change in the BCR's extracellular domains leading to BCR oligomerization and signaling.

P. Tolar and S.K. Pierce (✉)
Laboratory of Immunogenetics, National Institute of Allergy and Infectious Diseases, National Institutes of Health, Rockville, MD 20852, USA
e-mail: spierce@niaid.nih.gov

T. Saito and F.D. Batista (eds.), *Immunological Synapse*,
Current Topics in Microbiology and Immunology 340,
DOI 10.1007/978-3-642-03858-7_8, © Springer-Verlag Berlin Heidelberg 2010

We conclude that testing this model will require an in-depth understanding of the unique structural and organizational features of the BCR in the plasma membrane of living B cells in the presence and absence of antigen.

1   Introduction

A hallmark of adaptive immunity is the production of highly specific, high-affinity antibodies that serve to eliminate pathogens from the host. The production of antibodies is triggered by direct recognition of antigens by the clonally distributed B cell antigen receptors (BCRs) expressed on B cell surfaces. Once bound to antigens, the BCR triggers a sequence of intracellular signaling events and the internalization of antigens, which ultimately result in B cell proliferation and differentiation into plasma cells secreting antibodies (Reth 1992). In addition to the antigen-induced initiation of antibody responses, the BCR also generates what are believed to be antigen-independent signals that are important for the development and homeostasis of B cells. In pre-B cells, the expression of the pre-BCR, containing a surrogate light chain, leads to clustering of the pre-BCR and the commencement of the development of the pre-B cells into mature B cells (Bankovich et al. 2007; Ohnishi and Melchers 2003). In resting mature B cells, the BCR produces continuous low level "tonic signals" that are critical for B cell survival (Campbell 1999; Monroe 2006). With such a wide range of functions of the BCR, the molecular mechanism of initiation of BCR signaling is likely to be both intricate and interesting.

The BCR is a multichain receptor composed of a membrane form of immunoglobulin (mIg) and a heterodimer of Igα and Igβ accessory chains (Reth 1992). Although the mIg binds antigens, its short cytoplasmic tails do not directly connect to the B cells signaling machinery. The all-important intracellular signaling and internalization of the antigen–BCR complex are the function of the cytoplasmic domains of the Igα and Igβ chains. Over the last several years, many of the components of the B cell's intracellular signaling cascades have been characterized in considerable detail (Kurosaki 1999). The first proteins that are activated and recruited to the BCR-following antigen binding are members of the Src-family kinases, namely Lyn, Blk, and Fyn (Dal Porto et al. 2004). Src kinases phosphorylate essential tyrosines in the intracellular domains of Igα and Igβ. These tyrosines are part of the immunoreceptor tyrosine-based activation motives (ITAMs), and once phosphorylated they bind the SH2 domains of the kinase Syk. The activation of the Src-kinases and Syk triggers signaling cascades that involve the activation of at least four major signaling pathways, including phospholipase C, the Rho family of GTPases, Ras, and phosphatidylinositol-3-kinase (Campbell 1999; Kurosaki 1999). In addition, the initial signaling also triggers internalization of the BCR–antigen complex into intracellular compartments where the antigen is processed and presented on MHC class II molecules.

Although the downstream signaling pathways that connect the phosphorylated BCR Igα and Igβ chains to B cell activation are becoming well characterized, the initial molecular events that follow antigen binding to the BCR and lead to ITAM phosphorylation still remain largely obscured. Understanding the molecular mechanisms by which antigen binding to the BCR ectodomains is transduced to the intracellular domains of the BCR's Igα and β chains to initiate ITAM phosphorylation is essential to fully comprehend the function and regulation of the BCR both in antibody responses and in development. The key aspects of B cell biology that are inherently dependent on the function of the BCR include the ability of B cells to recognize and respond to the universe of foreign antigen structures that confront the immune system; the ability of B cells to discriminate the affinity of antigen binding to promote the development of high-affinity B cells; the modulation of BCR signaling by coreceptors; and the BCR's generation of antigen-independent tonic signals.

The first unique aspect of the BCR is that it is a clonally distributed receptor with an extraordinary diverse repertoire generated by random recombination of V region genes encoding the antigen-binding domains of the mIg. Through this diverse repertoire, B cells are able to respond to an enormous array of antigen structures ranging from components of the bacterial cell wall to small chemical compounds. The ability to respond to such a variety of ligands differing in their structure, size, and valency is a unique property of B cell immunity and is critical for antibody function. However, this property of the BCR raises a fundamental question concerning the mechanism by which signaling is initiated: namely, how does the binding of the universe of foreign antigens by BCRs ultimately engage the common mechanism of ITAM phosphorylation? In this context, understanding the mechanism of BCR activation may provide a molecular basis for the broad recognition of antigens by the BCRs.

A second unique aspect of the B cell response to antigen is the B cells' ability to discriminate the affinity of the interaction of the antigen with the BCR (Batista and Neuberger 1998). Affinity discrimination is essential for the affinity maturation of antibodies through iterative cycles of somatic hypermutation and antigen-driven selection, ensuring that antibodies have sufficient affinity for the pathogens or their products to prevent disease. The affinities that BCRs can discriminate are in the range of 10^{-6}–10^{-10} M (Batista and Neuberger 1998). Presumably, BCR signaling is sensitive to the affinity of the BCR–antigen interaction because the longer the half-life of the BCR–antigen complex, the longer the time the cytoplasmic domains have to initiate intracellular signaling. However, the mechanism by which the BCR discriminates such a wide range of affinities is not clear. It is particularly puzzling how affinity maturation occurs in response to multivalent antigens. The avidity of the binding of the bivalent BCR to multivalent antigens that contain many epitopes will provide a large advantage during affinity maturation over BCR binding to monovalent antigens containing only a single epitope. However, the high-avidity interaction may quickly reach the ceiling of the affinity discrimination range, leading to lower than desired affinities of the IgG secreted antibodies that cannot benefit from the avidity effect. Thus, understanding the mechanism of BCR activation will likely have important consequences for our understanding of the generation of high-affinity antibodies and ultimately aid in vaccine design.

Third, B cell responses appear to be both positively and negatively regulated at multiple levels. B cell coreceptors that interact with the BCRs on the cell surface and modulate BCR signaling, depending on the context of the antigen or the state of the B cell, play an important role for this regulation. Recent studies focusing on CD19 and the FcγRIIB (Depoil et al. 2008; Sohn et al. 2008a) illustrated that to understand how coreceptors interact with the BCR, we will need to understand the localization and structure of the activated BCR and as well as that of the coreceptors on the B cell surface. A clearer understanding of this process may reveal new strategies to modulate BCR signaling.

Fourth, an essential feature of the BCR is its ability to propagate tonic signals required for B cell survival in the apparent absence of antigen binding. In this pro-survival signaling, the BCR cooperates with the BAFF receptor (Stadanlick et al. 2008). Abrogation of either the BCR or the BAFF receptor leads to B cell death (Thompson et al. 2000; Kraus et al. 2004; Batten et al. 2000). Conversely, excessive signaling from the BAFF receptor leads to B cell hyperplasia and autoimmunity (Thien et al. 2004). It is possible that a similar dysregulation of the BCR's pro-survival signaling may lead to diseases. For example, there are indications that BCR signaling is required for the survival of certain types of B cell lymphomas (Shaffer et al. 2002). Presumably, a better understanding of the mechanisms by which the BCR initiates tonic signals could provide opportunities to regulate B cell fate under pathological conditions.

Collectively, these examples illustrate that knowledge of the molecular mechanisms that underlie the activation of the BCR will ultimately be required to gain an in-depth understanding of how B cells develop and how antibody responses are generated. An important step in our effort to understand BCR signaling is to learn more about how B cells recognize antigens in vivo and how the binding of the antigens to the BCR in living B cells leads to intracellular signaling. Here we describe a new picture of BCR activation that is emerging from the use of recently developed imaging technologies. By looking at living B cells both in vivo in lymphoid tissue and as single cells in vitro, these new approaches offer a view of the activation of B cells that was not possible before. Hopefully, learning about the BCR activation in live B cells in real time will lend insights into how the BCR functions in development and how antigen binding activates the BCR and triggers antibody responses.

2 How B Cells See Antigens In Vivo

Although a considerable amount has been learned about the mechanisms of BCR activation from studies of B cells stimulated with soluble antigens in vitro, studying B cell interacting with antigens in vivo in specialized microenvironments of the lymphoid tissues will be essential to gain a full understanding of how B cells recognize and are activated by antigens. B cells enter lymph nodes through the high endothelial venules in the paracortex and then rapidly move through cortex and B cell follicles localized underneath the lymph node capsule (Tarlinton and Lew 2007). Recently, using two-photon intravital imaging techniques, several groups were able to look inside lymph nodes and directly observe B cells engaging their antigens. Within minutes of injection of fluorescently labeled small soluble antigens in the periphery, the antigens were detected in B cell follicles, suggesting that small, soluble antigens have the ability to specifically enter the follicles and activate follicular B cells (Pape et al. 2007). In contrast, particulate antigens, such as virions and immune complexes, trafficking through the lymph were efficiently captured by a subset of macrophages lining the floor of the subcapsular sinus. Translocating the antigens from the subcapsular sinus into the lymph node cortex, the macrophages presented the antigens to B cells migrating through the cortex. This resulted in rapid accumulation and activation of B cells at the subcapsular sinus (Carrasco and Batista 2007; Phan et al. 2007; Junt et al. 2007).

In addition to the contacts with the subcapsular macrophages, B cells were also seen to engage antigens that had been carried into the lymph node by dendritic cells (DCs) (Qi et al. 2006). It is well established that DCs arriving from the periphery present processed antigens to T cells in the T-cell zone of the lymph node. However, unprocessed native antigen was also detected on the DC surfaces and these DC were able to stimulate B cells that migrated through the T-cell zone after they entered the lymph node through the high endothelial venules. These remarkable findings collectively indicate that antigen presenting cells (APCs) actively assist B cells in antigen recognition in vivo. Although at present we do not know how the antigens are captured and presented to B cells by APCs, it is likely that the B cell–APC contact represents a critical step in B cell activation in vivo, at least for some forms of antigens. These observations point to the importance of understanding how B cells respond to antigens presented in cellular contacts with APCs.

3 Imaging B cell Interactions with Antigen In Vitro: Defining the B cell Immune Synapse

Earlier work from Batista and colleagues showed that B cells avidly respond to antigens presented on the surface of APCs (Batista et al. 2001). When binding membrane antigens, B cells form a highly organized contact area called the immunological synapse that resembles synapses observed in T cells and NK cells engaging their APC or target cells. The B cell immunological synapse is composed of a central aggregate of the antigen-engaged BCRs, called the cSMAC. Surrounding the cSMAC is a ring of adhesion molecules called the pSMAC, which includes the LFA-1–ICAM-1 pair. Evidence was also provided that during formation of the immunological synapse, B cells are not only activated to signal but also to extracted and internalized antigen from the presenting cells. These seminal findings suggested that the organization of the BCR in the immunological synapse is important for BCR activation and antigen internalization.

In more recent studies, Batista et al. showed that B cell activation and immune synapse formation can also be observed in B cells interacting with antigens anchored to planar lipid bilayers, providing an experimental system that offered better resolution of the initial steps of the contact of the B cell with the antigen (Carrasco et al. 2004; Fleire et al. 2006; Weber et al. 2008). These studies showed that after B cells touch antigen-containing bilayers in a few contact points, they initiate a BCR-signaling-and actin-dependent spreading that allows the B cells to reach over the antigen-containing bilayer and collect a large number of antigens. The first contact and spreading of the B cells results in the formation of micro-clusters containing the antigen-engaged BCR. The BCR microclusters stream along actin fibers to the center of the synapse, where they accumulate to form the cSMAC. The spreading of the B cells is short-lived, however, and is quickly followed by contraction that collects all the BCR-bound antigen to the cSMAC. These remarkable observations indicated that the recognition of antigens presented by APCs is a much more active process than previously thought. Because the amount of antigen that the B cells engages depends on the spreading, which in turn is fueled by BCR signaling, B cell spreading provides a positive feedback on the BCR-mediated collection of antigens. This feedback amplifies the differences in the collection of antigens of variable affinity for the BCR and improves the B cell's ability to discriminate between low- and high-affinity antigens (Fleire et al. 2006).

Detailed observations of BCR microclusters as they first formed showed that they assembled almost exclusively at the sites of initial contact of the B cell with the antigen-containing membrane and in the peripheral lamellopodia of the spreading B cells (Fleire et al. 2006; Tolar et al. 2009). This is despite the fact that there are BCRs available on the B cell body and antigen available on the corresponding areas of the presenting membrane. In the case of lamellopodia, the new contacts occurred through the cycles of lamellopodia lifting, protruding, and adhering with the antigen-presenting membrane. It is possible that the curvature of the membrane in the contact sites leads to confinement of the BCRs bound to antigens at a certain distance from the presenting membrane. Diffusion of new BCRs into this contact point and their binding would thus create a high concentration of the engaged BCRs promoting BCR clustering.

Although the resolution to observe microcluster formation has been achieved only for imaging B cells in vitro, it is reasonable to think that similar mechanisms promote BCR microclustering in B cells engaging antigen on APC in vivo as they migrate through lymphoid tissues. Likely, the spreading of B cells is similar to the common mechanism by which cells form adhesion contacts. The mechanical activity of the lamellopodia is a result of a coordination of actin polymerization and actin–myosin contraction (Giannone et al. 2007). Eventually, pulling on the adhesion sites results in strengthening of the adhesion sites, and a similar effect may result in compacting the BCRs in microclusters (Smith et al. 2008). Consistent with this idea, disruption of the actin cytoskeleton in lymphocytes reduces the ability of the immunoreceptors to form microclusters (Arana et al. 2008).

4   Models for the Mechanisms by Which BCRs Cluster

The observation that BCRs form microclusters in the first steps of the immune synapse formation suggests that BCR microclusters may be the B cell's elementary signaling units. Indeed, imaging of intracellular signaling molecules in living B cells showed that the formation of the BCR microclusters is followed within seconds by recruitment of Lyn and Syk to the clusters and the initiation of calcium signaling through PLCγ$_2$ (Fleire et al. 2006; Weber et al. 2008; Sohn et al. 2008b). The proposal that the BCR microclusters are the structures in which BCR signaling occurs begs the questions as to how these structures are formed and what we can learn about the initiation of BCR signaling from the mechanism of their formation.

The current prevailing model for BCR clustering and activation is one we will refer to as the "crosslinking model." A shared feature of soluble antigens that are able to stimulate B cells is that they are multivalent, containing multiple BCR epitopes (Brezski and Monroe 2008). Although there is some controversy (Kim et al. 2006), most data confirm that for responses to soluble antigens, the BCRs must be crosslinked by the engagement of multiple binding sites on the antigen molecules (Metzger 1992). These data suggest that binding of multivalent antigens crosslinks the BCRs inducing clustering of the cytoplasmic domains of the BCRs. Proximity of the cytoplasmic domains of two or more clustered BCRs would allow recruitment of Src-kinases and phosphorylation of the ITAMs by mechanisms that have yet to be delineated. The notion that BCR crosslinking by multivalent antigen initiates signaling was reinforced by the crystal structures of antibodies showing that binding of soluble antigens does not propagate any conformational changes from the antigen binding site to the constant domains that could initiate signaling of the BCR. In addition, the requirement for crosslinking of the BCR to initiate signaling was compatible with the ability of related ITAM containing receptors to signal only after crosslinking by multivalent ligands (Metzger 1992). However, in the case of the BCR, the requirement for crosslinking does not explain B cell responses to small, relatively soluble antigens, such as toxins. Also, B cells produce antibodies to rapidly diffusing cell membrane components, such as phospholipids, that cannot directly crosslink the BCR for any significant period of time. In addition, not all oligomeric antigens may be able to crosslink the BCR into a configuration that would bring the cytoplasmic domains of the clustered BCRs into physical proximity (Reth et al. 2000).

In the context of these limitations of the crosslinking model, an alternative explanation of the requirement for multivalency of soluble antigens warrants consideration. Reth and colleagues proposed that multivalent antigens disrupt an auto-inhibited configuration of the BCR present in preformed BCR clusters (Reth et al. 2000). According to this "permissive geometry" model (Minguet and Schamel 2008), the binding of the antigens reorganizes the BCRs in the clusters into an active geometry. In this model, the individual BCRs do not change conformation but rather reorient one to another to trigger signaling. Alternatively, it is possible that the binding of antigen leads to a conformational change in the BCR

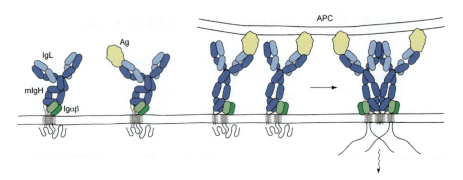

Fig. 1 Schematic illustration of the "conformation-induced oligomerization" model for B cell receptor (BCR) signaling. The BCR is preferentially in a closed, inactive conformation in resting cells. Binding of monovalent soluble antigen does not change the conformation of the BCR and does not induce signaling. Binding of membrane antigens pulls the BCR's ectodomains into an active conformation exposing an oligomerization interface in the membrane proximal region of the membrane immunoglobulin. Assembly of the BCR oligomer leads to perturbations of the local lipid environment, opening of the cytoplasmic domains and the initiation of signaling

ectodomains on the cell surface that promotes oligomerization, clustering, and signaling. We refer to this model as the "conformation-induced oligomerization" model (Fig. 1). In the following sections we discuss this model in greater detail and describe new single molecule imaging techniques that are providing evidence in support of the model. We then discuss how this model accommodates key aspects of B cell biology.

5   Insights into the Mechanism of BCR Microcluster Formation from Single Molecule Imaging

To analyze the molecular mechanism by which the BCRs assemble into microclusters in more detail, we recently developed imaging techniques to observe individual BCRs during microcluster formation (Tolar et al. 2009). To observe single BCR molecules, we labeled a small proportion of the BCR on the surface of B cells with fluorescent Fab fragments of Ig-specific antibodies. Under these conditions, individual labeled BCR could be observed in B cells spreading on bilayers containing antigens by total internal reflection microscopy (TIRF). The BCRs could be tracked for up to a few seconds, which is long enough to observe their behavior as they form microclusters. Using this imaging technique, we found that BCRs in resting cells were mostly mobile on the cell surface. However, during spreading of the B cells on the antigen-coated bilayers, BCRs immobilized as they formed microclusters. Surprisingly, the immobilization of the clustered BCRs was observed even after the BCR bound to monomeric antigen on the fluid lipid bilayers. This finding indicates that the microclusters form without the need for physical crosslinking of the BCRs. By combining fluorescence resonance energy transfer (FRET) between BCRs tagged in their cytoplasmic domains with FRET donor and acceptor fluorescent proteins with TIRF microscopy, we showed that within the first seconds of microcluster formation the BCRs come into close molecular proximity even though the BCRs were not physically crosslinked by antigen (P. Tolar, unpublished observation).

It is possible that the immobilization of the BCR as it forms microclusters reflects attachment of the BCR to the membrane cytoskeleton or to large complexes of intracellular signaling molecules. However, we found that the immobilization of the BCR in the microclusters was completely independent of the cytoplasmic domains of the BCR or of the presence of the Igαβ subunit (Tolar et al. 2009). Thus, the microclusters are composed of immobile oligomeric arrays of the BCR formed solely through intrinsic properties of the extracellular and transmembrane of domains the mIg. To search for the minimal requirements for the microclustering of the mIg, we carried out mutational studies and showed that the immobilization of the mIg in microclusters induced by antigen binding depends on the presence of the Cμ4 domain as well as on a WTxxST motif in the transmembrane region. Cμ4 is the membrane proximal domain that forms a homodimer at the bottom of the canonical Fc structure shared in all Ig molecules (Herr et al. 2003; Wan et al. 2002; Huber et al. 1976). The WTxxST motif in the N-terminal part of the transmembrane domains is predicted to line the side of the transmembrane helix that is opposite of the putative Igαβ interaction site. Notably, the WTxxST motif-containing side of the transmembrane domain has been previously implicated in the formation of BCR oligomers observed after lysis of B cells with limiting amounts of detergents (Schamel and Reth 2000).

Single molecule imaging showed that the mIgM molecules that lacked the Cμ4 domain and had the mutation of the WTxxST motif still accumulated and were confined in their movement inside of structures similar to microclusters (Tolar et al. 2009). However, they could not immobilize in the microclusters, suggesting that they could not form the oligomeric structures. Measurement of signaling activity of a chimeric receptor consisting of the mutated IgM and intracellular domains of Igα or Igβ showed that the constructs were significantly compromised in the tyrosine phosphorylation in the synapses as well as in the upregulation of CD69. Conversely, the expression of the Cμ4 domain alone, but not larger parts of the Fc region of the mIg, led to spontaneous clustering of the construct. Similar clustering was observed after expression of Cγ3, the membrane proximal domain of IgG. In addition, when expressed with the Igαβ heterodimer, clustering of the Cμ4 domain led to spontaneous recruitment of Syk into these clusters and upregulation of CD69.

These findings are consistent with a model of microcluster formation in which the Cμ4 and the transmembrane region contain a homotypic clustering interface that is not accessible in the mIg in resting B cells. Binding of membrane antigen confines the BCR in the contact areas with the presenting membrane and unmasks the clustering interface in the Cμ4 domain, which together lead to the formation of a BCR oligomer that promotes signaling from the cytoplasmic domains. As mentioned above, we refer to this model as to the "conformation-induced oligomerization model" (Fig. 1).

6   Is There Evidence for Conformation-Induced Oligomerization Predicted by the Model?

How can monovalent membrane antigens binding to the BCRs unmask a clustering interface? As mentioned above, structural studies suggest that it is unlikely that the binding of the antigen propagates conformational changes to the Fc through a direct allosteric mechanism (Metzger 1974). Structural studies as well as electron microscopy also provided no evidence for the clustering of soluble antibodies engaged by soluble antigens (Løset et al. 2004), although the Fc region of antibodies has some role in the formation of immunoprecipitates (Møller and Christiansen 1983; Møller 1979). Nevertheless, it is possible that the binding of a membrane antigen to the BCR induces a change in the Fc region of the Ig indirectly. Stretched by the antigen binding between the B cell membrane and the APC, the BCR could be subjected to a pulling or twisting force. The force could induce conformational changes within the $C\mu4$ and transmembrane domains, leading to formation of a clustering interface as depicted in Fig. 1. Alternatively, the force could induce a reorientation of the $C\mu3$ to allow access to a preformed clustering interface in $C\mu4$ and the transmembrane domains. It is also possible that similar activating changes in the BCR could be induced by soluble multivalent antigens, in which case the force would come from the binding of several BCRs to a single antigen object.

Although the structure of the Fc region of the IgM is not available, numerous structures have been solved of the Fc regions of IgG, IgE, and IgA (Herr et al. 2003; Wan et al. 2002; Huber et al. 1976). The canonical Fc region is composed of two angled Ig domains that pair to form a rhombus. In principle, the Fc region can undergo changes of the interdomain angle, leading to opening and closing of the top of the structure. In the available structures, the opening of the interdomain angle has been observed after binding to Fc receptors (Wurzburg et al. 2000; Radaev et al. 2001). Although these conformational changes are relatively subtle in IgG binding to $Fc\gamma Rs$, they are substantial in IgE binding to $Fc\varepsilon RI$, where the opening is potentially associated with a reorientation of the $C\varepsilon2$ domains (Wan et al. 2002). Interestingly, the changes of the angle between $C\varepsilon3$ and $C\varepsilon4$ domains are propagated to the AB and EF loops of the $C\varepsilon4$ at the bottom and side of the $Fc\varepsilon$. However, whether similar changes may be induced in the IgM and IgG BCR remains unknown. Likely, studying the Ig structure in the context of the full BCR complex will be necessary to better understand these issues.

7   Implications of the "Conformation-Induced Oligomerization" Model for B cell Biology

Although we do not currently understand the structural changes in the BCR that could initiate BCR oligomerization in the microclusters, there are interesting implications of the conformation-induced clustering model that are relevant for B cell biology. Importantly, the presence of a clustering interface in the BCR suggests that microcluster formation is independent of the antigen valency. The homotypic interaction of the membrane proximal and transmembrane domains may thus potentially be important for B cell responses to antigens that do not directly cross-link the BCR, or to antigens that crosslink the BCR into a configuration that does not directly bring the cytoplasmic domains of the BCR into an active configuration. Separately engaged BCRs would in this case associate laterally on the cell surface and bring the BCR into an active conformation by the interaction of their $C\mu4$ domains leading to efficient signaling. Thus, the clustering interface in the BCR could broaden B cell responses to a wider range of antigens. The ability of BCRs to oligomerize and signal following monovalent binding to antigen would also alleviate the problem of avidity in the B cell's discrimination of antigen affinity.

The specific structure of the oligomeric BCR may also contribute to BCR's interaction with membrane signaling adaptors and BCR coreceptors that modulate B cell activation. For example, recent studies showed that the coengagement of the BCR and $Fc\gamma RIIb$ during recognition of membrane-bound immune complexes blocks B cell spreading and the interactions of BCR microclusters with signaling components, suggesting that the $Fc\gamma RIIb$ blocks early steps of BCR activation in the microclusters (Sohn et al. 2008a). In addition, B cell spreading and intracellular signaling in response to membrane antigens requires the recruitment of the positively signaling transmembrane adaptor CD19 (Depoil et al. 2008). CD19 amplifies BCR signaling by recruiting intracellular signaling proteins such as Vav and PI3 kinase to the plasma membrane. While in response to soluble antigens CD19 interacts with the BCR as a part of the CD19–CD21–CD81–TAPA-1 complex that recognizes complement-tagged antigens, the involvement of CD19 in B cell responses to membrane antigens is independent of complement binding and occurs through dynamic interactions of the CD19 directly with BCR microclusters. These examples raise the possibility that the oligomeric BCR is the structure that interacts with positive and negative coreceptors to provide regulation of the earliest steps in B cell activation. Understanding how coreceptors interact with BCR microclusters may lead to new ways to modulate dysregulated B cell responses, particularly in autoimmune diseases.

The intrinsic ability of the BCR to cluster suggests that there may be a low level of spontaneous BCR clustering in resting B cells that may underlie antigen-independent tonic signaling. It is the current prevailing view that tonic BCR signaling is a result of a "leaky" regulation of the BCR's signaling pathways that are inherently at a fine balance between receptor phosphorylation and dephosphorylation (Monroe 2006). However, it is also possible that the tonic signaling is generated from the spontaneous clustering of a small fraction of BCR due to conformational flexibility of the extracellular domains. If so, the tonic signaling would arise from transient, albeit structurally defined BCR clusters. Such spontaneously forming clusters would be of interest as they may be potentially the basis of exaggerated constitutive BCR signaling under pathological conditions. For example, in the rare heavy chain disease, somatic deletions in the V_H-$C\mu2$ region lead to constitutive signaling from the truncated BCR, resulting in a B cell proliferative disorder (Corcos et al. 1991, 1995). It is possible that the truncation of the mIg domains unmasks the clustering interface of the BCR, as we observed in the expression of the isolated Cμ4 domain. It will be interesting to investigate whether the mechanism of BCR clustering contributes to more common diseases such as B cell lymphomas. In this case, understanding the mechanism of formation of BCR clusters may provide a new target for the intervention of the pathological BCR signaling.

8   The Unsolved Problem of Transducing Conformational Changes in the BCR Ectodomains to the Cytoplasmic Domains

Collectively, the data reviewed here suggest that the transition of the resting BCR into its active state involves specific participation of the extracellular and transmembrane regions of the BCR. But how are changes induced by antigen binding in the extracellular domains transduced through the transmembrane domains to the intracellular domains? In vitro, peptides representing the intracellular domains of Igαβ are unstructured, providing little information as to what specific changes may lead to the recruitment of Src-kinases and the phosphorylation of the ITAMs (Sigalov et al. 2004). However, it is not known whether the cytoplasmic domains of the native BCR complex in living cells take on a more defined structure. Using FRET to measure the distance between the BCR's Ig, Igα, and Igβ cytoplasmic domains, we observed that the cytoplasmic domains of the BCRs come into close proximity in the first ~5 s of microcluster formation (Tolar et al. 2005). After that, the FRET between the intracellular domains rapidly drops to a level of FRET that is still higher than the FRET in resting cells. This FRET pattern was observed in cells expressing any combination of BCR chains containing donor and acceptor fluorescent proteins, reporting either inter- or intramolecular BCR chain interactions. The FRET pattern suggests that while the BCRs remained clustered, the cytoplasmic domains opened up. The opening required phosphorylation of the ITAMs, but was independent of the recruitment of Syk or other downstream molecules. Thus, it is possible that in resting BCRs, the cytoplasmic domains of Igα and Igβ are in a closed, folded conformation in which the tyrosines of the ITAMs are not accessible as depicted in Fig. 1. Binding of Src-kinases and/or phosphorylation of the ITAMs stabilizes a new open or unfolded conformation and allows the initiation of downstream signaling.

One mechanism by which the BCR may recruit Src-kinase in the first seconds of microcluster formation is by inducing changes in local lipid composition in the microclusters. Such lipid changes could be induced by perturbation of the membrane by the local concentration of the BCR transmembrane domains, leading to transient trapping of the myristoyl and palmitoyl fatty acid membrane anchor of Src-family kinases. We recently showed by FRET in living cells that the interaction of a probe containing this lipid anchor with the BCR occurs rapidly after the onset of microcluster formation and overlaps with the very initial recruitment of Lyn to the BCR (Sohn et al. 2006, 2008b). The interaction of the lipid probe was transient and limited to nascent microclusters in the periphery of the immune synapse, whereas Lyn interacted with the microclusters during their trafficking to the cSMAC, suggesting that protein–protein interactions, presumably mediated by the SH2 domains binding to phosphorylated ITAMs, stabilize Src-family interaction with the BCR to sustain signaling.

9   Conclusions

Although experimental data are far from providing a complete picture of the mechanisms by which antigen binding activates the BCR, they collectively suggest that our currently incomplete understanding of these mechanisms is due to gaps in our knowledge of the structure and organization of the full BCR complex in living B cells. It will be exciting to watch these gaps being filled in the near future as new technologies allows closer and closer views of the BCR on the B cell surface. Hopefully, the knowledge of the structure of the BCR in the B cell plasma membrane, together with a better understanding of B cell recognition of antigens during an immune response in vivo, will render a clearer picture of BCR activation and the early signaling steps. With much remaining to be learned, the near future may still bring many surprises.

References

Arana E, Vehlow A, Harwood NE, Vigorito E, Henderson R, Turner M, Tybulewicz VL, Batista FD (2008) Activation of the small GTPase Rac2 via the B cell receptor regulates B cell adhesion and immunological-synapse formation. Immunity 28:88–99

Bankovich AJ, Raunser S, Juo ZS, Walz T, Davis MM, Garcia KC (2007) Structural insight into pre-B cell receptor function. Science 316:291–294

Batista FD, Neuberger MS (1998) Affinity dependence of the B cell response to antigen: a threshold, a ceiling, and the importance of off-rate. Immunity 8:751–759

Batista FD, Iber D, Neuberger MS (2001) B cells acquire antigen from target cells after synapse formation. Nature 411:489–494

Batten M, Groom J, Cachero TG, Qian F, Schneider P, Tschopp J, Browning JL, Mackay F (2000) BAFF mediates survival of peripheral immature B lymphocytes. J Exp Med 192:1453

Brezski RJ, Monroe JG (2008) B-cell receptor. Adv Exp Med Biol 640:12–21

Campbell KS (1999) Signal transduction from the B cell antigen-receptor. Curr Opin Immunol 11:256–264

Carrasco YR, Batista FD (2007) B cells acquire particulate antigen in a macrophage-rich area at the boundary between the follicle and the subcapsular sinus of the lymph node. Immunity 27:160–171

Carrasco YR, Fleire SJ, Cameron T, Dustin ML, Batista FD (2004) LFA-1/ICAM-1 interaction lowers the threshold of B cell activation by facilitating B cell adhesion and synapse formation. Immunity 20:589–599

Corcos D, Iglesias A, Dunda O, Bucchini D, Jami J (1991) Allelic exclusion in transgenic mice expressing a heavy chain disease-like human mu protein. Eur J Immunol 21:2711–2716

Corcos D, Dunda O, Butor C, Cesbron JY, Lorès P, Bucchini D, Jami J (1995) Pre-B-cell development in the absence of lambda 5 in transgenic mice expressing a heavy-chain disease protein. Curr Biol 5:1140–1148

Dal Porto JM, Gauld SB, Merrell KT, Mills D, Pugh-Bernard AE, Cambier J (2004) B cell antigen receptor signaling 101. Mol Immunol 41:599–613

Depoil D, Fleire S, Treanor BL, Weber M, Harwood NE, Marchbank KL, Tybulewicz VL, Batista FD (2008) CD19 is essential for B cell activation by promoting B cell receptor-antigen microcluster formation in response to membrane-bound ligand. Nat Immunol 9:63–72

Fleire SJ, Goldman JP, Carrasco YR, Weber M, Bray D, Batista FD (2006) B cell ligand discrimination through a spreading and contraction response. Science 312:738–741

Giannone G, Dubin-Thaler BJ, Rossier O, Cai Y, Chaga O, Jiang G, Beaver W, Dobereiner H-G, Freund Y, Borisy G et al (2007) Lamellipodial actin mechanically links myosin activity with adhesion-site formation. Cell 128:561

Herr AB, Ballister ER, Bjorkman PJ (2003) Insights into IgA-mediated immune responses from the crystal structures of human Fc[alpha]RI and its complex with IgA1-Fc. Nature 423:614

Huber R, Deisenhofer J, Colman PM, Matsushima M, Palm W (1976) Crystallographic structure studies of an IgG molecule and an Fc fragment. Nature 264:415–420

Junt T, Moseman EA, Iannacone M, Massberg S, Lang PA, Boes M, Fink K, Henrickson SE, Shayakhmetov DM, Di Paolo NC et al (2007) Subcapsular sinus macrophages in lymph nodes clear lymph-borne viruses and present them to antiviral B cells. Nature 450:110

Kim YM, Pan JY, Korbel GA, Peperzak V, Boes M, Ploegh HL (2006) Monovalent ligation of the B cell receptor induces receptor activation but fails to promote antigen presentation. Proc Natl Acad Sci USA 103:3327–3332

Kraus M, Alimzhanov MB, Rajewsky N, Rajewsky K (2004) Survival of resting mature B lymphocytes depends on BCR signaling via the Igalpha/beta heterodimer. Cell 117:787–800

Kurosaki T (1999) Genetic analysis of B cell antigen receptor signaling. Annu Rev Immunol 17:555–592

Løset GA, Roux KH, Zhu P, Michaelsen TE, Sandlie I (2004) Differential segmental flexibility and reach dictate the antigen binding mode of chimeric IgD and IgM: implications for the function of the B cell receptor. J Immunol 172:2925–2934

Metzger H (1974) Effect of antigen binding on the properties of antibody. Adv Immunol 18:169–207

Metzger H (1992) Transmembrane signaling: the joy of aggregation. J Immunol 149:1477–1487

Minguet S, Schamel WW (2008) Permissive geometry model. Adv Exp Med Biol 640:113–120

Møller NP (1979) Fc-mediated immune precipitation. I. A new role of the Fc-portion of IgG. Immunology 38:631–640

Møller NP, Christiansen G (1983) Fc-mediated immune precipitation. III. Visualization by electron microscopy. Immunology 48:469–476

Monroe JG (2006) ITAM-mediated tonic signalling through pre-BCR and BCR complexes. Nat Rev Immunol 6:283–294

Ohnishi K, Melchers F (2003) The nonimmunoglobulin portion of lambda5 mediates cell-autonomous pre-B cell receptor signaling. Nat Immunol 4:849–856

Pape KA, Catron DM, Itano AA, Jenkins MK (2007) The humoral immune response is initiated in lymph nodes by B cells that acquire soluble antigen directly in the follicles. Immunity 26:491–502

Phan TG, Grigorova I, Okada T, Cyster JG (2007) Subcapsular encounter and complement-dependent transport of immune complexes by lymph node B cells. Nat Immunol 8:992–1000

Qi H, Egen JG, Huang AY, Germain RN (2006) Extrafollicular activation of lymph node B cells by antigen-bearing dendritic cells. Science 312:1672–1676

Radaev S, Motyka S, Fridman WH, Sautes-Fridman C, Sun PD (2001) The structure of a human type III Fcgamma receptor in complex with Fc. J Biol Chem 276:16469–16477

Reth M (1992) Antigen receptors on B lymphocytes. Annu Rev Immunol 10:97–121

Reth M, Wienands J, Schamel WW (2000) An unsolved problem of the clonal selection theory and the model of an oligomeric B-cell antigen receptor. Immunol Rev 176:10–18

Schamel WW, Reth M (2000) Monomeric and oligomeric complexes of the B cell antigen receptor. Immunity 13:5–14

Shaffer AL, Rosenwald A, Staudt LM (2002) Lymphoid malignancies: the dark side of B-cell differentiation. Nat Rev Immunol 2:920

Sigalov A, Aivazian D, Stern L (2004) Homooligomerization of the cytoplasmic domain of the T cell receptor ζ chain and of other proteins containing the immunoreceptor tyrosine-based activation motif. Biochemistry 43:2049–2061

Smith A, Sengupta K, Goennenwein S, Seifert U, Sackmann E (2008) Force-induced growth of adhesion domains is controlled by receptor mobility. Proc Natl Acad Sci USA 105:6906

Sohn HW, Tolar P, Jin T, Pierce SK (2006) Fluorescence resonance energy transfer in living cells reveals dynamic membrane changes in the initiation of B cell signaling. Proc Natl Acad Sci USA 103:8143–8148

Sohn HW, Pierce SK, Tzeng SJ (2008a) Live cell imaging reveals that the inhibitory FcgammaRIIB destabilizes B cell receptor membrane-lipid interactions and blocks immune synapse formation. J Immunol 180:793–799

Sohn HW, Tolar P, Pierce SK (2008b) Membrane heterogeneities in the formation of B cell receptor-Lyn kinase microclusters and the immune synapse. J Cell Biol 182:367–379

Stadanlick JE, Kaileh M, Karnell FG, Scholz JL, Miller JP, Iii WJQ, Brezski RJ, Treml LS, Jordan KA, Monroe JG et al (2008) Tonic B cell antigen receptor signals supply an NF-l[kappa]lB substrate for prosurvival BLyS signaling. Nat Immunol 9:1379

Tarlinton D, Lew A (2007) Antigen to the node: B cells go native. Immunity 26:388–390

Thien M, Phan TG, Gardam S, Amesbury M, Basten A, Mackay F, Brink R (2004) Excess BAFF rescues self-reactive B cells from peripheral deletion and allows them to enter forbidden follicular and marginal zone niches. Immunity 20:785–798

Thompson JS, Schneider P, Kalled SL, Wang LC (2000) BAFF binds to the tumor necrosis factor receptor-like molecule B cell maturation antigen and IS. J Exp Med 192:129–135

Tolar P, Sohn HW, Pierce SK (2005) The initiation of antigen-induced B cell antigen receptor signaling viewed in living cells by fluorescence resonance energy transfer. Nat Immunol 6:1168

Tolar P, Hanna J, Krueger P, Pierce SK (2009) The constant region of the membrane immunoglobulin mediates B-cell receptor clustering and signaling in response to membrane antigens. Immunity 30:44–55. doi:10.1016/j.immuni.2008.11.007

Wan T, Beavil RL, Fabiane SM, Beavil AJ, Sohi MK, Keown M, Young RJ, Henry AJ, Owens RJ, Gould HJ et al (2002) The crystal structure of IgE Fc reveals an asymmetrically bent conformation. Nat Immunol 3:681–686

Weber M, Treanor B, Depoil D, Shinohara H, Harwood NE, Hikida M, Kurosaki T, Batista FD (2008) Phospholipase C-{gamma}2 and Vav cooperate within signaling microclusters to propagate B cell spreading in response to membrane-bound antigen. J Exp Med 205:1243

Wurzburg BA, Garman SC, Jardetzky TS (2000) Structure of the human IgE-Fc C epsilon 3-C epsilon 4 reveals conformational flexibility in the antibody effector domains. Immunity 13:375–385

Co-Receptors and Recognition of Self at the Immunological Synapse

Nicholas R.J. Gascoigne, Tomasz Zal, Pia P. Yachi, and John A.H. Hoerter

Contents

N.R.J. Gascoigne (✉), T. Zal, P.P. Yachi, and J.A.H. Hoerter
Department of Immunology and Microbial Science, The Scripps Research Institute, 10550 North
Torrey Pines Rd., La Jolla, CA 92037, USA
e-mail: Gascoigne@scripps.edu

Department of Immunology, University of Texas MD Anderson Cancer Center, 7455 Fannin,
Houston, TX 77030, USA

T. Saito and F.D. Batista (eds.), *Immunological Synapse*,
Current Topics in Microbiology and Immunology 340,
DOI 10.1007/978-3-642-03858-7_9, © Springer-Verlag Berlin Heidelberg 2010

Abstract The co-receptors CD4 and CD8 are important in the activation of T cells, primarily because of their ability to interact with the proteins of the MHC, enhancing recognition of the MHC–peptide complex by the T cell receptor (TCR). An antigen-presenting cell presents a small number of antigenic peptides on its MHC molecules, in the presence of a much larger number of endogenous, mostly nonstimulatory, peptides. Recent work has demonstrated that these endogenous MHC–peptide complexes have an important role in modulating the sensitivity of the TCR. But the role of the endogenous nonstimulatory MHC–peptide complexes differs in MHC class I and class II-restricted T cells. This chapter discusses the data on the role of CD4 or CD8 co-receptors in T cell activation at the immunological synapse, and the role of non stimulatory MHC–peptide complexes in aiding antigen recognition.

1   Introduction

The CD4 and CD8 proteins have long been known to be important in antigen recognition, and in the discrimination between antigens presented by MHC class I or class II molecules. Their precise role has been more difficult to elucidate. Recent data suggest that endogenous MHC–peptide complexes are involved in the activation of T cells by antigen, making the T cells more sensitive to low quantities of the antigen. The means by which these endogenous peptides aid in antigen recognition appear to be different in MHC class I and class II-restricted T cells. In this chapter, we review the data on CD4 and CD8 in the immunological synapse, and their apparently different modes of action in aiding TCR activation by limited antigen quantity in the presence of endogenous, nonstimulatory, MHC–peptide complexes.

2   Co-Receptors in the Immunological Synapse

2.1   MHC Recognition by Co-Receptors

CD4 and CD8 can bind to MHC class II or class I respectively, and over-expression of CD4 or CD8 on one cell type allows cell–cell binding to another cell type that overexpresses the relevant MHC molecule (Doyle and Strominger 1987; Norment et al. 1988). However, CD4 and CD8 are not usually thought to have an important role in adhesion in the absence of overexpression. Their main role is believed to be in their ability to act as co-receptors, to bind the MHC at the same time as TCR, and thus stabilize the TCR–MHCp complex. However, while there is clear evidence of this role for CD8, there is no similar evidence for CD4.

Because both CD4 and CD8 bind to the Src-family kinase Lck through their intracellular tails, this causes Lck to be brought into proximity with a TCR that is recognizing antigen, where it kick-starts the signaling cascade. CD4 is believed to be much more efficient at this function by virtue of a stronger interaction with Lck (Hurley et al. 1989).

Although both CD4 and CD8 interact with nonpolymorphic parts of the different MHC molecule classes (König et al. 1992; Moebius et al. 1993; Potter et al. 1989; Salter et al. 1990), they are radically divergent in structure: CD4 has a single polypeptide chain consisting of four immunoglobulin-like domains, of which the most amino-terminal membrane distal domain binds to MHC class II (Wang et al. 2001; Wu et al. 1997). There is some evidence that CD4 molecules can form noncovalent dimers through their membrane-proximal domains, which would result in a protein with the predicted ability to bind and therefore to cross-link two MHC class II proteins (Moldovan et al. 2002; Wu et al. 1997). In contrast, CD8 is an obligate dimer that can consist of $\alpha\alpha$ or $\alpha\beta$ chains, covalently bound to each other. These dimers form a binding site for a single MHC class I protein (Gao et al. 1997; Kern et al. 1998). It is commonly believed that a co-receptor and TCR interact with the same MHC–peptide molecule, but as yet no structure of a complete TCR–MHC–peptide–co-receptor complex has been obtained. The X-ray crystal structures of TCR–MHC–peptide leave room for the TCR to bind; similarly, CD4–MHC–peptide and CD8–MHC–peptide structures also leave room for TCR binding.

The cytoplasmic domain of CD4 has a site for palmitoylation (Crise and Rose 1992), which allows it to associate with lipid microdomains (Balamuth et al. 2004), where Lck is preferentially found. CD8β also has a palmitoylation site, but CD8α does not, so the CD8$\alpha\alpha$ dimer is less likely to associate with lipid microdomains and therefore come into contact with Lck than CD8$\alpha\beta$ (Arcaro et al. 2001). This combination of motif and opportunity may partially explain why CD8$\alpha\beta$ is a stronger co-receptor than CD8$\alpha\alpha$, even though they bind equally well to MHC class I (Garcia et al. 1996).

2.2 Co-Receptor Recruitment to the Immunological Synapse

CD4 and CD8 are recruited to the immunological synapse during antigen recognition (Krummel et al. 2000; Kupfer et al. 1987; Zal et al. 2002) (Fig. 1). This recruitment occurs very fast – within seconds – during antigen recognition, and the movement of co-receptor within the T-cell–APC contact area can be very dynamic (Zal et al. 2002). There is evidence of the co-receptor leaving the synapse while TCR accumulates (Krummel et al. 2000). Although the recruitment of Lck to the synapse requires its interaction with CD4 or CD8, activation of Lck as measured by phosphorylation occurs predominantly at the periphery of the synapse, rather than in the central region (Lee et al. 2002). There is strong evidence that during recognition of strong antigens, TCR forms microclusters in the peripheral synapse. This is where signaling is initiated, with TCR being endocytosed in the central synapse (Varma et al. 2006). However, with weaker stimulation, activated Lck is found in the central regions of the synapse (Cemerski et al. 2008).

In our early experiments on CD4 and TCR movement, we found that CD4 could move to the synapse between a T cell and an antigen presenting cell even when antigen was not available (Fig. 1d) (Zal et al. 2002). Thus the CD4 concentration in the synapse must have been due to the CD4 interaction with class II, irrespective of

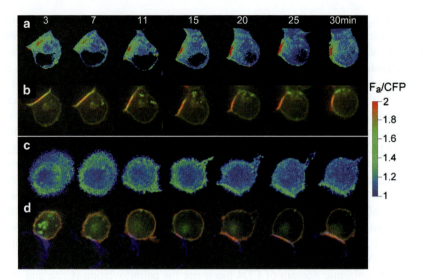

Fig. 1 CD4 co-receptor recruitment to the immunological synapse and FRET between TCR and CD4. (**a**), (**b**) show a time course of interaction between T cell and an APC presenting antigenic peptide. (**c**), (**d**) show the same with an APC that does not present the antigenic peptide. (**a**), (**c**) show the FRET response between CD3ζ–CFP and CD4–YFP, using a heat scale (Zal et al. 2002). (**b**), (**d**) show the fluorescence of the CD3ζ–CFP (*green*) and CD4–YFP (*red*). Only the antigenic stimulation causes close interaction between TCR and CD4, as reported by FRET between CD3ζ–CFP and CD4–YFP (**a** versus **c**), though both APCs recruited CD4 to the immunological synapse (**b** and **d**). Recruitment was much slower in the absence (**d**) versus the presence (**d**) of antigen. Reproduced with permission from Zal et al. (2002)

the peptide presented. This is referred to as noncognate MHC recognition, in contrast to the cognate recognition that is found between TCR and its specific MHC–peptide complex. The noncognate recruitment of CD4 was considerably slower than CD4 recruitment in the presence of antigen (Fig. 1b, d), and did not occur with all antigen-presenting cell types (Gascoigne and Zal 2004; Zal et al. 2002). In contrast, the noncognate recruitment of CD8 showed little difference between the presence and absence of specific antigen (Yachi et al. 2005). This indicated that the noncognate CD8–MHC class I interaction was sufficient to recruit CD8 and presumably MHC class I to the synapse.

3 Co-Receptor Interaction with NonCognate MHC Class I in Antigen Recognition

3.1 NonStimulatory Peptides Aid MHC Class I-Restricted Antigen Recognition by T Cells

Several studies have demonstrated that endogenous nonstimulatory peptides can enhance recognition of antigenic peptides (Krogsgaard et al. 2005; Yachi et al.

2005, 2007). This is particularly noticeable when the antigen is in limiting quantity, and in fact can explain why T cells are sensitive to tiny amounts of antigen – T cells have been reported to respond to a single antigenic peptide (Irvine et al. 2002; Sykulev et al. 1996), with full activation with as little as three (Purbhoo et al. 2004). The mechanism by which the endogenous peptides aid recognition appears to differ between MHC class I and class II-restricted T cells (Gascoigne 2008; Yachi et al. 2005, 2007). Here we will first deal with class I-restricted cells.

The RMA-S cell line is deficient in the *Tap2* gene so peptides are not loaded into the MHC class I molecule as it is folded. In the presence of exogenously added peptides, though, the class I is correctly folded (Ljunggren et al. 1989; Townsend et al. 1989), and at low temperature (~30°C) the class I molecules are folded and expressed at the cell surface without peptide. If the temperature is raised to 37°C, they fall apart (Ljunggren et al. 1990). This phenomenon has been used to load specific peptides onto class I molecules in the presence of very few other peptides – the RMA-S cells are cultured for a period at 30°C, the peptide of interest is added, and culture continued. This allows the peptide to associate with the class I molecule. The temperature is then raised to 37°C to destroy the class I molecules that have not bound peptide. We used this method to load RMA-S cells with titrated amounts of an antigenic peptide. We were able to measure the amount of antigenic class I–peptide complexes by using a specific antibody recognizing this complex (Porgador et al. 1997).

We found that the ability to stimulate T cells, as measured by a number of different parameters, declined steeply as the amount of antigen was reduced (Yachi et al. 2005, 2007). When the titration of antigen was performed in the presence of excess nonstimulatory peptides, the curve was shifted substantially, such that stimulation occurred at much lower concentrations of antigen than in the absence of the nonstimulatory peptides (Fig. 2). Using T hybridoma cells, this was true for the formation of conjugates between the T cells and antigen presenting cells (APCs), for TCR downregulation, and for the induction of close interactions between the TCR–CD3 complex and the co-receptor CD8 using Foerster Resonance Energy Transfer (FRET) microscopy (Yachi et al. 2005). Immature pre-positive selection thymocytes and naïve primary CD8$^+$ T cells also showed lower activation by a given amount of antigen on its own, compared to activation in the presence of nonstimulatory peptides (Yachi et al. 2007). We tested a number of different peptides that are known to bind to the MHC class I molecule (H2–K^b), including a peptide from a virus that does not stimulate the TCR that we tested, and several that are natural endogenously produced K^b–binding peptides that do not stimulate T cells or thymocytes bearing this TCR (Santori et al. 2002). Remarkably, each of the ~10 different peptides that we tested showed roughly equivalent ability to aid in antigen recognition (Yachi et al. 2005, 2007). This ability was demonstrated most strikingly when we loaded the RMA-S cells with a very small amount of antigen and then titrated in the nonstimulatory peptides: the stimulation of the responding T cells correlated with the amount of MHC class I expressed on the RMA-S cell surface (Fig. 3). Indeed, all our data led to the conclusion that

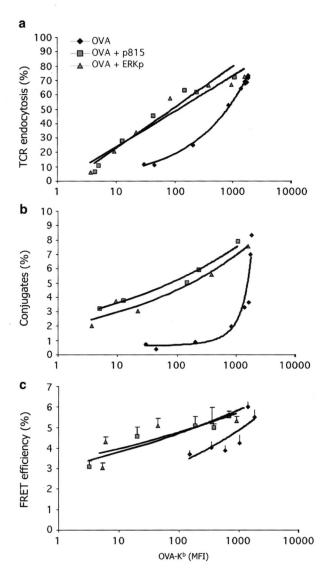

Fig. 2 Increased T-cell activation by endogenous nonstimulatory peptides at limiting antigen quantities. (**a**) shows the amount of TCR endocytosis at differing quantities of antigen OVA–K^b expressed on the cell surface of RMA-S cells, either alone or with added nonstimulatory peptides derived from VSV, Erk, or the P815 tumor antigen. Erk and P815 are natural endogenous K^b– binding peptides (Santori et al. 2002). (**b**) shows the percentage of T cells in conjugates with RMA-S cells treated as in (**a**). (**c**) shows the interaction between TCR and CD8 by the FRET signal between CD3ζ–CFP and CD8β–YFP. Used with permission from Yachi et al. (2005)

the important factor in the role of the endogenous/nonstimulatory peptides in aiding antigen recognition is in fact due to the expression of the MHC class I protein, rather than to the specific peptide that it presents.

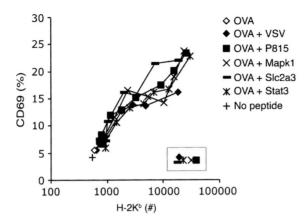

Fig. 3 The ability of nonstimulatory MHC–peptide ligands to enhance antigen recognition depends on their quantity rather than their sequence. A small amount of antigen was added to RMA-S cells (OVA). This resulted in very low expression of the epitope for the anti-OVA–K^b. Other nonstimulatory peptides were titrated in to increase the overall amount of K^b expression. This increased expression of K^b correlated with increased activation of thymocytes. Used with permission from Yachi et al. (2007)

Evidence from other labs also supports these findings. Early data showed an adhesion function of mouse CD8 in binding to noncognate MHC class I, after antigenic stimulation (O'Rourke et al. 1990), and this was recently confirmed for human CD8–MHC class I interactions (Varghese and Kane 2008). Interestingly, the effector memory cells and activated CTL, but not the naïve $CD8^+$ T cells, showed this antigen-enhancement of CD8–class I binding (Varghese and Kane 2008).

In a different experimental system, MHC class I–peptide complexes were bound as arrays of about ten molecules to quantum dots (Anikeeva et al. 2006). These were able to activate CTL as long as at least one of the class I molecules presented the antigenic peptide. If all ten had a nonstimulatory peptide, then there was no activation. The role of the nonstimulatory MHC–peptide complexes was to bind to CD8, as they did not promote recognition of a single antigenic MHC–peptide if they were mutated at the CD8 binding site (Anikeeva et al. 2006).

It must be noted that there are some reports that failed to show an effect of the endogenous MHC class I in aiding T-cell activation by antigen. In an experiment similar to our own, Sporri and Reis e Sousa (2002) compared T-cell activation by the Tap-sufficient RMA parental line with Tap-deficient RMA-S. The responses to RMA-S were strong enough and the authors concluded that the lack of endogenous peptides on the RMA-S cells did not affect stimulation by antigenic peptide (Sporri and Reis e Sousa 2002). When we performed the same experiment, we found significant difference between activation by RMA-S and RMA – the RMA cells induced stronger activation of T cells than did the RMA-S cells for the same amount of antigenic peptide (Fig. 4) (Yachi et al. 2007). Our main set of experiments, however, was to compare RMA-S cells with antigen plus or minus nonstimulatory peptides. Thus we were comparing the same cells, using the

Fig. 4 Endogenous peptides on RMA cells support antigen recognition. RMA and RMA-S cells were incubated with titrated amounts of antigen (OVA peptide) and used to stimulate naïve CD8$^+$ T cells expressing the OT-I anti-OVA–K^b TCR. CD69 upregulation was assessed as a function of expression of the OVA–K^b epitope recognized by the 25-D1.16 mAb (Porgador et al. 1997). Used with permission from Yachi et al. (2007)

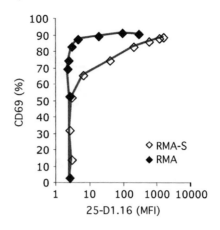

anti-K^b–peptide antibody (Porgador et al. 1997) to measure the amount of antigenic MHC–peptide on the cell surface, comparing the response to the same amount of antigen in the presence or absence of other exogenously added nonstimulatory peptides. This is probably a better way to assay the role of the nonstimulatory peptides than relying on the endogenously produced peptides of the RMA cells. Also, the RMA and RMA-S cells have been separated for over 20 years and may have other, more subtle, differences.

We conclude that the nonstimulatory peptides have a real effect on MHC class I-antigen recognition. It may have been overlooked in some studies because of the high sensitivity of the responding T cells which can show a response to small quantities of antigenic peptide alone. This may be because of the small but real number of endogenous peptides – derived from signal peptidase activity on nascent transmembrane and secreted proteins – that are expressed on the RMA-S cells.

3.2 The FRET Response Between CD8 and TCR–CD3, and What It Tells Us About the Role of Endogenous Peptides in T-Cell Activation

Our studies on T-cell activation by low amounts of antigen in the presence or absence of endogenous/nonstimulatory peptides included the rather surprising result that FRET between the fluorescently labeled CD3ζ–CFP and CD8β–YFP was enhanced by the presence of these nonstimulatory peptides (Fig. 2) (Yachi et al. 2005). This FRET response, like that between CD3ζ–CFP and CD4–YFP in an MHC class II-restricted T cell, is a measure of the close apposition of the CD4 or CD8 co-receptor to the TCR/CD3 complex – presumably the TCR that is interacting with the antigenic MHC–peptide complex (Gascoigne and Zal 2004; Yachi et al. 2005, 2006; Zal and Gascoigne 2004a,b; Zal et al. 2002). This means that the

Fig. 5 Models of co-receptor function in T-cell activation. For consistency, these are all drawn using CD8 as the co-receptor. However, the pseudodimer model (**b**) is derived from studies of CD4+ MHC class II-restricted T cells (Krogsgaard et al. 2005). (**a**) The "classical" model where the co-receptor stabilizes the interaction between TCR and antigenic MHC–peptide. (**b**) The "pseudodimer" model, where co-receptor cross-links two TCRs, one interacting with antigenic MHC–peptide, and the other interacting with endogenous MHC–peptide. (**c**) The "pre-concentration" model, where the co-receptor interaction with antigenic or nonstimulatory MHC–peptide causes concentration of MHC–peptide, co-receptor, and Lck to the synapse

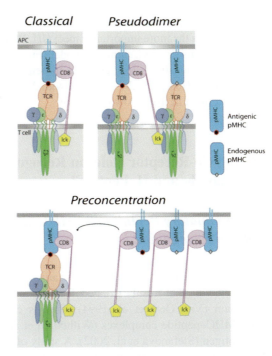

noncognate CD8–MHC class I interaction was somehow enhancing the cognate TCR–CD8 interaction induced by antigen (Fig. 2) (Yachi et al. 2005).

This suggested to us that the role of the noncognate CD8–MHC class I interaction is to concentrate the MHC class I and the CD8 (and therefore also Lck) proteins ("Pre-concentration model," Fig. 5). Either of these would have the overall effect of increasing antigen recognition and the cognate TCR–CD3–CD8 interaction. Concentration of MHC class I molecules would make it quicker and more efficient for the TCR to "find" the antigenic MHC class I–peptide amongst the mass of the nonstimulatory class I proteins. The on rate of the interaction is concentration-dependent, and the k_{on} of a TCR–MHC–peptide interaction (as measured in solution) can have a significant effect on the biological outcome of TCR recognition, even if the k_{off} has a larger influence overall (Alam et al. 1996, 1999; Gascoigne et al. 2001; Rosette et al. 2001; Stone et al. 2009). Thus the TCR would bind to MHC–peptide at a faster rate, the off rate remaining unchanged, so the TCR would sort through the available MHC–peptide complexes until it associates with one to which it binds more strongly. Looking at this pre-concentration model from the point of view of concentration of the CD8–Lck, the CD8 is more available to stabilize the TCR interaction with antigenic MHC–peptide, and the Lck similarly is more available to start the signaling cascade. Obviously, these two mechanisms are not mutually exclusive. We have some preliminary data indicating that the concentration of CD8/Lck is the more important aspect (JH, PPY and NRJG, unpublished).

We believe that this pre-concentration model (Fig. 5) is sufficient to explain our data on endogenous/nonstimulatory peptides in helping T-cell activation by small amounts of peptide. However, the situation with MHC class II-restricted cells is different, as described in the following sections.

4 Differing Co-Receptor Roles in Recognition of Endogenous MHC Class I– and II–Peptide?

4.1 NonStimulatory Peptides Aid MHC Class II-Restricted Antigen Recognition by T Cells

The initial idea of aid for antigen recognition caused by endogenous peptides came from studies showing that freshly isolated T cells show partial phosphorylation of the CD3ζ chain (Van Oers et al. 1994). This is caused by interactions with endogenous MHC–peptide complexes (Witherden et al. 2000), and enhances recognition of antigen (Stefanova et al. 2002). A study of the immunological synapse found that during antigen recognition, endogenous as well as antigenic MHC class II–peptide complexes became concentrated at the synapse (Wulfing et al. 2002).

This finding was greatly extended by showing that a set of endogenous nonstimulatory peptides were concentrated to the synapse during antigen recognition (Krogsgaard et al. 2005). Soluble dimers of MHC class II molecules bound to these endogenous peptides did not stimulate the T cells to flux Ca^{2+}, whereas dimers of the antigenic peptide did stimulate the T cells. When mixed MHC class II dimers were made with one antigenic peptide and one endogenous peptide, stimulation was achieved by a subset of the endogenous peptides, indicating that these endogenous peptides were able to enhance recognition of the antigen. Similar results were obtained with peptides added to cells expressing "empty" MHC class II molecules, to which peptides were added in a manner analogous to the RMA-S experiments described for class I experiments above (Krogsgaard et al. 2005). These data, like those obtained for the MHC class I-restricted response, indicated that recognition of endogenous nonstimulatory peptides aids antigen recognition. However, there is a fundamental difference in that only a subset of the endogenous nonstimulatory MHC class II–peptide complexes worked in this way (Krogsgaard et al. 2005), whereas all of the tested endogenous nonstimulatory MHC class I–peptide complexes functioned to help antigen recognition (Yachi et al. 2005; Yachi et al. 2007). There synapse-recruitment of the endogenous nonstimulatory MHC class II–peptide complexes was TCR rather than CD4-dependent (Wulfing et al. 2002), whereas our data show it to be CD8 rather than TCR-dependent for the class I system.

Krogsgaard also tested the importance of the CD4–MHC class II interaction in stimulation by antigen plus endogenous peptide, finding that when they mutated the

CD4-binding site of MHC class II for the molecule presenting antigen, stimulation was abolished. When they mutated this site on the endogenous peptide-presenting molecule, stimulation was not abolished. Taking account of these data and the finding that a single antigenic peptide can stimulate T cells (in the presence of endogenous peptides on an APC) (Irvine et al. 2002), these authors proposed a "pseudodimer" model for T-cell activation (Fig. 5). In this model, the extracellular, membrane-distal, domains of CD4 bind to the antigenic MHC peptide complex, which is bound by a TCR. The intracellular region of CD4, with Lck, is associated with the intracellular portion of another TCR molecule, in this case interacting with the nonstimulatory endogenous MHC–peptide complex. Thus the CD4 bridges two TCRs bound to two different species of MHC class II–peptide complexes. This model suggests that the TCR that is bound to the endogenous MHC–peptide, rather than the one bound to the antigenic MHC–peptide, is the one that will be phosphorylated.

4.2 Predictions and Tests of the Pseudodimer and Pre-Concentration Models

The pseudodimer model of T-cell activation predicts that the strength of agonist affects the ability of the endogenous nonstimulatory peptides to aid its recognition. Thus, the weaker the agonist (i.e., the faster the off rate of the TCR–MHC–peptide interaction), the smaller the proportion of the different endogenous peptides that would be able to act as co-agonists (Krogsgaard et al. 2005; Li et al. 2004). In contrast, the pre-concentration model predicts that the ability of the endogenous nonstimulatory peptides to aid recognition will not be reduced as the agonist strength decreases, as pre-concentration requires only that the co-receptor–MHC–peptide interaction be active.

Evidence has been forthcoming to support the prediction of the pseudodimer model in an MHC class II-restricted system. More of the tested endogenous peptides were able to help recognition of a strong agonist than were able to help recognition of a weaker agonist (Krogsgaard et al. 2005; Li et al. 2004). We performed a similar experiment in our MHC class I-restricted system. Recognition of the original antigen (as the strong agonist) was compared to three weaker agonists of varying strengths. We found that the recognition of each of the weaker agonists was aided by all of the different nonstimulatory peptides that we tested (Fig. 6) (Yachi et al. 2007). Indeed, we found that recognition of weak ligands was more reliant on recognition of the nonstimulatory MHC–peptides. These data indicate that for $CD8^+$ cells, the role of the endogenous nonstimulatory peptides is not through formation of a TCR pseudodimer, although we have not formally ruled out any contribution from the TCR interaction with the nonstimulatory MHC–peptide complexes. As noted above (Fig. 3), the endogenous nonstimulatory peptides seem to work in RMA-S cells by their ability to stabilize expression of MHC class I proteins.

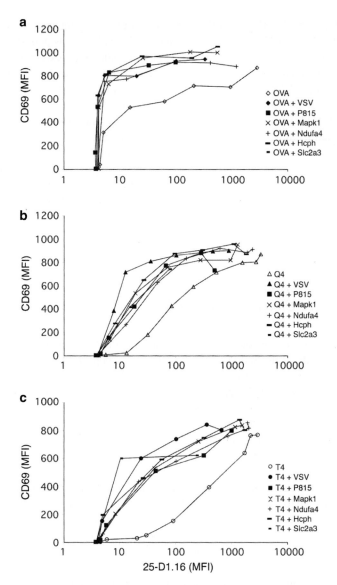

Fig. 6 The ability of nonstimulatory peptides to enhance antigen-recognition is independent of agonist strength. RMA-S cells were loaded with titrated amounts of antigen (OVA; **a**), a weaker agonist (Q4; **b**) or a very weak agonist (T4; **c**) in the absence or presence of various endogenous K^b-binding, OT-I nonstimulatory peptides (Santori et al. 2002). The upregulation of CD69 on pre-positive selection thymocytes from OT-I transgenic Tap$^{-/-}$ mice was assessed and expressed in relation to the expression of the OVA–K^b epitope of mAb 25-D1.16 mAb (Porgador et al. 1997). Used with permission from Yachi et al. (2007)

We are now taking an approach to studying the nonstimulatory peptides where single-chain MHC class I–peptide complexes (Yu et al. 2002) are used in the absence of other class I molecules. This allows us to mutate the CD8-binding site or a TCR-binding site in the antigenic or the nonstimulatory MHC class I–peptide complex. Our preliminary data indicate that the nonstimulatory MHC class I–peptide complex must be able to interact with CD8 for it to aid in antigen recognition, and also that reactivity to antigenic peptide on a nonCD8–binding MHC class I molecule can occur with high expression of a nonstimulatory CD8–binding class I–peptide complex (JH, PPY, NRJG, in progress).

This information leads us to the conclusion that for MHC class I-restricted T cells, at least, the data are adequately explained by the pre-concentration model (Yachi et al. 2005, 2007). As this is simpler than the pseudodimer model, Ockham's razor causes us to prefer the pre-concentration model. In any event, data from the MHC class I-restricted system do not follow the predictions of the pseudodimer model. Results from an MHC class II system seem to support the pseudodimer model, however. This suggests a fundamental difference between the role of the co-receptors in the MHC class I and class II-restricted cells.

4.3 Different Roles for CD4 and CD8 Co-Receptors in Endogenous Peptide Recognition

CD8 has a higher affinity for MHC class I than CD4 has for MHC class II. Most workers have been unable to measure the CD4–class II interaction, while that of CD8–class I is relatively well defined (Gao et al. 1997; Garcia et al. 1996; Kern et al. 1998; van der Merwe and Davis 2003). Experiments on binding of MHC tetramers to T cells find that the CD8–MHC class I interaction enhances tetramer-binding, but no CD4–class II interaction is detectable in this manner (Boniface et al. 1998; Bosselut et al. 2000; Crawford et al. 1998; Daniels and Jameson 2000; Kerry et al. 2003). Can this explain the difference in the role of the endogenous nonstimulatory peptides?

In thymocyte development, the tipping-point of affinity where the weakest negative-selecting ligands turn into positive selecting ligands (Alam et al. 1996) appears to be similar to the affinity of the CD8–MHC class I interaction (Daniels et al. 2006; Naeher et al. 2007). This has led to the suggestion that the affinity of the CD8–MHC class I interaction, being higher than that of the TCR interaction with nonstimulatory endogenous ligands, is the "affinity driver" for the molecular interactions in the synapse, with the implication that it occurs before the TCR–class I interaction (Gascoigne 2008). In contrast, the affinity of the class II-restricted TCR for the nonstimulatory MHC class II–peptide (being stronger than the CD4–class II interaction) is the affinity driver, implying that the TCR–class II interaction would occur before CD4–class II. Certainly, the TCR has some affinity for MHC proteins that is encoded in the CDR1 and CDR2 of the α- and β-chains (Dai et al. 2008; Sim et al. 1996, 1998; Zerrahn et al. 1997).

4.4 Does Co-Receptor–MHC Interaction Precede or Follow TCR Recognition of pMHC?

The noncognate CD8–MHC class I interaction has been shown to be enhanced by initial recognition of cognate antigen-MHC by the TCR (O'Rourke et al. 1990; Varghese and Kane 2008). However, we found that CD8 became concentrated at the synapse between a T cell and an APC in the absence of any antigenic stimulation (Yachi et al. 2005, 2006). We could even find CD8 recruitment to the synapse when we used a T-cell hybridoma lacking TCR (P.P.Y., unpublished). When we titrated the amount of peptide on the RMA-S cells - whether antigenic or nonstimulatory - we found that the amount of CD8 concentrated to the synapse correlated with the number of MHC class I molecules (Yachi et al. 2005). This data suggested that the CD8 interaction with MHC class I occurs independently of TCR recognition of antigen. Structural data (Gao et al. 1997; Kern et al. 1998) and the fact that noncognate MHC class I tetramers can bind to T cells, albeit weakly (Bosselut et al. 2000; Daniels et al. 2006), support this idea. Recent fluorescence correlation measurements of lateral diffusion rates indicate that the TCR interaction with antigenic MHC class I–peptide is preceded by the CD8–MHC class I interaction and that this aids in binding of MHC class I–peptide to TCR (Gakamsky et al. 2005).

In the case of the CD4 class II interaction, we also demonstrated that CD4 becomes concentrated at the immunological synapse and that this occurred without the presence of antigen, although its recruitment was more efficient when antigen was present (Fig. 1b, d) (Zal et al. 2002).

It is possible that recognition of antigen causes a qualitatively different interaction between CD8 and MHC class I to occur. In the past we suggested that the CD4–MHC class II interaction could set up an energetic barrier to TCR interaction with the class II molecule, such that only a TCR with a higher affinity than the CD4–class II interaction would be able to displace CD4 and therefore make the antigen-specific interaction (Gascoigne and Zal 2004; Zal et al. 2002). This could explain data showing that CD4 becomes excluded from the synapse even while TCR becomes concentrated within the synapse (Krummel et al. 2000).

4.5 Adhesion and TCR Cross-Linking in T-Cell Activation

There are several studies that showed that T cells could be activated by monomeric antigenic MHC–peptide complexes (Delon et al. 1998; Doucey et al. 2003; Ma et al. 2008; Randriamampita et al. 2003), in marked contrast to other studies showing that cross-linking was necessary (Boniface et al. 1998; Cochran et al. 2000). These data can be reconciled by the observation that all studies showing activation by monomeric MHC–peptide used systems where the T cells were stimulated on immobilized substrates, whereas the studies demonstrating a requirement for cross-linking all used soluble MHC–peptide complexes (Randriamampita et al. 2003). The mechanism by which this works is that adhesion leads to a transient increase in cyclic AMP, which in turn leads to Erk activation, sensitizing the T cell for the monomeric MHC–peptide stimulation (Conche et al. 2009). Immobilization of MHC–peptide has also been shown to occur as a result of an interaction between MHC class I molecules and ICAM1, causing concentration of both antigenic and nonstimulatory MHC class I–peptide complexes in the immunological synapse, and leading to increased T cell activation (Segura et al. 2008). These data suggest that part of the role of the nonstimulatory MHC–peptide complexes is to aid in the cell adhesion, which in turn aids the priming of the T cells.

5 Concluding Remarks

The emergence of T-cell recognition of endogenous peptides in the activation of T cells by antigen is a fascinating aspect of the immune system's importance in distinguishing self from nonself. In the old "needle in the haystack" metaphor, it shows the importance of the haystack in the search for the needle, in that the individual straws of hay appear to enhance the ability of the T cell to be stimulated by the needle, when it is finally encountered. The mechanism by which this occurs appears to be different in MHC class I and class II-restricted T cells. In the former, the CD8–MHC interaction appears to drive the formation of complexes that allow faster scanning through the MHC–peptide complexes by the TCR, or better concentration of co-receptor and Lck, or both. In the latter, the TCR–MHC–peptide interaction seems to be stable enough to drive cross-linking of TCRs by CD4 in a pseudodimer.

Acknowledgments Work from this lab was funded by the NIH (R01GM065230 and AI074074 to N.R.J.G. and K22AI065688 to T.Z.). P.P.Y was supported by T32HL07195 and T.Z by T32AI07290. J.H. was supported by NIH T32AI007244 and the Irving S. Sigal Fellowship. This is TSRI manuscript number 20016.

References

Alam SM, Travers PJ, Wung JL, Nasholds W, Redpath S, Jameson SC, Gascoigne NRJ (1996) T cell receptor affinity and thymocyte positive selection. Nature 381:616–620
Alam SM, Davies GM, Lin CM, Zal T, Nasholds W, Jameson SC, Hogquist KA, Gascoigne NRJ, Travers PJ (1999) Qualitative and quantitative differences in T cell receptor binding of agonist and antagonist ligands. Immunity 10:227–237
Anikeeva N, Lebedeva T, Clapp AR, Goldman ER, Dustin ML, Mattoussi H, Sykulev Y (2006) Quantum dot/peptide-MHC biosensors reveal strong CD8-dependent cooperation between self and viral antigens that augment the T cell response. Proc Natl Acad Sci USA 103: 16846–16851

Arcaro A, Gregoire C, Bakker TR, Baldi L, Jordan M, Goffin L, Boucheron N, Wurm F, van der Merwe PA, Malissen B et al (2001) CD8β endows CD8 with efficient coreceptor function by coupling T cell receptor/CD3 to raft-associated CD8/p56(lck) complexes. J Exp Med 194:1485–1495

Balamuth F, Brogdon JL, Bottomly K (2004) CD4 raft association and signaling regulate molecular clustering at the immunological synapse site. J Immunol 172:5887–5892

Boniface JJ, Rabinowitz JD, Wulfing C, Hampl J, Reich Z, Altman JD, Kantor RM, Beeson C, McConnell HM, Davis MM (1998) Initiation of signal transduction through the T cell receptor requires the multivalent engagement of peptide/MHC ligands. Immunity 9:459–466

Bosselut R, Kubo S, Guinter T, Kopacz JL, Altman JD, Feigenbaum L, Singer A (2000) Role of CD8b domains in CD8 coreceptor function: importance for MHC I binding, signaling, and positive selection of CD8+ T cells in the thymus. Immunity 12:409–418

Cemerski S, Das J, Giurisato E, Markiewicz MA, Allen PM, Chakraborty AK, Shaw AS (2008) The balance between T cell receptor signaling and degradation at the center of the immunological synapse is determined by antigen quality. Immunity 29:414–422

Cochran JR, Cameron TO, Stern LJ (2000) The relationship of MHC-peptide binding and T cell activation probed using chemically defined MHC class II oligomers. Immunity 12:241–250

Conche C, Boulla G, Trautmann A, Randriamampita C (2009) T cell adhesion primes antigen receptor-induced calcium responses through a transient rise in adenosine 3′, 5′-cyclic monophosphate. Immunity 30:33–43

Crawford F, Kozono H, White J, Marrack P, Kappler J (1998) Detection of antigen-specific T cells with multivalent soluble class II MHC covalent peptide complexes. Immunity 8:675–682

Crise B, Rose JK (1992) Identification of palmitoylation sites on CD4, the human immunodeficiency virus receptor. J Biol Chem 267:13593–13597

Dai S, Huseby ES, Rubtsova K, Scott-Browne J, Crawford F, Macdonald WA, Marrack P, Kappler JW (2008) Crossreactive T Cells spotlight the germline rules for αβ T cell-receptor interactions with MHC molecules. Immunity 28:324–334

Daniels MA, Jameson SC (2000) Critical role for CD8 in T cell receptor binding and activation by peptide/major histocompatibility complex multimers. J Exp Med 191:335–346

Daniels MA, Teixeiro E, Gill J, Hausmann B, Roubaty D, Holmberg K, Werlen G, Hollander GA, Gascoigne NRJ, Palmer E (2006) Thymic selection threshold defined by compartmentalization of Ras/MAPK signalling. Nature 444:724–729

Delon J, Gregoire C, Malissen B, Darche S, Lemaitre F, Kourilsky P, Abastado J-P, Trautmann A (1998) CD8 expression allows T cell signaling by monomeric peptide-MHC complexes. Immunity 9:467–473

Doucey MA, Legler DF, Faroudi M, Boucheron N, Baumgaertner P, Naeher D, Cebecauer M, Hudrisier D, Ruegg C, Palmer E et al (2003) The β₁ and β₃ integrins promote T cell receptor-mediated cytotoxic T lymphocyte activation. J Biol Chem 278:26983–26991

Doyle C, Strominger JL (1987) Interaction between CD4 and class II MHC molecules mediates cell adhesion. Nature 330:256–259

Gakamsky DM, Luescher IF, Pramanik A, Kopito RB, Lemonnier F, Vogel H, Rigler R, Pecht I (2005) CD8 kinetically promotes ligand binding to the T-cell antigen receptor. Biophys J 89:2121–2133

Gao GF, Tormo J, Gerth UC, Wyer JR, McMichael AJ, Stuart DI, Bell JI, Jones EY, Jakobsen BK (1997) Crystal structure of the human CD8αα and HLA-A2. Nature 387:630–634

Garcia KC, Scott CA, Brunmark A, Carbone FR, Peterson PA, Wilson IA, Teyton L (1996) CD8 enhances formation of stable T-cell receptor/MHC class I molecule complexes. Nature 384:577–581

Gascoigne NRJ (2008) Do T cells need endogenous peptides for activation? Nat Rev Immunol 8:895–900

Gascoigne NRJ, Zal T (2004) Molecular interactions at the T cell-antigen-presenting cell interface. Curr Opin Immunol 16:114–119

Gascoigne NRJ, Zal T, Alam SM (2001) T-cell receptor binding kinetics in T-cell development and activation. Exp Rev Mol Med 2001:1–17 http://www.expertreviews.org/01002502h.htm

Hurley TR, Luo K, Sefton BM (1989) Activators of protein kinase C induce dissociation of CD4, but not CD8, from p56lck. Science 245:407–409

Irvine DJ, Purbhoo MA, Krogsgaard M, Davis MM (2002) Direct observation of ligand recognition by T cells. Nature 419:845–849

Kern PS, Teng MK, Smolyar A, Liu JH, Liu J, Hussey RE, Spoerl R, Chang HC, Reinherz EL, Wang JH (1998) Structural basis of CD8 coreceptor function revealed by crystallographic analysis of a murine CD8αα ectodomain fragment in complex with H-2K^b. Immunity 9: 519–530

Kerry SE, Buslepp J, Cramer LA, Maile R, Hensley LL, Nielsen AI, Kavathas P, Vilen BJ, Collins EJ, Frelinger JA (2003) Interplay between TCR affinity and necessity of coreceptor ligation: high-affinity peptide-MHC/TCR interaction overcomes lack of CD8 engagement. J Immunol 171:4493–4503

König R, Huang L-Y, Germain RN (1992) MHC class II interaction with CD4 mediated by a region analogous to the MHC class I binding site for CD8. Nature 356:796–798

Krogsgaard M, Li QJ, Sumen C, Huppa JB, Huse M, Davis MM (2005) Agonist/endogenous peptide-MHC heterodimers drive T cell activation and sensitivity. Nature 434:238–243

Krummel MF, Sjaastad MD, Wülfing C, Davis MM (2000) Differential clustering of CD4 and CD3ζ during T cell recognition. Science 289:1349–1352

Kupfer A, Singer SJ, Janeway CA Jr, Swain SL (1987) Coclustering of CD4 (L3T4) molecule with the T cell receptor is induced by specific direct interaction of helper T cells and antigen-presenting cells. Proc Natl Acad Sci USA 84:5888–5892

Lee KH, Holdorf AD, Dustin ML, Chan AC, Allen PM, Shaw AS (2002) T cell receptor signaling precedes immunological synapse formation. Science 295:1539–1542

Li QJ, Dinner AR, Qi S, Irvine DJ, Huppa JB, Davis MM, Chakraborty AK (2004) CD4 enhances T cell sensitivity to antigen by coordinating Lck accumulation at the immunological synapse. Nat Immunol 5:791–799

Ljunggren HG, Paabo S, Cochet M, Kling G, Kourilsky P, Karre K (1989) Molecular analysis of H-2-deficient lymphoma lines. Distinct defects in biosynthesis and association of MHC class I heavy chains and β2-microglobulin observed in cells with increased sensitivity to NK cell lysis. J Immunol 142:2911–2917

Ljunggren HG, Stam NJ, Ohlen C, Neefjes JJ, Hoglund P, Heemels MT, Bastin J, Schumacher TN, Townsend A, Karre K et al (1990) Empty MHC class I molecules come out in the cold. Nature 346:476–480

Ma Z, Sharp KA, Janmey PA, Finkel TH (2008) Surface-anchored monomeric agonist pMHCs alone trigger TCR with high sensitivity. PLoS Biol 6:e43

Moebius U, Pallai P, Harrison SC, Reinherz EL (1993) Delineation of an extended surface contact area on human CD4 involved in class II major histocompatibility complex binding. Proc Natl Acad Sci USA 90:8259–8263

Moldovan MC, Yachou A, Levesque K, Wu H, Hendrickson WA, Cohen EA, Sekaly RP (2002) CD4 dimers constitute the functional component required for T cell activation. J Immunol 169:6261–6268

Naeher D, Daniels MA, Hausmann B, Guillaume P, Luescher I, Palmer E (2007) A constant affinity threshold for T cell tolerance. J Exp Med 204:2553–2559

Norment AM, Salter RD, Parham P, Engelhard VH, Littman DR (1988) Cell-cell adhesion mediated by CD8 and MHC class I molecules. Nature 336:79–81

O'Rourke AM, Rogers J, Mescher MF (1990) Activated CD8 binding to class I protein mediated by the T cell receptor results in signalling. Nature 346:187–189

Porgador A, Yewdell JW, Deng Y, Bennink JR, Germain RN (1997) Localization, quantitation, and in situ detection of specific peptide–MHC class I complexes using a monoclonal antibody. Immunity 6:715–726

Potter TA, Rajan TV, Dick RF II, Bluestone JA (1989) Substitution at residue 227 of H-2 class I molecules abrogates recognition by CD8-dependent, but not CD8-independent, cytotoxic T lymphocytes. Nature 337:73–75

Purbhoo MA, Irvine DJ, Huppa JB, Davis MM (2004) T cell killing does not require the formation of a stable mature immunological synapse. Nat Immunol 5:524–530

Randriamampita C, Boulla G, Revy P, Lemaitre F, Trautmann A (2003) T cell adhesion lowers the threshold for antigen detection. Eur J Immunol 33:1215–1223

Rosette C, Werlen G, Daniels MA, Holman PO, Alam SM, Travers PJ, Gascoigne NRJ, Palmer E, Jameson SC (2001) The impact of duration versus extent of TCR occupancy on T cell activation: a revision of the kinetic proofreading model. Immunity 15:59–70

Salter RD, Benjamin RJ, Wesley PK, Buxton SE, Garrett TPJ, Clayberger C, Krensky AM, Norment AM, Littman DR, Parham P (1990) A binding site for the T-cell co-receptor CD8 on the α3 domain of HLA-A2. Nature 345:41–46

Santori FR, Kieper WC, Brown SM, Lu Y, Neubert TA, Johnson KL, Naylor S, Vukmanovic S, Hogquist KA, Jameson SC (2002) Rare, structurally homologous self-peptides promote thymocyte positive selection. Immunity 17:131–142

Segura JM, Guillaume P, Mark S, Dojcinovic D, Johannsen A, Bosshard G, Angelov G, Legler DF, Vogel H, Luescher IF (2008) Increased mobility of major histocompatibility complex I-peptide complexes decreases the sensitivity of antigen recognition. J Biol Chem 283:24254–24263

Sim B-C, Zerva L, Greene MI, Gascoigne NRJ (1996) Control of MHC restriction by TCR Vα CDR1 and CDR2. Science 273:963–966

Sim B-C, Lo D, Gascoigne NRJ (1998) Preferential expression of TCR Vα regions in CD4/CD8 subsets: class discrimination or co-receptor recognition? Immunol Today 19:276–282

Sporri R, Reis e Sousa C (2002) Self peptide/MHC class I complexes have a negligible effect on the response of some CD8+ T cells to foreign antigen. Eur J Immunol 32:3161–3170

Stefanova I, Dorfman JR, Germain RN (2002) Self-recognition promotes the foreign antigen sensitivity of naive T lymphocytes. Nature 420:429–434

Stone JD, Chervin AS, Kranz DM (2009) T-cell receptor binding affinities and kinetics: impact on T-cell activity and specificity. Immunology 126:165–176

Sykulev Y, Joo M, Vturina I, Tsomides TJ, Eisen HN (1996) Evidence that a single peptide-MHC complex on a target cell can elicit a cytolytic T cell response. Immunity 4:565–571

Townsend ARM, Öhlén C, Bastin J, Ljunggren H-G, Foster L, Karre K (1989) Association of class I major histocompatibility heavy and light chains induced by viral peptides. Nature 340:443–448

van der Merwe PA, Davis SJ (2003) Molecular interactions mediating T cell antigen recognition. Annu Rev Immunol 21:659–684

Van Oers NSC, Killeen N, Weiss A (1994) ZAP-70 is constitutively associated with tyrosine-phosphorylated TCR z in murine thymocytes and lymph node T cells. Immunity 1:675–685

Varghese JC, Kane KP (2008) TCR complex-activated CD8 adhesion function by human T cells. J Immunol 181:6002–6009

Varma R, Campi G, Yokosuka T, Saito T, Dustin ML (2006) T cell receptor-proximal signals are sustained in peripheral microclusters and terminated in the central supramolecular activation cluster. Immunity 25:117–127

Wang JH, Meijers R, Xiong Y, Liu JH, Sakihama T, Zhang R, Joachimiak A, Reinherz EL (2001) Crystal structure of the human CD4 N-terminal two-domain fragment complexed to a class II MHC molecule. Proc Natl Acad Sci USA 98:10799–10804

Witherden D, van Oers N, Waltzinger C, Weiss A, Benoist C, Mathis D (2000) Tetracycline-controllable selection of CD4(+) T cells: half-life and survival signals in the absence of major histocompatibility complex class II molecules. J Exp Med 191:355–364

Wu H, Kwong PD, Hendrickson WA (1997) Dimeric association and segmental variability in the structure of human CD4. Nature 387:527–530

Wulfing C, Sumen C, Sjaastad MD, Wu LC, Dustin ML, Davis MM (2002) Costimulation and endogenous MHC ligands contribute to T cell recognition. Nat Immunol 3:42–47

Yachi PP, Ampudia J, Gascoigne NRJ, Zal T (2005) Nonstimulatory peptides contribute to antigen-induced CD8-T cell receptor interaction at the immunological synapse. Nat Immunol 6:785–792 PMCID: PMC1352171

Yachi PP, Ampudia J, Zal T, Gascoigne NRJ (2006) Altered peptide ligands induce delayed and reduced CD8-TCR interaction – a role for CD8 in distinguishing antigen quality. Immunity 25:203–211

Yachi PP, Lotz C, Ampudia J, Gascoigne NRJ (2007) T cell activation enhancement by endogenous pMHC acts for both weak and strong agonists but varies with differentiation state. J Exp Med 204:1747–2757 PMCID: PMC2118480

Yu YY, Netuschil N, Lybarger L, Connolly JM, Hansen TH (2002) Cutting edge: single-chain trimers of MHC class I molecules form stable structures that potently stimulate antigen-specific T cells and B cells. J Immunol 168:3145–3149

Zal T, Gascoigne NRJ (2004a) Photobleaching-corrected FRET efficiency imaging of live cells. Biophys J 86:3923–3939 PMCID: PMC1304294

Zal T, Gascoigne NRJ (2004b) Using live FRET imaging to reveal early protein-protein interactions during T cell activation. Curr Opin Immunol 16:418–427

Zal T, Zal MA, Gascoigne NRJ (2002) Inhibition of T-cell receptor-coreceptor interactions by antagonist ligands visualized by live FRET imaging of the T-hybridoma immunological synapse. Immunity 16:521–534

Zerrahn J, Held W, Raulet DH (1997) The MHC reactivity of the T cell repertoire prior to positive and negative selection. Cell 88:627–636

Vesicle Traffic to the Immunological Synapse: A Multifunctional Process Targeted by Lymphotropic Viruses

Andrés Alcover and Maria-Isabel Thoulouze

Contents

Abstract The site of contact between T lymphocytes and antigen-presenting cells becomes, upon antigen recognition, an organized junction named the immunological synapse. Various T cell organelles polarize, together with microtubules, toward the antigen-presenting cell. Among them, intracellular vesicular compartments, such as the Golgi apparatus, the recycling endosomal compartment, or cytotoxic granules help to build the immunological synapse and ensure effector functions, such as polarized secretion of cytokines by helper T cells, or exocytosis of lytic granules by cytotoxic T cells. Lymphotropic retroviruses, such as the human immunodeficiency virus type 1, the human T cell leukemia virus type 1, or the *Herpesvirus saimiri*, can subvert some of the vesicle traffic mechanisms impeding

---

A. Alcover (✉) and M.-I. Thoulouze
Institut Pasteur, Unité de Biologie Cellulaire des Lymphocytes, Département d'Immunologie, CNRS, URA1961, 28, rue Docteur Roux, F-75724, Paris Cedex 15, France
e-mail: andres.alcover@pasteur.fr; marie-isabelle.thoulouze@pasteur.fr

T. Saito and F.D. Batista (eds.), *Immunological Synapse*,
Current Topics in Microbiology and Immunology 340,
DOI 10.1007/978-3-642-03858-7_10, © Springer-Verlag Berlin Heidelberg 2010

the generation and function of the immunological synapses. This review focuses on the polarization of vesicle traffic, its regulation, and its role in maintaining the structure and function of the immunological synapse. We discuss how some lymphotropic viruses target the vesicle traffic in T lymphocytes, inhibiting the formation of immunological synapses and modulating the response of infected T cells.

1 Introduction

Seminal work from the 1980s provided the initial evidence of asymmetrical organelle distribution in helper T cells encountering antigen-bearing B lymphocytes, or in cytotoxic T cells (CTLs) encountering target cells. The T lymphocyte microtubule organizing center (MTOC) and the Golgi apparatus were found oriented to the antigen-presenting cell (APC). T-cell helper cytokines and cytotoxic granules appeared to be secreted toward the B cell and the target cell, respectively (Geiger et al. 1982; Kupfer and Dennert 1984; Kupfer et al. 1986, 1991, 1994; Kupfer and Singer 1989a, b; Yanelly et al. 1986). These studies set the bases for understanding the intimate physical and functional interactions between the two main types of T lymphocytes and their respective APCs.

The rapid development and accessibility of microscopy imaging technology further helped to define the spatial and temporal organization of the T cell–APC contact zone and lead to the notion of immunological synapse (Grakoui et al. 1999; Monks et al. 1998). During the last decade, a plethora of reports contributed to the current understanding of the mechanism of generation, the spatial and temporal organization, and the diversity of functions of immunological synapses. It appears clear today that immunological synapses are highly organized and dynamic cell–cell contacts where T cell activation is initiated and tuned, and where effector functions can be targeted to specific APCs or target cells (i.e., recent reviews Dustin 2008; Huse et al. 2008; Stinchcombe and Griffiths 2007).

The generation and function of immunological synapses involve a complex set of molecular transport mechanisms that engage at least four types of intracellular membrane compartments: the Golgi apparatus, secretory lysosomes, the early recycling endosomal compartment, and the late endosomal–lysomal compartment. The orchestrated action of several of these vesicle traffic mechanisms helps to maintain the concentration of key signaling molecules at the synapse and guarantees secretory mechanisms related to effector functions, like polarized secretion of cytokines or cytotoxic granules.

Human lymphotropic retroviruses, such as the human immunodeficiency virus type 1 (HIV-1), the human T leukemia virus type 1 (HTLV-1), and the Herpesvirus saimiri (HVS), target key T cell signaling molecules vesicle traffic, impairing the formation and function of the immunological synapses and hence modulating the response of the infected T lymphocytes.

2 Polarized Vesicle Traffic to the Immunological Synapse

2.1 Polarization of the Microtubule Cytoskeleton

Intracellular vesicle transport mechanisms are intimately linked to the microtubule cytoskeleton. Microtubules and their associated proteins direct and organize vesicle traffic to particular sites of the polarized cells. Likewise, polarized vesicle traffic to the immunological synapse occurs *via* the polarization of the microtubule cytoskeleton. Soon after contact with Ag-bearing APCs, the MTOC reorients toward the stimulatory contact zone (Fig. 1a). MTOC reorientation depends on TCR signaling and is regulated by posttranslational modifications of tubulin and by microtubule-based molecular motors. These issues have been previously reviewed (Pais-Correia et al. 2007; Rey et al. 2007; Valenzuela-Fernandez et al. 2008; Vicente-Manzanares and Sanchez-Madrid 2004) and will not be developed here. Microtubules project from the MTOC toward the periphery of the immunological synapse where they appear to anchor (Kuhn and Poenie 2002), while the MTOC closely apposes to the plasma membrane in a central area of the synapse (Stinchcombe et al. 2006). Several protein complexes may facilitate the anchoring and movement of microtubules at the periphery of the immune synapse pulling the MTOC close up to the contact zone. Microtubule-based molecular motors, such as dynein (Combs et al. 2006; Martin-Cofreces et al. 2008), the Rac1, and Cdc42 effector IQGAP (Stinchcombe et al. 2006), and members of the formin family of cytoskeletal regulators (Gomez et al. 2007) were shown to be necessary for MTOC polarization to the immunological synapse. Their individual contribution to this phenomenon is however still poorly understood.

2.2 Polarization of the Golgi Apparatus and the Secretory Vesicle Traffic

The Golgi apparatus is associated with the MTOC and reorients together with it following microtubule reorganization (Fig. 1b). Although the Golgi apparatus might release several secreted proteins, one of the main functions of Golgi polarization to the immunological synapse is thought to be the polarized secretion of helper cytokines, such as interleukin (IL)2, IL3, IL4, or interferon gamma (IFNγ), toward the APC in order to perform the T cell regulatory functions (Barcia et al. 2008; Depoil et al. 2005; Huse et al. 2006; Kupfer et al. 1991, 1994; Reichert et al. 2001). Interestingly, whereas vesicle compartments containing helper cytokines remain associated with the MTOC and polarize toward the synapse, the vesicles carrying inflammatory cytokines, such as the tumor necrosis factor, or the chemokine CCL3, distribute in a nondirectional manner (Huse et al. 2006). These two vesicular compartments could be distinguished by the presence of vesicle traffic

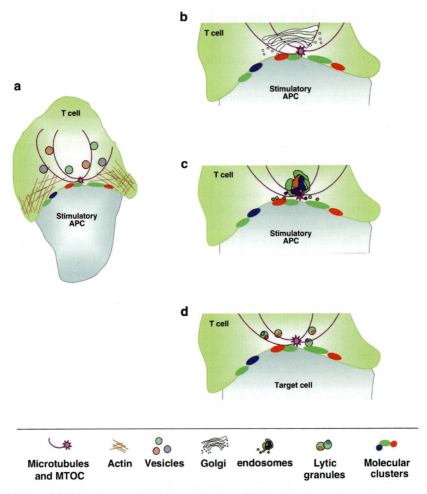

Fig. 1 Polarized vesicle traffic to the immunological synapse. (**a**) Antigen recognition triggers the rapid reorganization of the actin and microtubule cytoskeleton at the APC contact site. This leads to the polarization of the MTOC that positions close to the contact site and drives the polarization of several membrane compartments, like the Golgi apparatus (**b**), the endosomal compartment (**c**), and the secretory lysosomes (**d**). Vesicle traffic from these different compartments is therefore directed to the immunological synapse, helping its organization and function

regulators, such as Rab3d and Rab19, which were displayed by helper cytokine vesicles, or by the presence of the SNARE protein syntaxin-6, which was mainly present in vesicles containing inflammatory cytokines. Vesicles carrying helper and inflammatory cytokines can also display some common vesicle traffic regulators, but none of them expressed Rab27a, which controls cytotoxic granule transport (see below). Therefore, different proteins seem to regulate the transport of cytokines and lytic granules to the synapse. Worth noting, T cells contacting various APCs displaying different concentration of antigen make a choice and polarize their helper cytokine intracellular compartment toward the APC presenting the stronger stimulus (Depoil et al. 2005).

2.3 Polarization of Cytotoxic Granules

Among the different vesicle transport studied in T lymphocytes, the polarized secretion of lytic granules by CTLs has been the best studied and extensively reviewed by others (Stinchcombe and Griffiths 2007). Lytic granules are a particular type of lysosomes called secretory lysosomes (Bossi and Griffiths 2005). They carry perforin, granzymes, and Fas ligand, and rapidly polarize and fuse in a precise zone of the synapse of CTLs with target cells causing the rapid destruction of the target (Stinchcombe et al. 2001b). The study of several human genetic diseases causing immunodeficiency and albinism helped in the characterization of proteins that regulate the polarized traffic of lytic granules to the immunological synapse, and the melanocytes secretion required for pigmentation (Clark and Griffiths 2003; Stinchcombe and Griffiths 2007). Some of these proteins are also altered in particular mutant mouse strains. For instance, the protein LYST causes the Chediak–Higashi Syndrome and determines the Beige phenotype in mice (Barbosa et al. 1997; Perou et al. 1997). The GTPase Rab27a causes the Griscelli syndrome (Menasche et al. 2000) and the *ashen* mice phenotype (Wilson et al. 2000). Moreover, mutations in the Rab geranylgeranyl transferase leading to dysfunction of Rab27a are responsible for *gunmetal* mice (Detter et al. 2000). Both types of Rab27a alterations inhibit lytic granule delivery to the immunological synapse although at different stages (Stinchcombe et al. 2001a). Munc13-4 was identified as the protein defective in patients with familial hemophagocytic lymphohistiocytosis (HLH) (Feldmann et al. 2003). Munc13-4 can interact with Rab27a, likely connecting lytic granule movement and docking. It controls the late steps of lytic granule maturation and exocytosis in CTLs and mast cells (Menager et al. 2007; Neeft et al. 2005). The lack of the adapter protein AP-3 in patients of Hermansky–Pudlak syndrome leads to altered transport of lytic granules along the microtubules in CTLs (Clark et al. 2003). It is at present unknown whether AP3 is directly required for lysosome transport on microtubules, or allows the transport of other proteins involved in this process (Stinchcombe and Griffiths 2007). Noteworthy, when T cells establish simultaneous contacts with several target cells, they polarize most of their lytic granules toward the target cell that attracts the MTOC, and much less to the other ones. Nevertheless, both targets can be lysed (Wiedemann et al. 2006).

2.4 Polarization of Endosomal Compartments

Endosomal compartments are formed by a complex assembly of intermingled tubules and vesicles that sort internalized proteins, reorienting them either to a recycling pathway back to the plasma membrane, or to lysosomes for degradation. Both recycling endosomes and late endosomes/lysosomes polarize to the immunological synapse (Fig. 1b). The recycling endosomal compartment rapidly polarizes together with the MTOC to the T cell–APC contact zone and can transport membrane proteins that are being constitutively internalized and recycled back to the plasma membrane, such as the TCR (Alcover and Alarcón 2000; Das et al. 2004). Inhibition of endocytosis, polarization, recycling, or endosome fusion with the plasma membrane strongly reduces TCR accumulation in the synapse. Therefore, endosomal transport is essential to target TCRs and likely other molecules to the APC contact site, facilitating their accumulation in the immunological synapse (Das et al. 2004). The vSNARE VAMP-3, the t-SNAREs syntaxin-4 and SNAP-23 (Das et al. 2004), and the GTPase Rab35 (Patino-Lopez et al. 2008) are involved in this process. The negative regulator of T-cell activation CTLA4 is also transported *via* endosomes to the immune synapse (Linsley et al. 1996).

Late endosomes different from lytic granules also seem to polarize to the immunological synapse. A marker of this compartment, the lipid LBPA (lysobisphosphatidic acid) was found very close to the center of the immunological synapse (c-SMAC) of helper T cells, suggesting that receptors clustered in the c-SMAC may be sorted to a degradation pathway. This may be part of a mechanism that drives the extinction of TCR signals at the synapse (Varma et al. 2006). This process requires some endocytic adaptors such as CD2AP whose absence delays the disappearance of TCRs from the synapse and prolongs T-cell activation (Lee et al. 2003). It is at present unknown whether only TCRs, or also signaling molecules, could be sorted for degradation at the immunological synapse.

2.5 Polarization of Vesicular Compartments Carrying Signal Transduction Proteins

Some membrane associated signal transduction proteins, such as the protein tyrosine kinase Lck, or the adaptor LAT, also transit through vesicular compartments that are organized around the MTOC. These compartments polarize toward the APC contact site, and appear to release their cargo at the immunological synapse favoring Lck and LAT synaptic accumulation (Bonello et al. 2003; Ehrlich et al. 2002; Montoya et al. 2002). The nature of these vesicular compartments is at present unknown. Although an overlap between these compartments and transferrin-containing endosomes was reported, higher resolution images showed that Lck and LAT intracellular compartments were intermingled with, but distinct from, transferrin[+] endosomes (Thoulouze et al. 2006; M-I, unpublished observations). Lck is contained in vesicles expressing the traffic regulator protein MAL, a component of the specialized machinery for apical protein targeting. Moreover, in T cells lacking MAL, Lck is retained in intracellular vesicles and does not access the cell cortex or detergent resistant microdomains. MAL effect was specific for

Lck, since the fate of Fyn was not altered (Anton et al. 2008). MAL-deficient cells were activated to a lower extent, indicating that Lck vesicle transport is essential for the Lck localization required for efficient T-cell activation. It is at present unknown how the intracellular traffic of Fyn and LAT is controlled and whether they share some regulatory mechanisms with Lck.

2.6   The Immunological Synapse, an Active Zone for Vesicle Docking and Fusion

Vesicles from the different compartments cited above converge at the immunological synapse under the control of TCR signaling. Thus, different types of vesicles need to dock and fuse at the right place and time, and in a regulated manner. The site of vesicle docking and fusion at the immunological synapse appears to be located between the cSMAC and the p-SMAC (Das et al. 2004; Stinchcombe et al. 2001b). This suggests that, like in neural synapses, immunological synapses may contain active zones in which regulated docking and fusion of vesicles take place. In neural synapses, vesicle docking and fusion is mediated by a set of proteins that orchestrate the different stages of this complex process. Briefly, SNARE complexes formed between one v-SNARE, VAMP-1/synaptobrevin-1, present in the transport vesicle and two t-SNAREs, syntaxin-1, and SNAP-25, present in the target membrane bring vesicles and plasma membrane together ensuring membrane fusion. In addition, the Munc18-1 protein control SNARE complex formation and may be involved in fusion, whereas Munc13 and RIMs are important for vesicle priming. Finally, synaptotagmins are Ca^{2+}-sensitive proteins that control stimulus dependent vesicle fusion processes (Rizo and Rosenmund 2008). Similar regulators are involved in immune synapse formation and function. Thus, two t-SNAREs, Syntaxin-4 and SNAP-23 accumulate at the immunological synapse of CD4 T cells and a v-SNARE, VAMP-3, is present in recycling endosomes and is necessary for TCR accumulation in the synapse (Das et al. 2004). Moreover, Munc13-4 is necessary for lytic granule fusion in CTLs (Feldmann et al. 2003; Menager et al. 2007). Finally, some synaptotagmin-like proteins Slp1 and Slp2 contribute to lytic granule secretion in CTLs (Holt et al. 2008). It is at present unknown whether the different vesicle fusion processes that take place at the immunological synapse involve common or specific fusion regulatory machineries.

3   Infection by Lymphotropic Viruses Modulates Intracellular Molecular Trafficking to the Immunological Synapse and T-Cell Signaling

As strict parasites, viruses hijack the cellular machineries of infected cells to replicate and/or persist. Concomitantly, they have to evade innate and adaptive immune responses to establish infection and disseminate in vivo. For some lymphotropic viruses, infection leads to important alterations of T lymphocyte biology that contribute both to T-cell dysfunctions and to viral dissemination. As in any viral reservoir, several components of the lymphocyte machineries are first enlisted for viral progeny production. Moreover, by interfering with intracellular protein trafficking, modulating receptor signal transduction, or modifying cytoskeleton integrity, virus infection can impair the physiological immune synapse, and as a consequence, the initiation of an appropriate adaptive immune response.

Three lymphotropic retroviruses infecting CD4 T cells were reported to target trafficking or signaling mechanisms involved in immunological synapses formation, HIV-1, HTLV-1, and HVS (Fig. 2). They share the ability to target early T-cell signaling molecules, such as the protein tyrosine Lck or the adaptor LAT. Both molecules traffic toward the immune synapse via intracellular vesicles (see Sect. 2.5). Understanding how these viruses target vesicle traffic of signaling molecules may help us to better define the process of virus infection and decipher the importance of these traffic mechanisms for the generation and function of immunological synapses.

3.1   HIV-1

HIV-1 infection leads to severe CD4 T lymphocyte dysfunctions that take place during AIDS pathology. Infected T cells lose their capacity to control T-cell activation mechanisms and cannot balance the processes of T-cell proliferation and effector function versus those leading to apoptosis.

HIV-1 impairs the capacity of T lymphocytes to form immunological synapses. Conjugate formation and TCR and Lck clustering at the synapse are strongly inhibited. This is due, at least in part, to the effect of HIV-1 on TCR and Lck intracellular trafficking. In HIV-1-infected T cells, Lck accumulates in the endosomal compartment, whereas TCR traffic is slowed down at both the endocytosis and recycling steps. The HIV-1-encoded protein Nef is necessary and sufficient to cause both effects, but the molecular mechanism is still unknown (Thoulouze et al. 2006). Nef interacts with several intracellular trafficking adaptors and Rab proteins (Burtey et al. 2007; Schaefer et al. 2008) that could be involved in Lck or TCR traffic. Moreover, Nef alters the intracellular traffic and cell surface expression of several membrane molecules, including CD4 and CD28 (reviewed in Das and Jameel 2005; Piguet et al. 1999), that could affect immune synapse formation. The effect of Nef on Lck accumulation in endosomes is however not mediated by Nef-induced CD4 downregulation (Thoulouze et al. 2006), and it could result either from molecular interaction of Nef with Lck (molecular targeting) (Baur et al. 1997; Dutartre et al. 1998), or from a Nef-mediated effect on the intracellular compartment carrying Lck (compartment targeting). Recent studies indicate that Nef effect on Lck intracellular traffic involves the Nef domain that mediates the interaction with Pak2, but it is independent of actin remodeling (Haller et al. 2007). Worth noting, Nef distinctly affects molecules sharing the endosomal trafficking pathway,

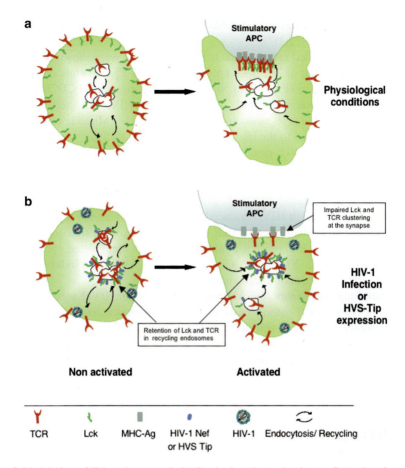

Fig. 2 Modulation of T lymphocyte polarization by lymphotropic viruses. Some lymphotropic viruses, like HIV-1 and HVS, subvert endosomal traffic in the T cell, impeding the formation of the immunological synapse and modulating TCR signaling. (**a**) Under physiological conditions T cells polarize the endosomal trafficking toward the APC contact site, targeting receptors (i.e., TCR) and signaling molecules (i.e., Lck) to the immunological synapse and contributing to their clustering at the synapse. (**b**) Expression of the HIV-1-encoded protein Nef and the HVS-encoded protein Tip is necessary and sufficient to induce TCR and Lck retention in endosomes impairing the formation of T cell–APC conjugates, the clustering of molecules at the synapse, and TCR signaling. It remains unknown whether both viral proteins effects involve the same mechanism

like the transferrin receptor and the TCR (Das et al. 2004; Thoulouze et al. 2006), suggesting that Nef targets the traffic of particular molecules rather than that of the whole endosomal compartment. Finally, contrary to Nef encoded by HIV-1, Nef proteins encoded by non pathogenic lentiviruses like HIV-2, or simian immunode-ficiency virus (SIV), induced TCR downregulation. It was therefore proposed that the ability of Nef to downregulate TCR surface expression and to inhibit T-cell activation was related with lower viral pathogenesis (Schindler et al. 2006).

No differences were found among these Nef proteins in their capacity to collapse Lck traffic (Haller et al. 2007).

Other HIV-1 encoded products, such as Vpu and Vpr were shown to modulate intracellular trafficking of key T-cell molecules. Thus, Vpu downmodulates CD4 expression (Nomaguchi et al. 2008), whereas Vpr downregulates CD28 and upregulates CTLA4 (Venkatachari et al. 2007). Finally, in HIV-1 infected T cells, the HIV-1 Env protein shares its vesicular traffic with CTLA4 (Miranda et al. 2002), a molecule that is targeted to the immune synapse *via* intracellular vesicles (Linsley et al. 1996). Thus, HIV-1 developed different mechanisms to impair immune synapse formation, targeting *via* several accessory molecules the intracellular traffic and the functions of the TCR, various costimulatory receptors, and some signaling molecules.

Interestingly, although HIV-1-induced inhibition of immune synapse formation is concomitant with defective early TCR signaling, downstream signaling pathways leading to IL2 production are not inhibited, but rather upregulated (Fenard et al. 2005; Thoulouze et al. 2006). This suggests that HIV-1 infection induces opposite effects at different stages of T-cell signaling.

The advantage of immunological synapse inhibition for HIV-1 survival, and the consequences for HIV-1 pathogenesis are not clear at present. HIV-1 may alter the natural balance between T-cell activation processes leading to proliferation and effector functions versus apoptosis, establishing a new balance that may favor viral replication while preventing the effectiveness of T-cell responses (Fackler et al. 2007).

3.2 HTLV-1

Contrary to HIV-1, HTLV-1 infection of CD4 T cells does not induce an over immuno-suppression, persisting in its host in the context of a normal immune response. HTLV-1 alters T cell physiology in various ways and may lead to T cell transformation and leukemia in a low percentage of infected individuals (Asquith and Bangham 2008).

Recent data indicate that HTLV-1 might affect the generation and function of immunological synapses. Thus, the HTLV-1-encoded accessory protein p12I enhances LFA-1-mediated T-cell adhesion, by inducing LFA-1 clustering on the plasma membrane. This would predict an increased capacity of HTLV-1-infected cells to form conjugates with APCs (Kim et al. 2006). Moreover, HTLV-1 infection, through the expression of the protein Tax, enhances the capacity of T cells to polarize in response to antigen-independent cell contacts, which could prime the infected T cell for rapid polarization (Nejmeddine et al. 2005). However, p12I was shown to affect the activation of T cells stimulated by APCs. P12I can interact with LAT and impair TCR signaling by inhibiting the phosphorylation of LAT, Vav, and PLCγ, as well as NFAT transcriptional activation. A pool of p12I accumulating with lipid rafts at the T cell–APC contact could be responsible for this inhibitory effect (Fukumoto et al. 2007). P12I could also act in a LAT-independent manner following TCR activation, leading to STAT5 and NFAT translocation to the nucleus (Nicot et al. 2001), increased IL-2 production (Ding et al. 2003), and decreased IL-2 requirement for T-cell proliferation (Nicot et al. 2001). These contrasting effects of p12I on T-cell activation are still poorly understood, but as for HIV-1, they may alter the natural balance between T-cell activation processes leading to proliferation and effector functions. It remains to be defined whether in the context of HTLV-1 infection, several HTLV-1-encoded proteins (i.e., p12I, Tax) cooperate to modulate immunological synapse generation and function in a way to favor virus adaptation to the host environment.

3.3 Herpesvirus saimiri

Like other Herpesviruses, HVS persists in its host through the ability to establish a latent infection with periodical reactivations that produce infectious virus.

The expression of the HSV-encoded protein Tip (tyrosine kinase interacting protein) was shown to modulate TCR signaling and impair the formation of the immunological synapses (Brinkmann and Schulz 2006; Cho et al. 2004). Tip is expressed primarily during viral latency, but it is not required for viral replication (Duboise et al. 1998), it is constitutively present in lipid rafts, and interacts with Lck. Tip inhibits early events of TCR signaling by sequestering Lck, TCRζ, and LFA-1 in an intracellular vesicular compartment (Cho et al. 2004, 2006; Jung et al. 1995; Park et al. 2003). Tip interacts with p80, a lysosomal protein that interacts with Lck and mediates Lck intracellular sequestration, sorting to lysosomes, and degradation (Park et al. 2002). In addition, Tip expression downregulates TCR and CD4 surface expression through distinct molecular mechanisms (Cho et al. 2006; Park et al. 2003).

Thus, HVS might inhibit immune synapse formation by encoding Tip, which collapses the traffic of Lck, LFA-1 and TCRζ, and downmodulates CD4 and TCR. A main difference with the effect of HIV-1 Nef is that Tip is mainly expressed during virus latency. It is tempting to speculate that signaling inhibition would prevent activation-induced apoptosis and prolong the life span of infected cells thus favoring virus latency.

In conclusion, modulation of immune synapse formation and TCR signaling appears as a common strategy employed by lymphotropic viruses to avoid host immune responses and T-cell activation during latency (Fig. 2). By expressing Nef and Tip, respectively, HIV-1 and HVS downregulate CD4 and Lck from the plasma membrane, accumulating them in endosomal compartments. By contrast, through p12I expression, HTLV-1 targets and inactivates the LAT adaptor - another signaling molecule known to traffic through intracellular vesicular compartments. Whether LAT is directly inactivated by p12I interaction or sequestered in intracellular compartments remains to be defined.

Neither HIV-1 Nef, nor HTLV-1 p12I downregulate TCR cell surface expression, whereas HVS Tip does. In this respect, HVS resembles SIV and HIV-2 which down-regulate TCR by means of their respective Nef proteins through a still undefined mechanism (Schindler et al. 2006). Interestingly, SIV and HIV-2 also collapse Lck intracellular traffic (Haller et al. 2007). TCR-down modulation could represent an additional mechanism to avoid immunological synapse formation and further modulate T-cell activation.

Therefore, the modulation of intracellular trafficking by these lymphotropic viruses appears as a subtle regulation of TCR signaling that may be favorable at various stages of these virus cycles. First, at the stage of virus replication, the modulation of T-cell activation may favor an equilibrium that ensures virus genome expression while reducing activation-induced apoptosis. Next, at the stage of latency, TCR signaling modulation may reduce virus genome expression ensuring the persistence of the virus reservoir. It is interesting that although these three different lymphotropic viruses adapted to the host environment by distinct means, all three target the same signaling pathway in the infected cell.

Finally, HIV-1 and HTLV-1 can subvert the mechanism of T-cell polarization involved in immune synapse formation and utilize cell–cell contacts to spread directly from cell to cell. By analogy to immunological synapses, these viral-induced cell–cell contacts were called virological synapses. They were characterized by the clustering of Gag and Env viral proteins in the infected cell side, and the transfer of viral RNA and proteins to the target cell (Igakura et al. 2003; Jolly et al. 2004; Sol-Foulon et al. 2007). Interestingly, recent data indicate that Lck facilitates assembly of HIV-1 at the T-cell plasma membrane (Strasner et al. 2008), and that ZAP-70 kinase regulates virological synapse formation between HIV-1-infected and target T lymphocytes (Sol-Foulon et al. 2007). This suggests that some molecular mechanisms involved in virus egress and virological synapse formation could interfere with those underlying immunological synapse formations, although this needs further investigation.

4 Conclusion and Remaining Questions

Multiple vesicular transport mechanisms are involved in the generation and function of helper and cytotoxic T-cell immunological synapses. Some lymphotropic viruses target these mechanisms, impairing the formation of immunological synapses, modulating early T-cell responses and using them to spread to other cells.

A number of important questions remain to be answered to elucidate both of these physiological and pathological processes. For instance:

- Which are the molecular mechanisms controlling the polarized traffic of the different types of vesicular organelles? Are they common or specific to the different organelles, or to the different cargo proteins?

- Do all these vesicular organelles utilize the same sites for vesicle docking and fusion at the immunological synapse? Do they all use the same fusion machinery and regulatory proteins?
- What is the importance of the endocytosis of receptors and signaling molecules at the immunological synapse, and their eventual sorting to lysosomes, for the negative modulation of T-cell signaling?
- Do viruses that perturb these trafficking processes target cargo proteins, or traffic regulators? Are they common for different viruses?
- More generally, is the targeting of T-cell intracellular traffic by viruses first dedicated to virus progeny generation and virus spread, or to the modulation of T-cell responses?

Acknowledgments Author's work is funded by Institut Pasteur (PTR 214), CNRS, Agence National de Recherche sur le SIDA (ANRS), Agence National de Recherche (ANR), and Association pour la Recherche sur le Cancer (ARC). We thank Drs H. Soares, V. Di Bartolo, and R. Lasserre for helpful discussions and critical reading of the manuscript.

References

Alcover A, Alarcón B (2000) Internalization and intracellular fate of TCR-CD3 complexes. Crit Rev Immunol 20:325–346

Anton O, Batista A, Millan J, Andres-Delgado L, Puertollano R, Correas I, Alonso MA (2008) An essential role for the MAL protein in targeting Lck to the plasma membrane of human T lymphocytes. J Exp Med 205:3201–3213

Asquith B, Bangham CR (2008) How does HTLV-I persist despite a strong cell-mediated immune response? Trends Immunol 29:4–11

Barbosa MD, Barrat FJ, Tchernev VT, Nguyen QA, Mishra VS, Colman SD, Pastural E, Dufourcq-Lagelouse R, Fischer A, Holcombe RF, Wallace MR, Brandt SJ, de Saint Basile G, Kingsmore SF (1997) Identification of mutations in two major mRNA isoforms of the Chediak-Higashi syndrome gene in human and mouse. Hum Mol Genet 6:1091–1098

Barcia C, Wawrowsky K, Barrett RJ, Liu C, Castro MG, Lowenstein PR (2008) In vivo polarization of IFN-gamma at Kupfer and non-Kupfer immunological synapses during the clearance of virally infected brain cells. J Immunol 180:1344–1352

Baur AS, Sass G, Laffert B, Willbold D, Cheng-Mayer C, Peterlin BM (1997) The N-terminus of Nef from HIV-1/SIV associates with a protein complex containing Lck and a serine kinase. Immunity 6:283–291

Bonello G, Blanchard N, Montoya MC, Aguado E, Langlet C, He HT, Nunez-Cruz S, Malissen M, Sanchez-Madrid F, Olive D, Hivroz C, Collette Y (2003) Dynamic recruitment of the adaptor protein LAT: LAT exists in two distinct intracellular pools and controls its own recruitment. J Cell Sci 117:1009–1016

Bossi G, Griffiths G (2005) CTL secretory lysosomes: biogenesis and secretion of a harmful organelle. Semin Immunol 17:87–94

Brinkmann MM, Schulz TF (2006) Regulation of intracellular signalling by the terminal membrane proteins of members of the Gammaherpesvirinae. J Gen Virol 87:1047–1074

Burtey A, Rappoport JZ, Bouchet J, Basmaciogullari S, Guatelli J, Simon SM, Benichou S, Benmerah A (2007) Dynamic interaction of HIV-1 Nef with the clathrin-mediated endocytic pathway at the plasma membrane. Traffic 8:61–76

Cho NH, Feng P, Lee SH, Lee BS, Liang X, Chang H, Jung JU (2004) Inhibition of T cell receptor signal transduction by tyrosine kinase-interacting protein of Herpesvirus saimiri. J Exp Med 200:681–687

Cho NH, Kingston D, Chang H, Kwon EK, Kim JM, Lee JH, Chu H, Choi MS, Kim IS, Jung JU (2006) Association of herpesvirus saimiri tip with lipid raft is essential for downregulation of T-cell receptor and CD4 coreceptor. J Virol 80:108–118

Clark R, Griffiths GM (2003) Lytic granules, secretory lysosomes and disease. Curr Opin Immunol 2003:516–521

Clark RH, Stinchcombe JC, Day A, Blott E, Booth S, Bossi G, Hamblin T, Davies EG, Griffiths GM (2003) Adaptor protein 3-dependent microtubule-mediated movement of lytic granules to the immunological synapse. Nat Immunol 4:1111–1120

Combs J, Kim SJ, Tan S, Ligon LA, Holzbaur EL, Kuhn J, Poenie M (2006) Recruitment of dynein to the Jurkat immunological synapse. Proc Natl Acad Sci USA 103:14883–14888

Das SR, Jameel S (2005) Biology of the HIV Nef protein. Indian J Med Res 121:315–332

Das V, Nal B, Dujeancourt A, Thoulouze MI, Galli T, Roux P, Dautry-Varsat A, Alcover A (2004) Activation-induced polarized recycling targets T cell antigen receptors to the immunological synapse; involvement of SNARE complexes. Immunity 20:577–588

Depoil D, Zaru R, Guiraud M, Chauveau A, Harriague J, Bismuth G, Utzny C, Muller S, Valitutti S (2005) Immunological synapses are versatile structures enabling selective T cell polarization. Immunity 22:185–194

Detter JC, Zhang Q, Mules EH, Novak EK, Mishra VS, Li W, McMurtrie EB, Tchernev VT, Wallace MR, Seabra MC, Swank RT, Kingsmore SF (2000) Rab geranylgeranyl transferase alpha mutation in the gunmetal mouse reduces Rab prenylation and platelet synthesis. Proc Natl Acad Sci USA 97:4144–4149

Ding W, Kim SJ, Nair AM, Michael B, Boris-Lawrie K, Tripp A, Feuer G, Lairmore MD (2003) Human T-cell lymphotropic virus type 1 p12I enhances interleukin-2 production during T-cell activation. J Virol 77:11027–11039

Duboise SM, Guo J, Czajak S, Desrosiers RC, Jung JU (1998) STP and Tip are essential for herpesvirus saimiri oncogenicity. J Virol 72:1308–1313

Dustin ML (2008) T-cell activation through immunological synapses and kinapses. Immunol Rev 221:77–89

Dutartre H, Harris M, Olive D, Collette Y (1998) The human immunodeficiency virus type 1 Nef protein binds the Src-related tyrosine kinase Lck SH2 domain through a novel phosphotyrosine independent mechanism. Virology 247:200–211

Ehrlich LIR, Ebert PJR, Krummel MF, Weiss A, Davis MM (2002) Dynamics pf p56lck translocation to the T cell immunological synapse following agonist and antagonist stimulation. Immunity 17:809–822

Fackler OT, Alcover A, Schwartz O (2007) Modulation of the immunological synapse: a key to HIV-1 pathogenesis? Nat Rev Immunol 7:310–317

Feldmann J, Callebaut I, Raposo G, Certain S, Bacq D, Dumont C, Lambert N, Ouachée-Chardin M, Chedeville G, Tamary H, Minard-Colin V, Vilmer E, Blanche S, Le Deist F, Fischer A, de Saint Basile G (2003) Munc-13-4 is essential for cytolytic granules fusion and is mutated in a form of familial hemophagocytic lymphohistiocytosis (FHL3). Cell 115:461–473

Fenard D, Yonemoto W, de Noronha C, Cavrois M, Williams SA, Greene WC (2005) Nef is physically recruited into the immunological synapse and potentiates T cell activation early after TCR engagment. J Immunol 175:6050–6057

Fukumoto R, Dundr M, Nicot C, Adams A, Valeri VW, Samelson LE, Franchini G (2007) Inhibition of T-cell receptor signal transduction and viral expression by the linker for activation of T cells-interacting p12I protein of human T-cell leukemia/lymphoma virus type 1. J Virol 81:9088–9099

Geiger B, Rosen D, Berke G (1982) Spatial relationships of microtubule-organizing centers and the contact area of cytotoxic T lymphocytes and target cells. J Cell Biol 95:137–143

Gomez TS, Kumar K, Medeiros RB, Shimizu Y, Leibson PJ, Billadeau DD (2007) Formins regulate the actin-related protein 2/3 complex-independent polarization of the centrosome to the immunological synapse. Immunity 26:177–190

Grakoui A, Bromley SK, Sumen C, Davis MM, Shaw AS, Allen PM, Dustin ML (1999) The immunological synapse: a molecular machine controlling T cell activation. Science 285:221–227

Haller C, Rauch S, Fackler OT (2007) HIV-1 Nef employs two distinct mechanisms to modulate Lck subcellular localization and TCR induced actin remodeling. PLoS ONE 2:e1212

Holt O, Kanno E, Bossi G, Booth S, Daniele T, Santoro A, Arico M, Saegusa C, Fukuda M, Griffiths GM (2008) Slp1 and Slp2-a localize to the plasma membrane of CTL and contribute to secretion from the immunological synapse. Traffic 9:446–457

Huse M, Lillemeier BF, Kuhns MS, Chen DS, Davis MM (2006) T cells use two directionally distinct pathways for cytokine secretion. Nat Immunol 7:247–255

Huse M, Quann EJ, Davis MM (2008) Shouts, whispers and the kiss of death: directional secretion in T cells. Nat Immunol 9:1105–1111

Igakura T, Stinchcombe JC, Goon PKC, Taylor GP, Weber JN, Griffiths GM, Tanaka Y, Osame M, Bangham CRM (2003) Spread of HTLV-1 between lymphocytes by virus-induced polarization of the cytoskeleton. Science 299:1713–1716

Jolly C, Kashefi K, Hollinshead M, Sattentau QJ (2004) HIV-1 cell to cell transfer across an Env-induced, actin-dependent synapse. J Exp Med 199:283–293

Jung JU, Lang SM, Jun T, Roberts TM, Veillette A, Desrosiers RC (1995) Downregulation of Lck-mediated signal transduction by tip of herpesvirus saimiri. J Virol 69:7814–7822

Kim SJ, Nair AM, Fernandez S, Mathes L, Lairmore MD (2006) Enhancement of LFA-1-mediated T cell adhesion by human T lymphotropic virus type 1 p12I1. J Immunol 176:5463–5470

Kuhn JR, Poenie M (2002) Dynamic polarization of the microtubule cytoskeleton during CTL-mediated killing. Immunity 16:111–121

Kupfer A, Dennert G (1984) Reorientation of the microtubule organizing center and the Golgi apparatus in cloned cytotoxic lymphocytes triggered by binding to lysable target cells. J Immunol 133:2762–2766

Kupfer A, Singer SJ (1989a) Cell biology of cytotoxic and helper T-cell functions: immunofluorescence microscopic studies of single cells and cell couples. Annu Rev Immunol 7:309–337

Kupfer A, Singer SJ (1989b) The specific interaction between T cells and antigen-presenting B cells. IV. Membrane and cytoskeletal reorganizations in the bound T cell as a function of antigen dose. J Exp Med 170:1697–1713

Kupfer A, Swain SL, Janeway CA Jr, Singer SJ (1986) The specific direct interaction of helper T cells and antigen-presenting B cells. Proc Natl Acad Sci USA 83:6080–6083

Kupfer A, Mosmann TR, Kupfer H (1991) Polarized expression of cytokines in cell conjugates of helper T cells and splenic B cells. Proc Natl Acad Sci USA 88:775–779

Kupfer H, Monks CRF, Kupfer A (1994) Small splenic B cells that bind to antigen-specific T helper (Th) cells and face the site of cytokine production in the Th cells selectively proliferate: immunofluorescence microscopic studies of Th-B antigen-presenting cell interactions. J Exp Med 179:1507–1515

Lee KH, Dinner AR, Tu C, Campi G, Raychaudhuri S, Varma R, Sims TN, Burack WR, Wu H, Wang J, Kanagawa O, Markiewicz M, Allen PM, Dustin ML, Chakraborty AK, Shaw AS (2003) The immunological synapse balances T cell receptor signaling and degradation. Science 302:1218–1222

Linsley PS, Bradshaw J, Greene J, Peach R, Bennett KL, Mittler RS (1996) Intracellular trafficking of CTLA-4 and focal localization towards sites of TCR engagement. Immunity 4:535–543

Martin-Cofreces NB, Robles-Valero J, Cabrero JR, Mittelbrunn M, Gordon-Alonso M, Sung CH, Alarcon B, Vazquez J, Sanchez-Madrid F (2008) MTOC translocation modulates IS formation and controls sustained T cell signaling. J Cell Biol 182:951–962

Menager MM, Menasche G, Romao M, Knapnougel P, Ho CH, Garfa M, Raposo G, Feldmann J, Fischer A, de Saint Basile G (2007) Secretory cytotoxic granule maturation and exocytosis require the effector protein hMunc13-4. Nat Immunol 8:257–267

Menasche G, Pastural E, Feldmann J, Certain S, Ersoy F, Dupuis S, Wulffraat N, Bianchi D, Fischer A, Le Deist F, de Saint Basile G (2000) Mutations in RAB27A cause Griscelli syndrome associated with haemophagocytic syndrome. Nat Genet 25:173–176

Miranda LR, Schaefer BC, Kupfer A, Hu Z, Franzusoff A (2002) Cell surface expression of the HIV-1 envelope glycoproteins is directed from intracellular CTLA-4-containing regulated secretory granules. Proc Natl Acad Sci USA 99:8031–8036

Monks CRF, Freiberg BA, Kupfer H, Sciaky N, Kupfer A (1998) Three-dimensional segregation of supramolecular activation clusters in T cells. Nature 395:82–86

Montoya MC, Sancho D, Bonello G, Collette Y, Langlet C, He HT, Aparicio P, Alcover A, Olive D, Sanchez-Madrid F (2002) Role of ICAM-3 in the initial interaction of T lymphocytes and APCs. Nat Immunol 3:159–168

Neeft M, Wieffer M, de Jong AS, Negroiu G, Metz CH, van Loon A, Griffith J, Krijgsveld J, Wulffraat N, Koch H, Heck AJ, Brose N, Kleijmeer M, van der Sluijs P (2005) Munc13-4 is an effector of rab27a and controls secretion of lysosomes in hematopoietic cells. Mol Biol Cell 16:731–741

Nejmeddine M, Barnard AL, Tanaka Y, Taylor GP, Bangham CRM (2005) Human T-lymphotropic virus type 1 Tax protein triggers micotubule reorientation in the virological synapse. J Biol Chem 280:29653–29660

Nicot C, Mulloy JC, Ferrari MG, Johnson JM, Fu K, Fukumoto R, Trovato R, Fullen J, Leonard WJ, Franchini G (2001) HTLV-1 p12(I) protein enhances STAT5 activation and decreases the interleukin-2 requirement for proliferation of primary human peripheral blood mononuclear cells. Blood 98:823–829

Nomaguchi M, Fujita M, Adachi A (2008) Role of HIV-1 Vpu protein for virus spread and pathogenesis. Microbes Infect 10:960–967

Pais-Correia AM, Thoulouze MI, Alcover A (2007) T cell polarization and the formation of the immunological synapse: from antigen recognition to virus spread. Curr Immunol Rev 3:107–188

Park J, Lee BS, Choi JK, Means RE, Choe J, Jung JU (2002) Herpesviral protein targets a cellular WD repeat endosomal protein to downregulate T lymphocyte receptor expression. Immunity 17:221–233

Park J, Cho NH, Choi JK, Feng P, Choe J, Jung JU (2003) Distinct roles of cellular Lck and p80 proteins in herpesvirus saimiri Tip function on lipid rafts. J Virol 77:9041–9051

Patino-Lopez G, Dong X, Ben-Aissa K, Bernot KM, Itoh T, Fukuda M, Kruhlak MJ, Samelson LE, Shaw S (2008) Rab35 and its GAP EPI64C in T cells regulate receptor recycling and immunological synapse formation. J Biol Chem 283:18323–18330

Perou CM, Leslie JD, Green W, Li L, Ward DM, Kaplan J (1997) The Beige/Chediak-Higashi syndrome gene encodes a widely expressed cytosolic protein. J Biol Chem 272:29790–29794

Piguet V, Schwartz O, Le Gall S, Trono D (1999) The downregulation of CD4 and MHC-1 by primate lentiviruses: a paradigm for the modulatioon of cell surface receptors. Immunol Rev 168:51–63

Reichert P, Reinhardt RL, Ingulli E, Jenkins MK (2001) Cutting edge: in vivo identification of TCR redistribution and polarized IL-2 production by naive CD4 T cells. J Immunol 166:4278–4281

Rey M, Sanchez-Madrid F, Valenzuela-Fernandez A (2007) The role of actomyosin and the microtubular network in both the immunological synapse and T cell activation. Front Biosci 12:437–447

Rizo J, Rosenmund C (2008) Synaptic vesicle fusion. Nat Struct Mol Biol 15:665–674

Schaefer MR, Wonderlich ER, Roeth JF, Leonard JA, Collins KL (2008) HIV-1 Nef targets MHC-I and CD4 for degradation via a final common beta-COP-dependent pathway in T cells. PLoS Pathog 4:e1000131

Schindler M, Munch J, Kutsch O, Li H, Santiago ML, Bibollet-Ruche F, Muller-Trutwin MC, Novembre FJ, Peeters M, Courgnaud V, Bailes E, Roques P, Sodora DL, Silvestri G,

Sharp PM, Hahn BH, Kirchhoff F (2006) Nef-mediated suppression of T cell activation was lost in a lentiviral lineage that gave rise to HIV-1. Cell 125:1055–1067

Sol-Foulon N, Sourisseau M, Porrot F, Thoulouze MI, Trouillet C, Nobile C, Blanchet F, di Bartolo V, Noraz N, Taylor N, Alcover A, Hivroz C, Schwartz O (2007) ZAP-70 kinase regulates HIV cell-to-cell spread and virological synapse formation. EMBO J 26:512–526

Stinchcombe JC, Griffiths GM (2007) Secretory mechanisms in cell-mediated cytotoxicity. Annu Rev Cell Dev Biol 23:495–517

Stinchcombe JC, Barral DC, Mules EH, Booth S, Hume AN, Machesky LM, Seabra MC, Griffiths GM (2001a) Rab27a is required for regulated secretion in cytotoxic T lymphocytes. J Cell Biol 152:825–834

Stinchcombe JC, Bossi G, Booth S, Griffiths GM (2001b) The immunological synapse of CTL contains a secretory domain and membrane bridges. Immunity 15:751–761

Stinchcombe JC, Majorovits E, Bossi G, Fuller S, Griffiths GM (2006) Centrosome polarization delivers secretory granules to the immunological synapse. Nature 443:462–465

Strasner AB, Natarajan M, Doman T, Key D, August A, Henderson AJ (2008) The Src kinase Lck facilitates assembly of HIV-1 at the plasma membrane. J Immunol 181:3706–3713

Thoulouze MI, Sol-Foulon N, Blanchet F, Dautry-Varsat A, Schwartz O, Alcover A (2006) Human immunodeficiency virus type-1 infection impairs the formation of the immunological synapse. Immunity 24:547–561

Valenzuela-Fernandez A, Cabrero JR, Serrador JM, Sanchez-Madrid F (2008) HDAC6: a key regulator of cytoskeleton, cell migration and cell-cell interactions. Trends Cell Biol 18:291–297

Varma R, Campi G, Yokosuka T, Saito T, Dustin ML (2006) T cell receptor-proximal signals are sustained in peripheral microclusters and terminated in the central supramolecular activation cluster. Immunity 25:117–127

Venkatachari NJ, Majumder B, Ayyavoo V (2007) Human immunodeficiency virus (HIV) type 1 Vpr induces differential regulation of T cell costimulatory molecules: direct effect of Vpr on T cell activation and immune function. Virology 358:347–356

Vicente-Manzanares M, Sanchez-Madrid F (2004) Role of the cytoskeleton during lymphocyte responses. Nat Rev Immunol 4:110–122

Wiedemann A, Depoil D, Faroudi M, Valitutti S (2006) Cytotoxic T lymphocytes kill multiple targets simultaneously via spatiotemporal uncoupling of lytic and stimulatory synapses. Proc Natl Acad Sci USA 103:10985–10990

Wilson SM, Yip R, Swing DA, O'Sullivan TN, Zhang Y, Novak EK, Swank RT, Russell LB, Copeland NG, Jenkins NA (2000) A mutation in Rab27a causes the vesicle transport defects observed in ashen mice. Proc Natl Acad Sci USA 97:7933–7938

Yanelly JR, Sullivan JA, Mandell JL, Egelhard VH (1986) Reorientation and fusion of cytotoxic T lymphocyte granules after interaction with target cells as determined by high resolution cinemigrography. J Immunol 136:377

Plasticity of Immunological Synapses

Salvatore Valitutti and Loïc Dupré

Contents

Abstract TCR engagement with peptide/MHC complexes displayed on the surface of the antigen-presenting cells is the crucial event in developing an adaptive immune response and occurs within specialized signaling areas named immunological synapses. Immunological synapses are diverse both in structure and function

S. Valitutti (✉)
INSERM, U563, Section Dynamique Moléculaire des Interactions Lymphocytaires, Toulouse, 31300, France
e-mail: salvatore.valitutti@inserm.fr

L. Dupré
Université Toulouse III Paul-Sabatier, Centre de Physiopathologie de Toulouse Purpan, Toulouse, 31400, France
e-mail: loic.dupre@inserm.fr

The authors declare that they have no competing financial interests.

T. Saito and F.D. Batista (eds.), *Immunological Synapse*,
Current Topics in Microbiology and Immunology 340,
DOI 10.1007/978-3-642-03858-7_11, © Springer-Verlag Berlin Heidelberg 2010

and exhibit a strikingly dynamic molecular organization. In this review, we focus on the diversity of immunological synapses and on their plasticity in response to stimulation. We discuss how the study of the adaptable features of immunological synapses can be instrumental to a better understanding of the complex regulation of adaptive immunity.

1 Introduction

T lymphocytes expressing the $\alpha\beta$ T cell receptor (TCR) are activated by the engagement of their TCR with peptide/MHC (pMHC) complexes displayed on the surface of antigen-presenting cells (APC). A distinct feature of T cell activation is that the TCR/pMHC interaction occurs in the context of a specialized signaling domain formed at the T cell/APC contact site: the immunological synapse (IS) (Dustin et al. 1998; Grakoui et al. 1999). The etymology of συναψι (*sunapsis*, connection) follows from the Greek words συν (*sun*, with) + απτω (*apto*, bind) = συναπτω, joint together. In neurophysiology, the term *synapse* indicates the functional connection between neurons for signal exchange. The term IS indicates that like neurons cells of the immune system can form specialized contacts for signal exchange (Dustin et al. 1998; Grakoui et al. 1999; Norcross 1984).

A decade ago, supra-molecular activation clusters (SMAC) have been described at the IS (Monks et al. 1998). SMAC are micrometer-scale molecular structures that assemble within a few minutes after T cell/APC encounter. They are composed of two concentric regions: the central SMAC (cSMAC) in which the TCR accumulates and the peripheral SMAC (pSMAC) in which the integrin LFA-1 is enriched. More recently, the term distal SMAC (dSMAC) has been proposed (Freiberg et al. 2002) and refers to the periphery of the IS, where large and heavily glycosylated molecules such as CD43 and CD45 are enriched (Huppa and Davis 2003). Concentric and symmetric molecular rearrangements were originally considered the hallmark of the prototypical IS. Conversely, it is now well established that, depending on the activation state of T lymphocytes, on the nature of the APC, and on the strength and quality of antigenic stimulation, IS can adopt different molecular compositions and three-dimensional architectures and can mediate different biological functions (Friedl et al. 2005; Trautmann and Valitutti 2003). Moreover, as we will discuss in this review, recent research showed that IS can exhibit a high degree of dynamism and adaptability since their structure and signaling characteristics can be remodeled in response to variable stimuli during the different phases of antigenic stimulation.

In the present survey of recent research on IS, we will first illustrate how much IS can be heterogeneous in shape and function. We will then focus on explaining the key role of the actin cytokeleton as a founding element of IS dynamic architecture.

Finally, we will discuss how IS behave as versatile and adaptable integrators of T cell activation.

2 Heterogeneity of Immunological Synapses

Immunological synapses exhibit a high degree of heterogeneity all along their "life cycle": from their assembly during initial T cell/APC contact to their mature stage as they assist T cell effector functions.

2.1 Antigen-Independent Initial Cell–Cell Contact

Both T cells and APC (such as dendritic cells (DC), B cells, and macrophages) exhibit an actin cytoskeleton-dependent mobility that allows them to migrate and to encounter a large number of cellular partners (Miller et al. 2002). Conjugation of T cells with APC is initially mediated by the interaction between adhesion molecules such as LFA-1 on the T cells and ICAM-1 on APC. This step does not require the TCR/pMHC interaction and is per se highly variable: frequency, rapidity, and stability of antigen-independent conjugate formation can significantly differ depending on the T cell activation state of and on the nature of the APC. Effector T cells are in general more efficient than naive T cells in forming conjugates with adjacent cells (including parenchymal cells in tissues) due to a higher expression level of adhesion molecules (Springer 1990). Among APC, mature DC are the most efficient in binding T cells and therefore tend to form conjugates with multiple T cells simultaneously. This is due to the large cellular surface of DC, their highly dynamic dendrites that probe the surrounding environment (Lindquist et al. 2004) and the expression of high levels of adhesion molecules on their surface (Benvenuti et al. 2004). Environmental factors also influence the frequency and duration of T cell/APC interactions. Kinetic observation of the T cell migration in tissues has established that the lymphoid organs and peripheral interstitial tissues provide a three-dimensional reticular network that governs cellular migration (Friedl et al. 2005; Germain et al. 2008). As a consequence, the microanatomy and the molecular composition of tissue conduits along which the T cell migration takes place can influence the frequency and the duration of initial cell–cell encounters (Bajenoff et al. 2006; Germain et al. 2008). Importantly, variations in the local concentrations of chemokines displayed along the reticular network can affect the opportunity of T cell/APC encounters. Along this line, it has been shown that antigen-presenting DC engaged with $CD4^+$ T cells are activated to secrete chemokines (CCL3/4) and attract $CCR5^+CD8^+$ T cells (Castellino et al. 2006).

2.2 Antigen-Driven Cell–Cell Contact Stabilization

Upon productive TCR/pMHC engagement, T cell adhesion to APC increases via an inside-out signaling resulting from the translation of TCR triggering into increased affinity and avidity of LFA-1/ICAM-1 binding (Alon and Dustin 2007). At the same time, the T cells undergo a shape remodeling and stop their progression via a mechanism dependent on $[Ca^{2+}]_i$ increase and on myosin II inactivation (Dustin et al. 1997; Jacobelli et al. 2004; Negulescu et al. 1996). The phase of antigen-driven cell–cell contact stabilization can be highly variable. The "stop signal" depends both on the T cell and APC functional characteristics and on the strength of antigenic stimulation. At saturating antigen concentrations in vitro, T cells are firmly bound to APC and exhibit only limited motility while undergoing sustained signaling (Espagnolle et al. 2007). Differently, at limiting antigen densities (that most likely reflect the strength of antigenic stimulation in physiological conditions), the "stop signal" is rather transient. Within a few minutes after conjugate formation, T cells start to move again and undergo sustained signaling while crawling on the APC surface (Valitutti et al. 1995). The stability of T cell/APC contacts can also be influenced by additional factors. It has been shown that CTLA-4 expression by the T cells inhibits the "stop signal" upon conjugation with cognate APC (Schneider et al. 2006). Moreover, the presence of the surrounding regulatory T cells (Treg) can affect in vivo the stability of naive T cell/DC conjugates (Tadokoro et al. 2006). Finally, it has been proposed that "costimulatory" chemokines secreted by the APC might increase the stability of the conjugates and the level of T cell activation. In contrast, "distracting" chemokines might compete with forces engaged during the "stop signal" and prevent formation of stable conjugates (Viola et al. 2006).

2.3 Molecular Segregation and Signal Transduction

The study of the relationship between molecular rearrangements at the IS and signal transduction in the T cells has yielded somewhat contradictory findings (Valitutti 2008). The cSMAC was initially seen as an area of signal integration/amplification responsible for the remarkable T cell sensitivity to antigenic stimulation (Monks et al. 1998; Grakoui et al. 1999). This view has been challenged by the observation that large-scale molecular segregation at the IS is dispensable for productive TCR engagement (Zaru et al. 2002). This observation together with the experimental evidence that signal transduction initiates in the periphery of the IS and precedes cSMAC formation (Lee et al. 2002) has established that signaling at the IS is not mechanistically linked to the formation of a central area of signal transduction.

A more recent model on the functional role of cSMAC/pSMAC segregation has been proposed. It predicts that the cSMAC and pSMAC regions have reversed roles as compared to the initial model: the periphery of the IS would be the area where productive engagement of the TCR takes place, while the cSMAC would be the area where the TCR and recruited signaling components are degraded, resulting in extinction of the signal transduction (Lee et al. 2003; Varma et al. 2006).

Studies combining the in silico and in vitro approaches contributed to further revise this paradigm and suggested that the cSMAC, by enhancing weak signals and attenuating strong ones, could function as an adaptive controller of T cell activation (Lee et al. 2003; Cemerski et al. 2007, 2008). The current view on signaling at the IS postulates that depending on the strength of antigenic stimulation, the rate of TCR degradation at the cSMAC and consequently the foci of sustained signaling evolve differently (Lee et al. 2003; Cemerski et al. 2008; Varma et al. 2006; Valitutti 2008). At strong antigenic stimuli, signal transduction occurs in the cSMAC (Cemerski et al. 2008; Leupin et al. 2000), however tyrosine phosphorylation events are barely detectable because of the high rate of degradation of TCR (Cemerski et al. 2008; Lee et al. 2003) and of recruited signaling components (Penna et al. 1999). For weak antigenic stimuli, the rate of TCR degradation is slower and thus the cSMAC becomes a preferential area of sustained signal transduction where TCRs accumulate and are engaged by MHC molecules also accumulated into the IS center (Monks et al. 1998; Grakoui et al. 1999). This view extends previous results indicating that TCR internalization and degradation may play a central role in extinguishing T cell responses (Cai et al. 1997; Valitutti et al. 1996b) as it posits a subtle role of the balance between signaling and degradation in fine-tuning T cell activation. All in all, IS signaling characteristics and their adaptability to stimulation support the notion that these signaling areas can be heterogeneous in structure and can exhibit versatile signaling characteristics.

2.4   Heterogeneous IS Support T Cell Biological Functions

IS heterogeneity interestingly reflects the variability of T cell biological functions. A typical example of how specific molecular patterning at the IS associates to specific T cell effector function is given by the IS forming at the CTL/target cell contact site. It is well established that CTL exhibit a dual activation threshold. Indeed, they can be triggered to lethal hit delivery by as few as three to five specific pMHC present at the IS (Purbhoo et al. 2004), whereas they require a strong antigenic stimulus to be activated to cytokine production (Valitutti et al. 1996a). Strong antigenic stimulation (sufficient to elicit both cytotoxicity and cytokine production) results in large-scale concentric molecular segregation reminiscent of the one seen in $CD4^+$ helper T cells (Faroudi et al. 2003a). Limiting antigen concentrations (sufficient to elicit cytotoxicity) however result in undetectable or rudimentary molecular segregation at the IS; yet individual CTL polarize their lytic granules toward target cells and annihilate them (Faroudi et al. 2003a). The terms *lytic* and *stimulatory* synapses have been coined to indicate these different synaptic phenotypes (Faroudi et al. 2003a). The structure of the segregated IS formed by CTL upon optimal antigenic stimulation does not fully resemble the one formed by $CD4^+$ T cells. It has been indeed described that at the CTL/target cell IS, two distinct domains are formed: a signaling domain (corresponding to a cSMAC) and a secretory domain where tubulin cytoskeleton and lytic granules converge (Stinchcombe et al. 2001).

It is interesting to note that naive CD8$^+$ T cells seem to be even less dependent than CTL on the formation of concentric IS for the activation of their biological response. Even when receiving a strong antigenic and costimulation stimulus, the naive CD8$^+$ T cells have been shown to be activated to IL-2 production and proliferation in the absence of a discrete cSMAC/pSMAC segregation at the IS (O'Keefe et al. 2004).

Another example in which the IS structure mirrors T cell biological function is given by the naive T cells/DC encounter under conditions leading to Th1 or Th2 commitment. Upon IS formation, T cells (in particular those from mice biased toward Th1 phenotype) show IFN-γ receptor enrichment at the IS (Maldonado et al. 2004). This enrichment is prevented in conditions antagonizing Th1 polarization such as the presence of IL-4 in the extracellular milieu (Maldonado et al. 2004).

Finally, also the step of negative selection in thymocytes appears to have its synaptic hallmark. It has been shown that the thymocytes undergoing negative selection form partially segregated IS in which TCRζ-chain is seen mostly at the periphery of the thymocyte/stromal cell contact site (Richie et al. 2002).

In conclusion, IS has have been shown to be highly heterogenic in their build-up, signaling characteristics, molecular composition, and three-dimensional structure. This high degree of diversity may result from a high degree of molecular dynamics occurring at the T cell/APC contact site allowing T cells to adopt IS structures that better adapt to stimulation conditions and optimally integrate the different stimuli.

3 Dynamics of IS Assembly and Signal Integration: Central Role of the Actin Cytoskeleton

It is well established that actin cytoskeleton integrity is required for productive T cell/APC encounter and for the assembly of key signaling networks at the T cell/ APC contact site (Billadeau et al. 2007). The actin cytoskeleton exerts multiple tasks during the T cell/APC interaction. As illustrated in Fig. 1, these tasks are thought to include: (a) morphological transition from elongated shape to round-up shape following adhesion to the APC (Negulescu et al. 1996; Valitutti et al. 1995); (b) formation of lateral membrane protrusions allowing scanning the surface of the APC (Tskvitaria-Fuller et al. 2003); (c) stabilization of the MTOC and secretory machinery polarization (Stinchcombe et al. 2006) ; (d) molecular segregation into signaling platforms (Campi et al. 2005); (e) centripetal motility of receptors and signaling platforms (Kaizuka et al. 2007; Varma et al. 2006);(f) receptor endocytosis (McGavin et al. 2001). Among the pleiotropic roles of the actin cytoskeleton in the T cell/APC cognate interaction and signaling, we focus in this section on the role of the actin cytoskeleton in IS molecular assembly and dynamics.

Actin remodelling at the IS

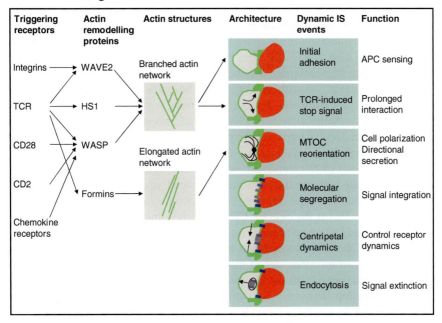

Fig. 1 Actin remodeling at the IS. Schematic representation of the pathways leading to actin nucleation in the T cells and of the IS life cycle stages controlled by actin cytoskeleton dynamics. The *arrows* indicate some of the molecular connections (e.g., between cell surface receptors and actin nucleators) described in the literature. The main IS molecular events thought to be dependent on actin cytoskeleton dynamics are depicted at the contact between a T cell (with actin in *green*) and an APC (*red*)

The build-up of IS molecular organization can be explained by two mechanisms that are most probably interconnected: cytoskeleton-driven movements and diffusion-trapping. The actin cytokeleton is highly enriched at the T cell/APC interface very early after contact. It follows a first outward swiping motion that widens the cellular interface and then a second phase of inward swiping motion (Tskvitaria-Fuller et al. 2003). This second phase may correspond to the actin waves centripetally converging toward the center of the IS, observed at the contact with planar lipid bilayers embedded with MHC and ICAM-1 (Kaizuka et al. 2007; Varma et al. 2006). Actin cytoskeleton integrity has been shown to be required for the formation of the TCR microclusters at the T cell/lipid bilayer contact site and for signaling within the TCR microclusters (Varma et al. 2006). It has also been established that both the TCR and LFA-1 microclusters are transported along the centripetal actin flow toward the cSMAC (Kaizuka et al. 2007). Interestingly, distinct patterns of cSMAC enrichment for the TCR and LFA-1 microclusters have been observed, possibly due to differential actin interactions (Kaizuka et al. 2007). The molecular links responsible for the anchorage of receptors and signaling components to the underlying actin filaments remain largely unknown to date.

In addition to contribute to the IS assembly by driving molecular movements through direct anchorage, the actin cytoskeleton could also provide a network for diffusion-trapping events. Surface receptors and intracellular molecules associated to the plasma membrane diffuse along the lipid bilayer and have a lateral motility determined by their molecular size, their interaction with defined membrane domains and their association within molecular clusters (Harder et al. 2007). Upon cognate interaction with an APC, the diffusion pattern of surface molecules can be affected, for example, through interactions with molecular partners with reduced mobility. Actin-anchored molecular platforms and the actin network itself may serve as molecular traps affecting the diffusion of IS components such as receptors and signaling molecules.

The interactions of IS components with the actin cytoskeleton may be dynamic and may alternate between different modes. Indeed, upon T cell activation, some molecules appear to transit from a state of actin cytoskeleton anchorage to a diffusion mode. This is the case for CD43, which is anchored to the actin-binding protein moesin in resting conditions. As a result of the TCR activation, the CD43 is uncoupled from the actin cytoskeleton and follows a free diffusion mode that drags it out of the IS. As a further step of transition, the CD43 is reanchored to moesin following its exclusion from the IS center (Delon et al. 2001).

The relationship between actin cytoskeleton polymerization and signaling in T cells is presently not fully clear. It is commonly assumed that the networks of polymerized actin and actin-binding proteins are implicated in T cell signaling by providing the framework for the build-up of signaling platforms. We favor the idea that a bidirectional cross-talk between actin cytoskeleton organization and TCR mediated signaling could lead to IS assembly and signal integration. In support of this idea, induction of a rise in $[Ca^{2+}]_i$ has been shown to reduce the overall mobility of TCR on the T cell surface via a mechanism dependent on actin cytoskeleton polymerization (Dushek et al. 2008). This observation suggests that although actin polymerization is usually considered to be required for signaling at the IS, reverse mechanisms (signaling events required for actin polymerization) exist as well. It is tempting to speculate that a TCR induced $[Ca^{2+}]_i$ increase, by enhancing actin polymerization, could in turn modulate TCR mobility. This might be instrumental in regulating the supply of TCR to the IS during sustained T cell/APC interaction (Dushek et al. 2008) and in promoting the formation of signaling structures enriched in polymerized actin such as TCR micro-clusters (Varma et al. 2006). Along the same lines, a recent study has shown that engagement of the integrin VLA-4 retards the dynamics of inward actin flows at the IS. As a result, the persistence of phosphorylated SLP-76 within ZAP-70-containing microclusters at the periphery of the IS is increased, which promotes sustained signaling (Nguyen et al. 2008). These sets of results therefore illustrate how initial receptor engagement rapidly regulates actin cytoskeleton remodeling which in turn tunes receptor dynamics. This cross-talk therefore appears central to optimize local assembly of associated signaling cascades and to regulate the duration and intensity of T cell activation.

All in all, a large number of studies link the actin cytoskeleton to a direct role in the molecular build-up of the IS. The actin cytokeleton can therefore be seen as a founding element of the dynamic and polymorphic IS architecture. Importantly, the multitask activity of the actin cytoskeleton at the IS might reflect an ability to translate various stimuli at the plasma membrane into adapted remodeling patterns.

4   Actin Regulatory Proteins: Integrating MultiFactorial Stimulation into Adapted Actin Remodeling in Time and Space

Actin cytoskeleton remodeling during the T cell activation is controlled by multiple actin-regulatory proteins. The biochemical activities of these proteins include nucleation, bundling, stabilization, severing, and depolymerization of actin filaments. The confinement of the specific actin remodeling patterns and dynamics at the IS area is ensured by the local recruitment and activation of actin regulatory proteins by small GTPases of the Rho family, by phosphoinositides and by receptor-associated kinases and adaptors. Additional levels of local activation may be ensured by links between the actin and tubulin cytoskeletons, as well as by interaction with proteins promoting or sensing membrane deformation (Takenawa and Suetsugu 2007). Recent studies have started to unravel how the specific actin-regulatory proteins (mainly actin-nucleating proteins) regulate actin dynamics and thereby control the quality and intensity of T cell activation. An emerging concept is that individual actin regulatory proteins play specific roles in the build-up of IS and in the signaling pathways originating from the IS (Fig. 1, Billadeau et al. 2007).

The most studied actin-regulatory protein is the hematopoietic specific WASP (Wiskott–Aldrich syndrome protein). WASP is activated downstream of Cdc42 and nucleates actin through the Arp2/3 complex by forming new actin branches on the sides of existing actin filaments (Takenawa and Suetsugu 2007). WASP deficiency in humans, due to inherited mutations in the corresponding gene, causes the Wiskott–Aldrich syndrome, a rare and severe primary immune deficiency (Ochs and Thrasher 2006). WASP-deficient T cells exhibit consistent defects in IL-2 and Th1 cytokine production as well as in proliferation (Molina et al. 1993; Trifari et al. 2006). Following TCR triggering, WASP is rapidly recruited to the plasma membrane in association with lipid rafts and is activated by GTP-bound Cdc42 at the site of TCR stimulation (Cannon et al. 2001; Dupre et al. 2002; Krause et al. 2000; Sasahara et al. 2002).

It appears clear that WASP-driven actin nucleation at the nascent IS is dispensable for conjugate formation and firm adhesion (Krawczyk et al. 2002). However, controversial results have been obtained as whether WASP is required for IS assembly (Badour et al. 2004; Cannon and Burkhardt 2004; Dupre et al. 2002; Nolz et al. 2006). A recent study may reconcile the initially diverging sets of data

(Sims et al. 2007). This study shows that WASP defective naive T cells display normal initial IS formation, but are unable to reform IS after breaking of the IS symmetry. IS appear indeed to be subject to periodical destabilization and breaking of their symmetry, a phenomenon induced by PKCθ and inhibited by WASP. Controlled periodic destabilization of the IS would favor T cell activation and ultimately IL-2 secretion (Sims et al. 2007). The functional purpose of the PKCθ-driven continuous IS instability would be to increase the scanning activity of the T cells thus favoring signal collection on the APC surface. Conversely, it is tempting to speculate that WASP-driven stabilization of IS may favor asymmetric cell divisions important for memory/effector differentiation (Chang et al. 2007). This may favor a more robust skewing toward the Th1 effector cells in agreement with the observation that T cells from WASP-deficient patients have been shown to have defects in producing Th1 cytokines (Trifari et al. 2006).

The other members of the WASP family regulating actin nucleation through the Arp2/3 complex are N-WASP and the WAVE(1–3) isoforms (Takenawa and Suetsugu 2007). However, among them, mainly WAVE2 is expressed in T cells. WAVE2 activation is controlled by the Rho-GTPase Rac1. Knock-down of WAVE2 in Jurkat T cells suppresses actin polymerization at the IS (Nolz et al. 2006) and affects the T cell/APC conjugate formation. Therefore, actin nucleation in the T cells appears to be initiated by WAVE2, which mediates actin-rich membrane protrusions during adhesion to the APC and initiation of synapse formation. WASP-driven actin nucleation would be predominantly required in a second phase, to stabilize interactions between the T cells and APC.

A third important activator of the Arp2/3 complex in T cells is HS1, the hematopoietic lineage-restricted homolog of the actin-binding protein cortactin. HS1 may act in concert with WAVE2 and WASP since it appears to play a key role in stabilizing existing branched actin filaments by bridging the Arp2/3 complex with F-actin (Gomez et al. 2006). Through diverse interaction motifs, WASP, WAVE2, and HS1 can interact with multiple signaling molecules downstream of numerous IS-localized receptors Fig. 1. These include the TCR, CD28, CD2, chemokine receptors, and integrins. Therefore, these proteins appear to control T cell activation by integrating in a coordinated fashion signals originating from key activatory and regulatory receptors present at the IS.

It is tempting to speculate that actin cytoskeleton could contribute to IS diversity since distinct actin regulatory proteins may control the assembly and stability of different IS architectures endowed with different functions. An interesting illustration of this concept is the recently described role of formins at the IS of CTL (Gomez et al. 2007). Formins act as effectors for different small Rho-GTPases. However, in contrast to the Arp2/3-dependent actin nucleating proteins, formins nucleate and elongate nonbranched F-actin filaments, thereby structuring a distinct actin network. In CTL, the formins Diaphanous-1 (DIA1) and Formin-like-1 (FMNL1) are not involved in regulating F-actin accumulation at the IS, but instead they colocalize with the centrosome and control MTOC polarization and killing of target cells. Differently, Arp2/3 complex-depleted cells, which cannot form F-actin-rich lamellipodia, still polarize actin-based filopodia and are still capable of MTOC polarization. Therefore, by assembling distinct actin meshworks, Arp2/3 dependent nucleators (WAVE2 and WASP) and formins may control distinct functions at the IS, namely activation versus polarized secretion. This further suggests that distinct F-actin nucleators might be specialized in assembling distinct IS architectures in CTL. For instance, depending on the strength of antigenic stimulation they might be implicated in assembling *lytic* versus *stimulatory* IS at the CTL/target cell contact site, leading to distinct cellular functions (Faroudi et al. 2003a).

5 Immunological Synapses Are Adaptable Structures

On the basis of the initial in vitro descriptions, IS were originally viewed as *long-lived* and "*monogamous*" structures formed at the contact site between one T cell and one APC.

A first in situ study addressing this issue in explanted lymph nodes supported this view by showing that T cells form long-lasting contacts with antigen-presenting DC, while continuing to move over the DC surface (Stoll et al. 2002). Following the initial observation of prolonged contacts formed in situ (Stoll et al. 2002), several in vivo studies showed that sustained T cell/APC interaction is a central step in antigen recognition by T cells (Bousso and Robey 2003; Mempel et al. 2004; Celli et al. 2007; Miller et al. 2002).

Nevertheless, the notion of long-lived IS has evolved during the last few years. Indeed, additional in vivo studies have shown that during the first few hours after entry into lymph nodes, T cells typically make sequential and short-lived contacts with a number of cognate DC. Serial short-lived contacts are productive since they result in the upregulation of the activation marker CD69 in T cells (Mempel et al. 2004). Herickson et al. recently showed that the duration of this initial phase correlates inversely with the number of specific pMHC per DC and with the density of antigen-presenting DC in the lymphoid tissue (Henrickson et al. 2008). This suggests that the initial period of transient contacts allows the T cells to achieve a state of preactivation that is required only at limiting pMHC densities. At high pMHC densities, phase 1 becomes very short or even dispensable. This first phase is followed by a second phase during which prolonged contacts are established between T cells and antigen-presenting DC (Mempel et al. 2004). Long-lived contacts (phase 2) are followed by a third phase during which dividing T cells regain mobility (Mempel et al. 2004; Miller et al. 2004). Additional studies showed that during these late serial encounters in vivo, T cells can integrate signals from different APC resulting in sustained IL-2R expression and IFN-γ production (Celli et al. 2005).

Taken together, the observations made in vivo raise the question of whether long-lasting T cell/APC contacts are strictly required for T cell activation. A consistent interpretation is that different T cell responses may be more or less dependent on stable contacts. While the upregulation of activation markers such as

CD69 and CD25 in naive T cells and the production of IFN-γ in already activated T cells would be achieved or maintained by sequential T cell/APC encounters, the activation of naive T cells to IL-2 production and proliferation would require prolonged contacts between the T cells and APC.

In vitro studies corroborate this interpretation. Gunzer and Friedl showed that naive T cell/DC interactions within three-dimensional collagen matrices are short and sequential (Gunzer et al. 2000). This work provided the first indication that T cell activation can occur in vitro in conditions in which T cells preferentially form short-lived contacts. Furthermore, Faroudi et al. showed that individual human effector T cells integrate signals for IFN-γ production during sequential activation periods (Faroudi et al. 2003b). Finally, using time-lapse video microscopy to monitor activation of the individual naive T cells expressing a reporter transgene for IL-2, Weaver and colleagues showed that T cells establishing transient interactions with DC are activated (as detected by upregulation of CD25) but do not express IL-2. Only T cells establishing prolonged dynamic contacts with DC express IL-2 (Hurez et al. 2003).

Recent research has also revised the notion of *monogamous* synapses. Time-lapse video microscopy of the T cell/APC interactions in vitro and visualization of cellular dynamics in lymphoid tissues showed that both T cells and APC can simultaneously engage multiple cellular partners (Valitutti et al. 1995; Okada et al. 2005; Miller et al. 2004). These observations raise the question of how the T cells can sense signals derived from different contact sites and accordingly adjust their responses. A study in which helper T cells were simultaneously conjugated with APC displaying different densities of cognate pMHC provided a first answer to this question. Depoil et al. showed that during simultaneous interaction with different APC, the T cells form dominant foci of signal transduction at the contact site with the APC providing the strongest stimulus and rapidly polarize their secretory machinery toward these cognate cells. Interestingly, preformed IS between the T cell and the APC displaying low pMHC densities can be rapidly disassembled and reformed toward APC offering higher pMHC densities, indicating that extra-synaptic TCR detecting a stronger stimulus can outcompete the signals derived from intra-synaptic TCR and drive cellular reorientation (Fig. 2, Depoil et al. 2005).

Using a novel approach based on photo-activated pMHC, Huse et al. were able to detect the activation of signal transduction in the T cells with high time/space resolution. Their work shows that activation of different foci of signal transduction instantaneously drives the T cell repolarization responses (Huse et al. 2007). These recent findings support the notion that IS are dynamic and adaptable structures remodeled by changes in antigenic stimuli received from different APC.

The IS formed at the CTL/target cell interface also exhibits a high degree of flexibility. It has indeed been shown that in CTL interacting simultaneously with two target cells displaying similar pMHC densities, the MTOC oscillates between those two target cells (Kuhn and Poenie 2002). More recently, it has been shown that when the CTL interact simultaneously with multiple target cells offering different antigenic stimuli, they polarize their lytic granules (*lytic synapse*) in

a   **Signal strength discrimination at the T helper cell/APC contact site**

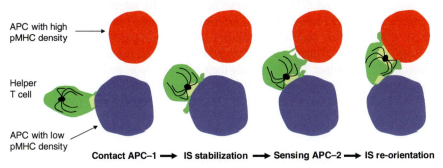

APC with high
pMHC density

Helper
T cell

APC with low
pMHC density

Contact APC–1 ➝ IS stabilization ➝ Sensing APC–2 ➝ IS re-orientation

b   **"Multiple killing" of target cells encountered simultaneously**

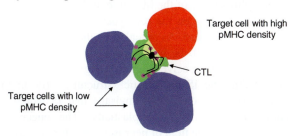

Target cell with high
pMHC density

CTL

Target cells with low
pMHC density

Fig. 2 Immunological synapses are versatile structures. (**a**) A helper T cell simultaneously in contact with two APC offering antigenic stimuli of different strength polarizes toward the APC offering the strongest stimulus. An IS is formed between a T cell and an APC displaying a low antigen density (APC 1, *blue*). Signal transduction takes place at this IS as detected by antiphosphotyrosine staining (*yellow*). Upon conjugation with a second APC (APC 2, *red*) displaying a stronger antigenic stimulus, a second IS begins to be formed at the contact site with the second APC while T-cell tubulin cytoskeleton (*black*), Golgi apparatus and mitochondria (not shown, (Depoil et al. 2005)) re-polarize toward the stronger stimulus. The first IS is progressively disassembled in parallel with the ongoing formation of the second one. (**b**) A CTL kills simultaneously multiple target cells offering antigenic stimuli of different strength. CTL form a *stimulatory synapse* with a target cell offering a strong antigenic stimulus (*red*) as represented by antiphosphotyrosine staining (*yellow*) and MTOC polarization (*black*). Lytic granules (*violet*) are secreted in the direction of this target cell as well as in the direction of additional adjacent targets offering weak antigenic stimuli (Wiedemann et al. 2006)

the direction of the different target cells and kill them simultaneously (Fig. 2, Wiedemann et al. 2006). Interestingly, in conjugation with a target cell offering an antigenic stimulus strong enough to induce the formation of a *stimulatory synapse* and a second target cell offering low antigenic stimulus, a CTL is able to establish simultaneously a *stimulatory* synapse with the first target and a *lytic* synapse with the second one (Fig. 2, Wiedemann et al. 2006).

All in all, the above discussed results demonstrate that the IS of both helper and cytotoxic T cells are not static and monogamous structures. On the contrary, they are dynamic and versatile signaling areas allowing the T cells to discriminate among different signals received simultaneously and to adjust their biological function accordingly. It is interesting to note that a basic difference exists between the helper T cells and CTL. While the helper T cells selectively polarize their secretory machinery toward the APC offering the strongest stimulus (Depoil et al. 2005), CTL polarize their lytic granules toward multiple target cells simultaneously, regardless of their stimulatory potential (Wiedemann et al. 2006). As a consequence, the helper T cells provide their help in a dedicated fashion, while the CTL are not selective in rapidly killing multiple cellular targets. These specific behaviors are both instrumental to the efficacy of adaptive immune responses.

6 On the "Raison d'être" of Immunological Synapse Plasticity

We have seen through this survey of the literature of the last decade that IS can be diverse and adaptable depending on the cell types considered and the nature and quality of the antigenic stimulation. As revealed by the active actin remodeling at the IS, these structures appear to be highly dynamic to allow a given T cell to optimally integrate the stimuli received during antigenic stimulation. Are those qualities enough to define the IS as "plastic" structures? By analogy with the function of neuronal synapses, one could envisage that IS would be the signal integrators regulating the process of T cell "plasticity." The concept of plasticity in biology has been developed in the field of neurosciences. It refers to the ability of a system (the brain) to achieve novel functions (learning, memory), by transforming its internal connectivity (neuron networks) in response to stimuli. It implies that a plastic system is not only based on preprogramed functions and transformations (Will et al. 2008). Following that definition, one may consider that the process of T cell differentiation and maturation following antigen encounter is endowed with some level of plasticity. It is clearly established that naive CD4$^+$ T cells bear the potential to differentiate into distinct lineages, including Th1, Th2, Th17, and inducible T-regulatory cells. Recent studies have brought to light the concept that the commitment to these T cell subsets is not solely genetically determined and is probably more plastic than previously thought. It was recently suggested that epigenetic mechanisms are underlying the plasticity of effector and regulatory T cells (Lee et al. 2009; Wei et al. 2009). In that context, it is tempting to speculate that the relative plasticity of T cell differentiation is at least in part mirrored by the highly tunable capacity of the IS to integrate and decode stimuli. During the navigation of a given naive T cell within the site of cognate antigen stimulation, the IS would integrate and decode the sequence of stimuli delivered. This includes pMHC stimulation as well as other membrane bound and soluble factors presented by the different APC encountered at the same time or sequentially. This integrative process would result in a specific tuning of the activation of a given T cell. As a result, T cells would indeed commit to well-defined differentiation paths, but a certain degree of flexibility and variability could be provided via the IS.

Another intriguing level of plasticity is linked to the notion that IS may serve as structural devices that simultaneously integrate stimuli and direct polarized secretion. We have seen that the CTL can assemble distinct IS structures (*lytic* versus *stimulatory*) depending on the strength of antigenic stimulation. Thus, they can functionally uncouple signal integration from polarized lytic granule secretion (Faroudi et al. 2003a; Wiedemann et al. 2006). An interesting question is to define how a *stimulatory* synapse can combine both signal integration and lytic granule exocytosis. It is likely that the spatial separation of signaling and secretory domains (Stinchcombe et al. 2001) and the temporal separation between secretory mechanisms (occurring within 2–3 min) and later signaling cascade assembly (Wiedemann et al. 2006) can contribute to allow *stimulatory* synapses to accomplish their multitask function. It is tempting to speculate that a multitask organization for signal integration and secretory events might also be at work in naive T cell and helper T-cell synapses to allow these cells to coordinate signal integration with secretory mechanisms.

Finally, IS plasticity can also be shaped by the context in which the T cell/APC encounter occurs. In vivo, in a context of a packed cellular environment such as a secondary lymphoid organ, a T cell engaged in a cognate interaction with an APC will most probably also be interacting with other cells that may influence the quality of the T/APC encounter. IS stability can be modulated by the local density of antigen-specific T cells that could therefore compete among them for conjugation with cognate APC. Accordingly, it has been shown that as T cells clonally expand and accumulate, they downregulate the ability of additional T cells to form long-lasting productive IS (Garcia et al. 2007). IS function may also be subverted by third-party cellular components. A relevant example is given by Treg, that can interfere with the Th cell/APC communication at the IS (Sumoza-Toledo et al. 2006), and in particular with the polarized secretion of IFN-γ toward the APC (Esquerre et al. 2008).

In conclusion, recent lines of evidence highlight IS plasticity as a key instrument of intercellular information transfer. Future research dedicated to the definition of molecular mechanisms regulating IS dynamics in vitro and to visualization of IS in situ, in different contexts of immune activation and regulation, will be instrumental to better understand IS plasticity. Furthermore, system biology approaches, by integrating multiple cellular and molecular parameters, will shed new light on how the plasticity of cell–cell communication at the IS contributes to the tuning of adaptive immunity.

Acknowledgments This work was supported by grants from la Ligue contre le Cancer ("Equipe labellisée 2009" to SV) and a Marie Curie Excellence grant (European Community contract MEXT-CT-2005-025032 to LD).

References

Alon R, Dustin ML (2007) Force as a facilitator of integrin conformational changes during leukocyte arrest on blood vessels and antigen-presenting cells. Immunity 26:17–27
Badour K, Zhang J, Shi F, Leng Y, Collins M, Siminovitch KA (2004) Fyn and PTP-PEST-mediated regulation of Wiskott-Aldrich syndrome protein (WASp) tyrosine phosphorylation is

required for coupling T cell antigen receptor engagement to WASp effector function and T cell activation. J Exp Med 199:99–112

Bajenoff M, Egen JG, Koo LY, Laugier JP, Brau F, Glaichenhaus N, Germain RN (2006) Stromal cell networks regulate lymphocyte entry, migration, and territoriality in lymph nodes. Immunity 25:989–1001

Benvenuti F, Lagaudriere-Gesbert C, Grandjean I, Jancic C, Hivroz C, Trautmann A, Lantz O, Amigorena S (2004) Dendritic cell maturation controls adhesion, synapse formation, and the duration of the interactions with naive T lymphocytes. J Immunol 172:292–301

Billadeau DD, Nolz JC, Gomez TS (2007) Regulation of T-cell activation by the cytoskeleton. Nat Rev Immunol 7:131–143

Bousso P, Robey E (2003) Dynamics of CD8+ T cell priming by dendritic cells in intact lymph nodes. Nat Immunol 4:579–585

Cai Z, Kishimoto H, Brunmark A, Jackson MR, Peterson PA, Sprent J (1997) Requirements for peptide-induced T cell receptor downregulation on naive CD8+ T cells. J Exp Med 185:641–651

Campi G, Varma R, Dustin ML (2005) Actin and agonist MHC-peptide complex-dependent T cell receptor microclusters as scaffolds for signaling. J Exp Med 202:1031–1036

Cannon J, Burkhardt J (2004) Differential roles for Wiskott-Aldrich syndrome protein in immune synapse formation and IL-2 production. J Immunol 173:1658–1662

Cannon J, Labno C, Bosco G, Seth A, McGavin H, Siminovitch K, Rosen M, Burkhardt J (2001) WASP recruitment to the T cell:APC contact site occurs independently of Cdc42 activation. Immunity 15:249–259

Castellino F, Huang AY, Altan-Bonnet G, Stoll S, Scheinecker C, Germain RN (2006) Chemokines enhance immunity by guiding naive CD8+ T cells to sites of CD4+ T cell-dendritic cell interaction. Nature 440:890–895

Celli S, Garcia Z, Bousso P (2005) CD4 T cells integrate signals delivered during successive DC encounters in vivo. J Exp Med 202:1271–1278

Celli S, Lemaitre F, Bousso P (2007) Real-time manipulation of T cell-dendritic cell interactions in vivo reveals the importance of prolonged contacts for CD4+ T cell activation. Immunity 27:625–634

Cemerski S, Das J, Locasale J, Arnold P, Giurisato E, Markiewicz MA, Fremont D, Allen PM, Chakraborty AK, Shaw AS (2007) The stimulatory potency of T cell antigens is influenced by the formation of the immunological synapse. Immunity 26:345–355

Cemerski S, Das J, Giurisato E, Markiewicz MA, Allen PM, Chakraborty AK, Shaw AS (2008) The balance between T cell receptor signaling and degradation at the center of the immunological synapse is determined by antigen quality. Immunity 29:414–422

Chang JT, Palanivel VR, Kinjyo I, Schambach F, Intlekofer AM, Banerjee A, Longworth SA, Vinup KE, Mrass P, Oliaro J et al (2007) Asymmetric T lymphocyte division in the initiation of adaptive immune responses. Science 315:1687–1691

Delon J, Kaibuchi K, Germain RN (2001) Exclusion of CD43 from the immunological synapse is mediated by phosphorylation-regulated relocation of the cytoskeletal adaptor moesin. Immunity 15:691–701

Depoil D, Zaru R, Guiraud M, Chauveau A, Harriague J, Bismuth G, Utzny C, Muller S, Valitutti S (2005) Immunological synapses are versatile structures enabling selective T cell polarization. Immunity 22:185–194

Dupre L, Aiuti A, Trifari S, Martino S, Saracco P, Bordignon C, Roncarolo MG (2002) Wiskott-Aldrich syndrome protein regulates lipid raft dynamics during immunological synapse formation. Immunity 17:157–166

Dushek O, Mueller S, Soubies S, Depoil D, Caramalho I, Coombs D, Valitutti S (2008) Effects of intracellular calcium and actin cytoskeleton on TCR mobility measured by fluorescence recovery. PLoS ONE 3:e3913

Dustin ML, Bromley SK, Kan Z, Peterson DA, Unanue ER (1997) Antigen receptor engagement delivers a stop signal to migrating T lymphocytes. Proc Natl Acad Sci USA 94:3909–3913

Dustin ML, Olszowy MW, Holdorf AD, Li J, Bromley S, Desai N, Widder P, Rosenberger F, van der Merwe PA, Allen PM, Shaw AS (1998) A novel adaptor protein orchestrates receptor patterning and cytoskeletal polarity in T-cell contacts. Cell 94:667–677

Espagnolle N, Depoil D, Zaru R, Demeur C, Champagne E, Guiraud M, Valitutti S (2007) CD2 and TCR synergize for the activation of phospholipase Cgamma1/calcium pathway at the immunological synapse. Int Immunol 19:239–248

Esquerre M, Tauzin B, Guiraud M, Muller S, Saoudi A, Valitutti S (2008) Human regulatory T cells inhibit polarization of T helper cells toward antigen-presenting cells via a TGF-beta-dependent mechanism. Proc Natl Acad Sci USA 105:2550–2555

Faroudi M, Utzny C, Salio M, Cerundolo V, Guiraud M, Muller S, Valitutti S (2003a) Lytic versus stimulatory synapse in cytotoxic T lymphocyte/target cell interaction: manifestation of a dual activation threshold. Proc Natl Acad Sci USA 100:14145–14150

Faroudi M, Zaru R, Paulet P, Muller S, Valitutti S (2003b) Cutting edge: T lymphocyte activation by repeated immunological synapse formation and intermittent signaling. J Immunol 171:1128–1132

Freiberg BA, Kupfer H, Maslanik W, Delli J, Kappler J, Zaller DM, Kupfer A (2002) Staging and resetting T cell activation in SMACs. Nat Immunol 3:911–917

Friedl P, den Boer AT, Gunzer M (2005) Tuning immune responses: diversity and adaptation of the immunological synapse. Nat Rev Immunol 5:532–545

Garcia Z, Pradelli E, Celli S, Beuneu H, Simon A, Bousso P (2007) Competition for antigen determines the stability of T cell-dendritic cell interactions during clonal expansion. Proc Natl Acad Sci USA 104:4553–4558

Germain RN, Bajenoff M, Castellino F, Chieppa M, Egen JG, Huang AY, Ishii M, Koo LY, Qi H (2008) Making friends in out-of-the-way places: how cells of the immune system get together and how they conduct their business as revealed by intravital imaging. Immunol Rev 221:163–181

Gomez TS, McCarney SD, Carrizosa E, Labno CM, Comiskey EO, Nolz JC, Zhu P, Freedman BD, Clark MR, Rawlings DJ et al (2006) HS1 functions as an essential actin-regulatory adaptor protein at the immune synapse. Immunity 24:741–752

Gomez TS, Kumar K, Medeiros RB, Shimizu Y, Leibson PJ, Billadeau DD (2007) Formins regulate the actin-related protein 2/3 complex-independent polarization of the centrosome to the immunological synapse. Immunity 26:177–190

Grakoui A, Bromley SK, Sumen C, Davis MM, Shaw AS, Allen PM, Dustin ML (1999) The immunological synapse: a molecular machine controlling T cell activation. Science 285:221–227

Gunzer M, Schafer A, Borgmann S, Grabbe S, Zanker KS, Brocker EB, Kampgen E, Friedl P (2000) Antigen presentation in extracellular matrix: interactions of T cells with dendritic cells are dynamic, short lived, and sequential. Immunity 13:323–332

Harder T, Rentero C, Zech T, Gaus K (2007) Plasma membrane segregation during T cell activation: probing the order of domains. Curr Opin Immunol 19:470–475

Henrickson SE, Mempel TR, Mazo IB, Liu B, Artyomov MN, Zheng H, Peixoto A, Flynn MP, Senman B, Junt T et al (2008) T cell sensing of antigen dose governs interactive behavior with dendritic cells and sets a threshold for T cell activation. Nat Immunol 9:282–291

Huppa JB, Davis MM (2003) T-cell-antigen recognition and the immunological synapse. Nat Rev Immunol 3:973–983

Hurez V, Saparov A, Tousson A, Fuller MJ, Kubo T, Oliver J, Weaver BT, Weaver CT (2003) Restricted clonal expression of IL-2 by naive T cells reflects differential dynamic interactions with dendritic cells. J Exp Med 198:123–132

Huse M, Klein LO, Girvin AT, Faraj JM, Li QJ, Kuhns MS, Davis MM (2007) Spatial and temporal dynamics of T cell receptor signaling with a photoactivatable agonist. Immunity 27:76–88

Jacobelli J, Chmura SA, Buxton DB, Davis MM, Krummel MF (2004) A single class II myosin modulates T cell motility and stopping, but not synapse formation. Nat Immunol 5:531–538

Kaizuka Y, Douglass AD, Varma R, Dustin ML, Vale RD (2007) Mechanisms for segregating T cell receptor and adhesion molecules during immunological synapse formation in Jurkat T cells. Proc Natl Acad Sci USA 104:20296–20301

Krause M, Sechi A, Konradt M, Monner D, Gertler F, Wehland J (2000) Fyn-binding protein (Fyb)/SLP-76-associated protein (SLAP), Ena/vasodilator-stimulated phosphoprotein (VASP) proteins and the Arp2/3 complex link T cell receptor (TCR) signaling to the actin cytoskeleton. J Cell Biol 149:181–194

Krawczyk C, Oliveira-dos-Santos A, Sasaki T, Griffiths E, Ohashi PS, Snapper S, Alt F, Penninger JM (2002) Vav1 controls integrin clustering and MHC/peptide-specific cell adhesion to antigen-presenting cells. Immunity 16:331–343

Kuhn JR, Poenie M (2002) Dynamic polarization of the microtubule cytoskeleton during CTL-mediated killing. Immunity 16:111–121

Lee KH, Holdorf AD, Dustin ML, Chan AC, Allen PM, Shaw AS (2002) T cell receptor signaling precedes immunological synapse formation. Science 295:1539–1542

Lee KH, Dinner AR, Tu C, Campi G, Raychaudhuri S, Varma R, Sims TN, Burack WR, Wu H, Wang J et al (2003) The immunological synapse balances T cell receptor signaling and degradation. Science 302:1218–1222

Lee YK, Turner H, Maynard CL, Oliver JR, Chen D, Elson CO, Weaver CT (2009) Late developmental plasticity in the T helper 17 lineage. Immunity 30:92–107

Leupin O, Zaru R, Laroche T, Muller S, Valitutti S (2000) Exclusion of CD45 from the T-cell receptor signaling area in antigen-stimulated T lymphocytes. Curr Biol 10:277–280

Lindquist RL, Shakhar G, Dudziak D, Wardemann H, Eisenreich T, Dustin ML, Nussenzweig MC (2004) Visualizing dendritic cell networks in vivo. Nat Immunol 5:1243–1250

Maldonado RA, Irvine DJ, Schreiber R, Glimcher LH (2004) A role for the immunological synapse in lineage commitment of CD4 lymphocytes. Nature 431:527–532

McGavin MK, Badour K, Hardy LA, Kubiseski TJ, Zhang J, Siminovitch KA (2001) The intersectin 2 adaptor links Wiskott Aldrich Syndrome protein (WASp)-mediated actin polymerization to T cell antigen receptor endocytosis. J Exp Med 194:1777–1787

Mempel TR, Henrickson SE, Von Andrian UH (2004) T-cell priming by dendritic cells in lymph nodes occurs in three distinct phases. Nature 427:154–159

Miller MJ, Wei SH, Parker I, Cahalan MD (2002) Two-photon imaging of lymphocyte motility and antigen response in intact lymph node. Science 296:1869–1873

Miller MJ, Safrina O, Parker I, Cahalan MD (2004) Imaging the single cell dynamics of CD4+ T cell activation by dendritic cells in lymph nodes. J Exp Med 200:847–856

Molina IJ, Sancho J, Terhorst C, Rosen FS, Remold-O'Donnell E (1993) T cells of patients with the Wiskott-Aldrich Syndrome have a restricted defect in proliferative responses. J Immunol 151:4383–4390

Monks CR, Freiberg BA, Kupfer H, Sciaky N, Kupfer A (1998) Three-dimensional segregation of supramolecular activation clusters in T cells. Nature 395:82–86

Negulescu PA, Krasieva TB, Khan A, Kerschbaum HH, Cahalan MD (1996) Polarity of T cell shape, motility, and sensitivity to antigen. Immunity 4:421–430

Nguyen K, Sylvain NR, Bunnell SC (2008) T cell costimulation via the integrin VLA-4 inhibits the actin-dependent centralization of signaling microclusters containing the adaptor SLP-76. Immunity 28:810–821

Nolz JC, Gomez TS, Zhu P, Li S, Medeiros RB, Shimizu Y, Burkhardt JK, Freedman BD, Billadeau DD (2006) The WAVE2 complex regulates actin cytoskeletal reorganization and CRAC-mediated calcium entry during T cell activation. Curr Biol 16:24–34

Norcross M (1984) A synaptic basis for T-lymphocyte activation. Ann Immunol (Paris) 135D:113–134

Ochs HD, Thrasher AJ (2006) The Wiskott-Aldrich syndrome. J Allergy Clin Immunol 117:725–738 quiz 739

Okada T, Miller MJ, Parker I, Krummel MF, Neighbors M, Hartley SB, O'Garra A, Cahalan MD, Cyster JG (2005) Antigen-engaged B cells undergo chemotaxis toward the T zone and form motile conjugates with helper T cells. PLoS Biol 3:e150

O'Keefe JP, Blaine K, Alegre ML, Gajewski TF (2004) Formation of a central supramolecular activation cluster is not required for activation of naive CD8+ T cells. Proc Natl Acad Sci USA 101:9351–9356

Penna D, Muller S, Martinon F, Demotz S, Iwashima M, Valitutti S (1999) Degradation of ZAP-70 following antigenic stimulation in human T lymphocytes: role of calpain proteolytic pathway. J Immunol 163:50–56

Purbhoo MA, Irvine DJ, Huppa JB, Davis MM (2004) T cell killing does not require the formation of a stable mature immunological synapse. Nat Immunol 5:524–530

Richie LI, Ebert PJ, Wu LC, Krummel MF, Owen JJ, Davis MM (2002) Imaging synapse formation during thymocyte selection: inability of CD3zeta to form a stable central accumulation during negative selection. Immunity 16:595–606

Sasahara Y, Rachid R, Byrne MJ, de la Fuente MA, Abraham RT, Ramesh N, Geha RS (2002) Mechanism of recruitment of WASP to the immunological synapse and of its activation following TCR ligation. Mol Cell 10:1269–1281

Schneider H, Downey J, Smith A, Zinselmeyer BH, Rush C, Brewer JM, Wei B, Hogg N, Garside P, Rudd CE (2006) Reversal of the TCR stop signal by CTLA-4. Science 313:1972–1975

Sims TN, Soos TJ, Xenias HS, Dubin-Thaler B, Hofman JM, Waite JC, Cameron TO, Thomas VK, Varma R, Wiggins CH et al (2007) Opposing effects of PKCtheta and WASp on symmetry breaking and relocation of the immunological synapse. Cell 129:773–785

Springer TA (1990) Adhesion receptors of the immune system. Nature 346:425–434

Stinchcombe JC, Bossi G, Booth S, Griffiths GM (2001) The immunological synapse of CTL contains a secretory domain and membrane bridges. Immunity 15:751–761

Stinchcombe JC, Majorovits E, Bossi G, Fuller S, Griffiths GM (2006) Centrosome polarization delivers secretory granules to the immunological synapse. Nature 443:462–465

Stoll S, Delon J, Brotz TM, Germain RN (2002) Dynamic imaging of T cell-dendritic cell interactions in lymph nodes. Science 296:1873–1876

Sumoza-Toledo A, Eaton AD, Sarukhan A (2006) Regulatory T cells inhibit protein kinase C theta recruitment to the immune synapse of naive T cells with the same antigen specificity. J Immunol 176:5779–5787

Tadokoro CE, Shakhar G, Shen S, Ding Y, Lino AC, Maraver A, Lafaille JJ, Dustin ML (2006) Regulatory T cells inhibit stable contacts between CD4+ T cells and dendritic cells in vivo. J Exp Med 203:505–511

Takenawa T, Suetsugu S (2007) The WASP-WAVE protein network: connecting the membrane to the cytoskeleton. Nat Rev Mol Cell Biol 8:37–48

Trautmann A, Valitutti S (2003) The diversity of immunological synapses. Curr Opin Immunol 15:249–254

Trifari S, Sitia G, Aiuti A, Scaramuzza S, Marangoni F, Guidotti LG, Martino S, Saracco P, Notarangelo LD, Roncarolo MG, Dupre L (2006) Defective Th1 Cytokine Gene Transcription in CD4+ and CD8+ T Cells from Wiskott-Aldrich Syndrome Patients. J Immunol 177:7451–7461

Tskvitaria-Fuller I, Rozelle AL, Yin HL, Wulfing C (2003) Regulation of sustained actin dynamics by the TCR and costimulation as a mechanism of receptor localization. J Immunol 171:2287–2295

Valitutti S (2008) Immunological synapse: center of attention again. Immunity 29:384–386

Valitutti S, Dessing M, Aktories K, Gallati H, Lanzavecchia A (1995) Sustained signaling leading to T cell activation results from prolonged T cell receptor occupancy. Role of T cell actin cytoskeleton. J Exp Med 181:577–584

Valitutti S, Muller S, Dessing M, Lanzavecchia A (1996a) Different responses are elicited in cytotoxic T lymphocytes by different levels of T cell receptor occupancy. J Exp Med 183:1917–1921

Valitutti S, Muller S, Dessing M, Lanzavecchia A (1996b) Signal extinction and T cell repolarization in T helper cell-antigen-presenting cell conjugates. Eur J Immunol 26:2012–2016

Varma R, Campi G, Yokosuka T, Saito T, Dustin ML (2006) T cell receptor-proximal signals are sustained in peripheral microclusters and terminated in the central supramolecular activation cluster. Immunity 25:117–127

Viola A, Contento RL, Molon B (2006) T cells and their partners: the chemokine dating agency. Trends Immunol 27:421–427

Wei G, Wei L, Zhu J, Zang C, Hu-Li J, Yao Z, Cui K, Kanno Y, Roh TY, Watford WT et al (2009) Global mapping of H3K4me3 and H3K27me3 reveals specificity and plasticity in lineage fate determination of differentiating CD4+ T cells. Immunity 30:155–167

Wiedemann A, Depoil D, Faroudi M, Valitutti S (2006) Cytotoxic T lymphocytes kill multiple targets simultaneously via spatiotemporal uncoupling of lytic and stimulatory synapses. Proc Natl Acad Sci USA 103:10985–10990

Will B, Dalrymple-Alford J, Wolff M, Cassel JC (2008) The concept of brain plasticity – Paillard's systemic analysis and emphasis on structure and function (followed by the translation of a seminal paper by Paillard on plasticity). Behav Brain Res 192:2–7

Zaru R, Cameron TO, Stern LJ, Muller S, Valitutti S (2002) Cutting edge: TCR engagement and triggering in the absence of large-scale molecular segregation at the T cell-APC contact site. J Immunol 168:4287–4291

APC, T Cells, and the Immune Synapse

Peter Reichardt, Bastian Dornbach, and Matthias Gunzer

Contents

Abstract CD4$^+$ T cells engage different activating cells during their generation in the bone marrow and thymus and during their homeostasis and activation in the periphery. During these processes, T cells or their precursors establish a molecular platform for communication in the interface between the two cells that is called immune synapse (IS). Here we review the current knowledge about those different IS. Apart from looking at the structure and signalling of the IS from the T cell region, we will also focus on the area of the IS partner, mostly antigen-presenting cells (APC). We will discuss the features of different APC and their role played in the control of the resulting activated or differentiated T cell. We will also demonstrate that despite 10 years of research into the subject, large areas of this field are yet to be explored. This will keep us busy for the years to come – new exciting results lie ahead of us.

P. Reichardt and M. Gunzer (✉)
Otto-von-Guericke University, Institute of Molecular and Clinical Immunology, Leipziger Str. 44, D-39120, Magdeburg, Germany
e-mail: matthias.gunzer@med.ovgu.de

B. Dornbach
Helmholtz Centre for Infection Research, Inhoffenstr. 7, D-38124 Braunschweig, Germany

T. Saito and F.D. Batista (eds.), *Immunological Synapse*,
Current Topics in Microbiology and Immunology 340,
DOI 10.1007/978-3-642-03858-7_12, © Springer-Verlag Berlin Heidelberg 2010

1   Introduction

A T cell interacts with many different cell types during its generation, functional maturation, and effector phase. During each event, it forms a synapse to decode the information provided by the opposite cell and to respond to it accordingly. For the developing and mature T cells, this structure would be called immune synapse (IS). The general concept of the IS will be described extensively in other chapters of this issue and we will not define it further here. The interested reader is referred to some extensive reviews on the subject (Friedl et al. 2005; Reichardt et al. 2007a; Bromley et al. 2001). For the sake of this review, we invite you to our tour through the life of a T cell thereby looking through a virtual "nano-camera" that always focuses on the currently formed synapse while we follow a T cell precursor from its birth place in the bone marrow to the thymus, the lymph node and, ultimately, the peripheral effector site. With this approach, we will provide an overview of what is currently known about the antigen-presenting cells (APC) or stimulating cells encountered during this developmental path, the peculiarities of the synapses formed and their impact on T cell function.

2   Generation of T cell Precursors in the Bone Marrow:
The Hematopoietic Synapse

The life of a T cell starts in the bone marrow. As all blood cells, T cells are derived from hematopoietic stem cells (HSC) that reside within the bone marrow. Single HSC are able to repopulate the entire system of blood cells in lethally irradiated recipients and thus transplantation of allogeneic or autologous HSC represent important options in the therapy of certain cancer or autoimmune diseases (Osawa et al. 1996).

Despite intensive research and successful clinical application, the basic biology of the HSC in the marrow is still not well known. HSC are very rare. Only 0.05–0.5% of all bone marrow cells are considered to be HSC in humans (Gunsilius et al. 2001). The place within the bone marrow cavity, where HSC reside, has been termed "niche" although the nature of the cell type actually forming the niche is still a matter of debate (Geiger et al. 2007; Kopp et al. 2005; Scadden 2006). Very recent imaging data suggest that osteoblasts, which had long been suspected to form the niche (Wilson and Trumpp 2006; Adams and Scadden 2006), are not in direct contact with transplanted HSC (Lo Celso et al. 2009). What is known and also supported by several independent groups is the fact that the niche is close to and in direct contact to the inner surface of the calcified bone, the endosteum (Lo Celso et al. 2009; Nilsson et al. 2001; Wilson and Trumpp 2006; Köhler et al. 2009).

The HSC have to perform two important tasks: the maintenance of their own numbers (self renewal) and the generation of mature blood cells (hematopoiesis). The central process for this function is a cell division event that generates two nonidentical daughter cells, a HSC and a cell that will differentiate into mature cells. Therefore, this process has been termed asymmetric division (Adams and Scadden 2006). The surface of the niche-forming cell is considered critical for the decision about which cell will remain an HSC and which will differentiate, but the defined ligands or molecular mechanisms that would govern this decision are still hypothetical (Wilson and Trumpp 2006).

Despite its importance for hematopoiesis in general and the T cell system in particular the synapse that forms when an HSC contacts a niche cell has not been investigated so far. Thus, the molecular structure of this synapse is undefined as is the difference in the structure of niches that foster asymmetric or symmetric divisions including those leading to the earliest bone-marrow-resident precursors of T cell development (see below). Promisingly, there are now systems available, that allow the direct imaging of symmetric and asymmetric division of HSC on stromal cells in cell-culture *in vitro* (Wu et al. 2007). Such models can be a first step towards the analysis of the structure of the cell–cell synapse. Since the system is based on the HSC-specific expression of GFP in transgenic animals, it might even allow identifying individual HSC in their niche in the marrow, an indispensable prerequisite for any approach towards an analysis of HSC-niche synapses *in situ*.

3   Generation of T cells in the Thymus: Thymic Synapses

The next step in the life of a T cell is its "education" from a non-committed bone-marrow precursor to a real T cell. This happens in the thymus. The thymus is the organ where thymocytes are scanned for the reactivity of their T cell receptors (TCR). Each thymocyte has a unique TCR that is generated in a chance process via somatic recombination from a set of genetic building blocks (Germain 2002). Thus, despite being able to generate TCR with a specificity against any possible foreign antigen, this process also bears the risk of generating TCRs with no useful affinity to function properly at all. More dangerous, however, is the risk of generating TCRs which are reactive against self structures. In a process called positive selection the thymus sorts out the fraction of thymocytes that have a non-reactive TCR. Negative selection is then used to delete self reactive cells. In addition, thymic selection defines which T cell subtype, CD4 or CD8, will be generated, as early thymocytes are not yet defined in this respect (von Boehmer et al. 2003).

Thymic development starts with the immigration of precursor cells from the bone marrow. The identity of these cells is still a matter of debate and it has even been discussed that HSC directly enter the thymus (Boehm and Bleul 2006). More recent data indicate that a very rare population of precursors characterized by the markers $Lin^-Sca-1^+c-Kit^+CCR9^+Flt-3^{low}$ leaves the bone marrow and directly seeds the thymus, then giving rise to all the later stages of thymic T cell development (Benz et al. 2008). The point of entry at the cortico-medullary junction of the thymus also forms the niche for these cells in a manner similar to the bone marrow niche for HSC. As in bone marrow biology the identity of the thymic niche cell is yet unclear. Discussed cell types are endothelial cells of the blood vessels at the exit site of the seeder cells or thymic epithelial cells in this area (Boehm and Bleul 2006).

It is clear that the thymus seeding cells which still have the principal capacity to also form B cells rapidly lose this ability after thymus entry. This is mediated by the receptor Notch1 on the thymus seeding cells as well as all the later stages of thymocytes which are triggered by the ligands Delta-1 or Jagged expressed on thymic stromal cells (Visan et al. 2006b). The signalling of this pathway already starts at the cortico-medullary junction and a competition of the seeder cells with more advanced stages of thymocyte development for the limited amounts of Notch-ligands seems to regulate the coverage of the niches and, thus, thymus size and cellularity (Tan et al. 2005; Visan et al. 2006b). It is not known, how long the thymus seeders are occupying a given niche site and how they are dislodged or whether they are more resident and constantly undergo asymmetric divisions to produce offspring that undergoes thymocyte development (Boehm and Bleul 2006). In any case, the contact of a thymus seeder cell with its niche can be considered the first T cell-specific synapse. To the best of our knowledge, the molecular structure of this synapse is unknown despite its critical importance for T cell biology. Given the rarity of the cell type (it was demonstrated, that only 200 cells form the entire repertoire of seeder cells in the thymus and are sufficient to generate all thymocytes (Spangrude and Scollay 1990)) it will be challenging to analyze the synapse within the organ itself, although individual cells have been visualized in situ (Lind et al. 2001). However, use of highly enriched precursors cultured in contact with bone marrow stromal cells transfected with the Notch-ligand Delta-like 1 might provide a first approach for an in vitro analysis of this synapse (Benz et al. 2008; Schmitt and Zuniga-Pflucker 2002).

T cell precursors generated from the niche-resident seeding cells move upwards to the subcapsular thymic area, thereby more and more committing to the T cell lineage (Lind et al. 2001). Again Notch-ligands are essential but cells which are contacted during this period are not well defined. The next critical synapse, and also the first which is well investigated is the IS leading to positive or negative selection of thymocytes (Ebert et al. 2008; Ehrlich et al. 2002). This synapse is also the first that uses peptide loaded MHC complexes as critical structure for the determination of a differential outcome of thymocyte activation. Presenting cells are cortical epithelial cells and medullary epithelial as well as dendritic cells (DC) (Germain 2002).

Historically, the first thymic synapse investigated was the one inducing negative selection of thymocytes which have rearranged their TCR and now express both CD4 and CD8 (double positive, DP) (Richie et al. 2002). A "classical" IS consists of a round interaction plane of 1–2 μm diameter which is organized in several structural areas termed SMACs (supra molecular activation clusters) by their discoverers (Monks et al. 1998). Conventionally, the central cSMAC is enriched in signalling components and peripheral pSMACs contain adhesion molecules (Monks et al. 1998), although meanwhile numerous deviations from this concept have been described (Friedl et al. 2005). In addition to imaging of the synapse itself (Reichardt et al. 2007b) we have described the cellular dynamics underlying the synapse formation and found, that T cells engaging DC during antigen presentation do interact in transient short contacts (Gunzer et al. 2000). This has later been confirmed by intravital imaging and was extended by the finding that, at later stages, contacts of T cells to DC or of thymocytes to selecting stromal cells are longer-lived (Bousso et al. 2002; Mempel et al. 2004).

When investigating the synapse formed by a DP cell with a negatively select-ing stromal cell, it came as a surprise that the important TCR-signalling mole-cules LCK and CD3ζ were selectively excluded from the cSMAC (Richie et al. 2002). This was partly an inherent feature of the thymocyte itself, because the same cells after being positively selected to naïve T cells and then stimulated to become mature T blasts made synapses with mostly central accumulation of LCK and CD3ζ. However, also the APC was important in this respect, because exchanging the thymus-derived stromal cell with a more peripheral type of APC (CH27 B cells) allowed thymocytes to establish a central accumulation of CD3ζ and thymic stromal cells inhibited this pattern when synapsing with peripheral blasts (Richie et al. 2002). Another important finding of the authors was the fact that the cells contacted a negative-selecting stromal cell in a very long-lasting manner. This was interpreted as a way of the stromal cell to ensure that the thymocyte could not escape before negative selection was completed (Richie et al. 2002).

In the same study positively selecting synapses were also investigated, unfortu-nately, however, only at one imaging plane that did not allow extracting informa-tion on the spatial organization of LCK or CD3ζ within the IS. The positively selecting synapses induced less efficient recruitment of LCK or CD3ζ to the interface with the selecting cell (Richie et al. 2002). The same group recently published a further analysis of positively and negatively selecting synapses. They found, that just two negatively selecting pMHC molecules in the interface were sufficient to induce almost complete cell death in reacting thymocytes. This was associated with complete and sustained nuclear recruitment of the key transcription factor NFATc in the thymocytes. At the same time, positively selected thymocytes could not form a clearly discernible synapse but instead established multiple short encounters with stromal cells that also led to a considerable nuclear import of NFATc. Interestingly, this reorientation of NFATc was dependent on the recogni-tion of self pMHC molecules on the selecting cell pointing to the fact that opposite to the negatively selecting event, the positive selection requires multiple short encounters with self pMHC that slightly tickle the TCR but do not lead to robust nuclear import of NFATc (Ebert et al. 2008).

In vivo, the synapses described above generate a set of T cells that are either CD4 or CD8, recognize self ligands well enough to be kept alive but not as efficiently as to be deleted. These surviving cells, only ~5% or all generated DP thymocytes, are now called naïve T cells and leave the thymus via the blood stream to enter peripheral lymphatic organs in their hunt for truly activating foreign ligands (Gunzer 2007).

4   Antigen Presentation in the Lymph Node Is Mainly Done by Dendritic Cells

At the end of their journey through the circulation, naïve T cells will regularly leave the blood vessels by entering secondary lymphoid organs, namely the spleen and the lymph nodes. It is in the lymph node, where T cells spend much of their life awaiting a specific, matching antigen to be presented to them. Thus, the lymph node is the "home" of the T cells, and immunologists termed the lymphocyte's behaviour to go to lymph nodes as "homing" (Goodnow and Cyster 1997).

Within the lymph node, there exist several distinct topographic zones with a specific microenvironment providing optimal conditions for cell development and cell–cell interaction. T cells will leave the blood vessels in specialized zones with comparatively enlarged diameter and thickened endothelial walls, termed high endothelial vessels or HEVs (Stamper and Woodruff 1976). The presence of entry receptors such as CD62L (L-Selectin) ensure that naïve-T cells enter the lymph node in a multi-step process right here (Springer 1994). HEVs are predominantly positioned close to paracortical T cell zones where T cells will immediately encounter antigen-loaded DC. This is where the "classical" T cell priming following contact to APC will occur (Mempel et al. 2004; von Andrian and Mempel 2003).

Full T cell activation is reached when a T cell encounters a mature DC. High levels of MHC-II and co-stimulatory molecules such as CD80, CD86 provide an efficient stimulating surface for the T cell (Banchereau and Steinman 1998). In case of infection and peripheral inflammation, maturation of immigrating DC will begin in (inflamed) peripheral tissues and while DC move through afferent lymphatic vessels to deliver their captured antigen to the lymph node (Itano et al. 2003). In addition, antigen can also float through afferent lymph and be captured by the lymph node resident DC (Sixt et al. 2005). Productive interactions between T cells and DC presenting a matching antigen will immediately lead to changes in the cytoskeletal architecture of the T cell, permitting cholesterol-enriched microdomains (lipid rafts) in the cell membrane to coalesce into a platform for intercellular adhesion molecules, signal-transduction molecules, and numerous TCR/MHC pairings (Friedl et al. 2005). The segregated clusters of TCR–MHC at the cell–cell interface between T cells and mature DC (which usually display an active cytoskeleton) are comparatively small, and are hence termed microcluster (Brossard et al. 2005). In addition, small clusters of co-stimulatory molecules such as CD28, and adhesion molecules such as LFA-1 are also present (Tseng et al. 2008). Thus, the basic components of larger, supramolecular clusters, as found between T cells and B cells ((Monks et al. 1998) and see below) are present. What the microclusters lack in size they make up in numbers: several tens of contact spots between T cells and DC were reported (Brossard et al. 2005). Larger segregational complexes leading to the picture of a mature IS with distinct cSMAC and pSMAC, respectively, develop by conflating microclusters, possibly driven by cytoskeletal forces (Tseng et al. 2008; Seminario and Bunnell 2008). However, in terms of functionality, it seems inappropriate to judge small, multifocal clusters as "immature" and large clusters as "mature" structures. In fact, microclusters may represent the basic form of a larger cSMAC–pSMAC-type of IS, and key signalling events are probably to be shared in both systems. Very simplified, TCR signalling and CD80 assembly in the central part are essential but not sufficient elements for effective signalling. CD28 also enriches at the cSMAC and drives recruitment of the protein kinase C theta (PKCθ), one of the key molecules of T cell signal transduction (Monks et al. 1997). Activated T cells will then differentiate into T effector cells.

At the level of the IS, a molecular distinction between the classical effector lines Th1 and Th2 was uncovered when it was found that the interferon-gamma receptor co-polarizes much more rapidly with engaged TCR in a Th1-prone mouse strain (C57BL/6) than in a Th2-prone strain (BALB/c) and that this co-polarization is prevented in the presence of IL-4, a cytokine directing T cells into a Th2 profile (Maldonado et al. 2004). Thus, a molecular link was established between TCR and cytokine signalling and it was shown how the physical conformation of the IS can direct T cell differentiation. A totally different role for the IS was proposed in a seminal paper from the group of Steven Reiner. They showed that synapsing T cells preparing to divide in the process of proliferation expressed an asymmetric composition of surface molecules. After division of the cells this asymmetric surface composition led to two differentiated cell types: an effector type of T cell (the daughter cell that contained the initial IS) and a memory type of cell (the daughter cell that was generated from the membrane part opposite of the synapse). Thus, IS might also have important influence on the future fate of T cells (Chang et al. 2007). Indeed, this observation bears all the components described above for asymmetric division of HSC in the bone marrow, with the "niche" being the surface of the APC itself. This example powerfully demonstrates how the APC can influence the overall outcome of a T cell response. Structural differences between naïve and memory CD4$^+$ T cells were also described in another study, where the IS of memory T cells was found to contain more pre-clusters of signalling molecules and an increased recruitment of the tyrosine phosphatase CD45 compared to naïve T cells (Watson and Lee 2004). However, apart from that, not a lot of information is available on IS formation in other effector lines such as Th17 cells or Treg (see below).

Once activated, the default pathway of T cells is to leave the lymph node. Upregulation of sphingosine-1-phosphate-receptor type 1 enhances T cell egress towards high levels of sphingosine-1-phosphate in deeper regions of the lymph node (Lo et al. 2005). In getting ready to leave, T cells pass through a last distinct zone of the lymph node, the medulla. Along medullary cords and crossing medullary sinus spaces T cells will reach efferent lymphatic vessels which will ultimately bring them back to the central blood circulation (Sanna et al. 2006; Wei et al. 2005). The medulla is characterized by a high number of B cells and macrophages (Krall and Braun 1992). Venous vessels in the medulla carry a somewhat differing repertoire of L-selectin ligands and may contribute to T cell homing to a small extent (M'Rini et al. 2003). The physiological importance of this is, however, unknown. Although the medulla is full of APC, solid experimental evidence is lacking that priming processes would occur in the medulla and that this might contribute to the immune response. Again, we have no knowledge of the existence or specific nature of IS formation by T cells in the lymph node medulla.

In general, the full activation of a CD4$^+$ T cell is, however, rare. Most T cells will die without ever meeting the right antigen and maturing into a full-blown, cytokine-producing and help-providing effector cell. Rather, the default situation of presentation to a T cell is absence of "danger" (Matzinger 2002). Thus, in a perfectly functioning, germ free body, encountered DC will exclusively present fragments of own, healthy cells and structures. The presenting DC will be an inactivated, immature (iDC), as no signs of inflammation or microbial attack flanked its way through afferent lymph vessels or are present in the T-zone's micromilieu. This can be judged by the surface marker DEC-205, which is expressed on most DC in the T zone of a non-inflamed lymph node (Witmer-Pack et al. 1995) and defines immature DC (Bonifaz et al. 2002). The majority of contacts between iDC and T cells will not lead to T cell activation. In fact, most have no effect on the differentiation profile of the T cells and they would remain naïve by definition. However, CD4$^+$ T cells depend on contacts to MHC-II molecules presenting self ligands for survival (Brocker 1997; Muranski et al. 2000; Stefanova et al. 2002). Is a synapse involved in this process? How does it look? We don't know. It probably resembles the synapse or merely absence of synapse that was described above for positive selection in the thymus. But more work is needed to really prove this point.

As soon as the strength of signalling elicited in the T cell reaches a certain threshold, by increasing affinity between TCR and peptide–MHC ligand and/or by increased co-stimulatory activity, the T cell will start to undergo a differentiation process. There are suboptimal signals which are too low to reach full effector potential. These signals are called sub-optimal, yet do induce a type of differentiation that is distinct from both pure survival and full effector function. In fact, suboptimal T cell activation, potentially also mediated, following contacts to self peptides, is currently discussed to be one major source of regulatory T cells (Treg) originating in the periphery (Hsieh et al. 2004; Shevach et al. 2006). Whether the formation of an IS during the induction of a Treg differs from an IS during regular, full T cell activation is unclear.

At the end of T cell activation, a specific T cell effector type has formed. Classical effector T cells will migrate to peripheral tissues to secrete stimulating cytokines such as IFNγ. Whether this also involves cell–cell contacts or the formation of an IS with a target cell, e.g. local macrophages, is not well known. However, physical interaction between macrophages/monocytes and local T cells have been demonstrated during granuloma formation in vivo (Egen et al. 2008). As for the function of Treg, there is evidence that many Treg, namely the Foxp3$^+$ natural Treg (nTreg) require direct cell–cell contact for them to become effective (Gondek et al. 2005). Still, a direct physical interference of Treg with the formation of classical T–DC has not been demonstrated yet. In contrast, Treg were shown to preferentially form clusters with DC *in vitro* and delay the maturation of DC (Serra et al. 2003; Onishi et al. 2008). Treg also interfere with the recruitment of signalling molecules such as PKCθ towards the IS in naïve T cells (Sumoza-Toledo et al. 2006). However, the specific composition of a putative regulatory IS between a Treg and a DC or between a Treg and a naïve T cell during regulation is completely unexplored.

5 B Cells as APC

Structure and molecular makeup of the IS can change completely, when a different type of APC than DC is involved. Still, few studies were undertaken to directly compare the IS formation following T cell contact to varying APC. As such, we have shown that the cellular interface between T cells and naïve B cells presenting a peptide specific for the TCR is characterized *in vitro* by a comparatively large, mature IS, which is stable for many hours (Reichardt et al. 2007b). B cells were known to always form stable cell pairs with T cells *in vitro* and *in vivo* (Gunzer et al. 2004; Okada et al. 2005). This was in contrast to DC, which contact T cells mostly in the range of minutes, at least during the early phases of T cell activation (Gunzer et al. 2000; Miller et al. 2004; Bryce et al. 2004). The long interaction between B cells and T cells was somewhat counterintuitive, as longer contacts are generally believed to be more effective (Celli et al. 2007; Scholer et al. 2008) while B cells, foremost naïve B cells, are very inefficient APC (Masten and Lipscomb 1999; Lassila et al. 1988). In contrast, the IS structure emerging from DC–T contacts is usually much smaller and transient, hence the terms microcluster or kinapse are appropriately used in describing them. These structures have been recently reviewed (Dustin 2008; Seminario and Bunnell 2008) and will also be covered in more detail in other chapters of this issue. Examples of the divergent IS structures found in pairs of T cells contacting naïve B cells or DC, respectively, are visualized in Fig. 1.

As for naïve B cell–T cell pairs, it came as another surprise when it was found that T cells following such extended contacts displayed an aberrant effector pheno-type with regulatory capacity. These B cell-generated Treg, TofB, were able to inhibit solid organ transplant rejection in the mouse (Reichardt et al. 2007b). Thus, it was possible to speculate, that the naïve-B cell–T cell–IS represents a novel type of IS, the regulatory IS. However, at present, the direct molecular link between the B–T–IS formation and Treg cell function is still unknown.

One characteristic feature of the B–IS is its prolonged, hour-long presence. However, a long-term stable IS induced by B cells may not necessarily reflect high signalling activity. Such, interference with actin polymerization in MHC-II triggered B cells abrogated activation of contacting T cells while B–T conjugate formation remained unaltered (Delaguillaumie et al. 2008). In contrast, active cytoskeletal reorganization was shown to be needed for IS formation in T–DC pairs (Al-Alwan et al. 2001). Thus, while actin assembles at the IS in both types of APC, it probably has distinct functions during antigen presentation and possibly IS formation. Conjugate formation, actin accumulation at the IS, and signalling

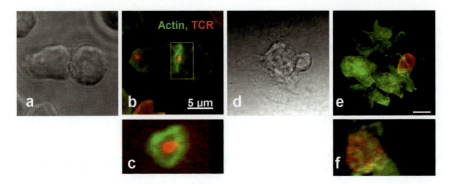

Fig. 1 Naïve CD4⁺ T cells form a mature immunological synapse when contacting specific antigen-presenting naïve B cells but not when contacting DC. Transmitted light (**a**, **d**) and two color confocal (**b**, **c**, **e**, **f**) microscopy. (**a–c**) Individual pairs of T cells and naive B cells, loaded with TCR-specific peptide demonstrate localization of the entire TCR signal (*red*) at the contact plane in direct view (**b**) and in *en face* 3D reconstruction (**c**). (**d–f**) In contrast, pairs between T cells and DC show TCR staining scattered over the cell body without preferential accumulation of TCR at the contact site to DC. For details on experimental conditions and imaging see Reichardt et al. (2007b)

intensity can well be separated events. Along the same line, B cells depend very much on LFA-1 for T cell binding and activation (Hosseini et al. 2009), while DC do not (Gunzer et al. 2004).

In fact, the interplay between Rap1, LFA-1, and the co-stimulatory molecules CTLA-4/CD28 in B cells vs. DC recently led us to comprise a model to link the observed differences in conjugate formation and differential T cell activation in DC–T vs. B–T pairs (Reichardt et al. 2007b). As co-stimulatory molecules are also one focus point in studying differentiation between effector and Treg cell pheno-type and potentially its respective IS structure, we will describe this in a little more detail below. Taken together, the cytoskeletal architecture of the cellular contact between T cell and APC can be one important parameter in determining the signalling pattern present in these contacts.

The second characteristic point of the B–T synapse is its large central part, the cSMAC. The role of the cSMAC is currently very incompletely understood. More complexity to the role of the cSMAC during T cell activation was added recently when it was found that the signalling activity in the cSMAC can significantly change throughout the persistence of the IS (Grakoui et al. 1999; Lee et al. 2002). In any case, the current concept of synapse function considers the cSMAC an area of TCR internalization and signal termination (Lee et al. 2003; Cemerski et al. 2008). Also, it is certainly possible that the amount of signalling is determined by the (TCR-matching) quality of the antigen (Cemerski et al. 2008). This might be particularly true when approaching from the lower side of TCR ligand affinity: many reports conclude that below a certain threshold, no (productive) physical contact will be established between APC and T cell. However, when low affinity TCR ligands are present, the outcome might depend on other factors, such as costimulation and activation of cytoskeleton (Al-Alwan et al. 2003). Taken together, the prolonged persistence of a mature IS, which is characterized by a clearly defined cSMAC, could "tip the balance" towards negative signalling and/or the possible induction of a regulatory phenotype.

6 T Cells Helping B Cells to Function

A very different case of B–T pairings emerges during the process of providing T cell help to B cells. Follicular helper T cells (T_{FH}) invade B cell zones of the lymph node in order to provide (CD40L–CD40-mediated) help to turn on the B cell's antibody-producing machinery (Breitfeld et al. 2000). The current view is that B cells receive a strong activation signal following uptake of specific antigen via their B cell receptor (BCR) and are enabled to migrate along a chemotactic gradient towards the T cell zone (Casamayor-Palleja et al. 2002; Reif et al. 2002). Thus, activated B cells will enrich at the border between B- and T-zone and be interaction partners for immigrating T_{FH} cells (Reif et al. 2002; Okada et al. 2005). The physiological aim of this interaction is to provide help to B cells and to ensure specificity of this process. The specificity is ensured by the peptide that is presented by the B cell via its many MHCII molecules to the T_{FH}. It is molecularly linked to the antigen, to which its BCR is binding, because this BCR mediated the uptake of the antigen (Goodnow et al. 2005). The B cell seeking help needs to "find" a T_{FH} that has previously been activated in the T zone by a DC towards the T cell epitopes of the same antigen. By this mechanism it is ensured that only those antigens that are present in large enough amounts to be presented by DC to T cells and also taken up by BCRs from specific B cells, will lead to full-blown antibody responses. An autoreactive B cell, that by chance generates a BCR which can take up and present self proteins, would normally not find a cognate T_{FH}, since this should have been deleted by thymic selection (Goodnow et al. 2005).

The synapse forming between a B cell and a T_{FH} is central for the development of high-affinity antibodies. By means of surface molecules such as ICOS or CD40-L, T_{FH} make sure that germinal centre B cells receive signals allowing them to transform into antibody secreting plasma cells. Tight control of these signals is required. Uncontrolled provision of follicular help as in the Roquin-defective mouse mutant *sanroque* can lead to severe autoimmunity (Vinuesa et al. 2005). In addition, a differing set of cytokines (Nurieva et al. 2008) as well as specific proteins such as signalling lymphocytic activation molecule-associated protein (SAP) are likely to play a role (Kamperschroer et al. 2008). In the light of these facts it is really striking that the synapse between a germinal centre B cell and a cognate T_{FH} has not been investigated so far. This gap in our knowledge should be closed in the next years.

7 IS and APC-Mediated Induction of Treg: Focus on Co-stimulatory Molecules

While the TCR ligand recognition displays a high specificity ensuring tailor-made immunes response at the clonotypic level, T cells of diverse phenotypes may result from APC contact depending on context and APC specification. As we have seen, the duration of specific APC–T cell contacts, such as in DC–T and B–T pairs, can vary strongly, and the duration by itself may not be a good parameter for judging the outcome of the T cell activation (Reichardt et al. 2007b). Such, stable interactions between T cells and DC were observed in vivo which precede both the outcome of tolerance or immunity (Shakhar et al. 2005). If duration is less of an issue, other factors in which DC and B cells are known to differ vastly may be of greater importance: co-stimulatory signals and cytoskeletal activity.

There is a long known role for co-stimulatory signals, in particular of the CD28/ICOS/CTLA-4/PD-1 family of co-stimulatory molecules, in the decision making of a T cell in developing full (pro-inflammatory) effector function versus regulation, anergy, or systemic tolerance. While CD28 is a molecule providing positive signals, CTLA-4 is a master negative switch of T cell activation (Rudd and Schneider 2003). The co-stimulatory molecules can differ in structural features yet share signalling motifs and compete for recruitment towards the cSMAC (Egen and Allison 2002). As such, the inducible co-stimulatory molecule, ICOS, shares similar binding motifs with CD28 in its cytosplamic tail (Fos et al. 2008). The PD-1/PD-L2 assembly exhibits distinct structural and organizational features. Even more co-stimulatory pathways are likely to be involved *in vivo*. In CD28 $^{-/-}$ mice, blockade of the CD40–CD40L and CD134 (OX-40)–CD134L interaction in combination was necessary to achieve prolonged transplant survival (Habicht et al. 2007).

The common signalling element downstream of all of these co-stimulatory (or rather co-modulatory) molecules is PI3K. Co-stimulatory signalling via PI3K results in recruitment of PKCθ to the cSMAC. PKCθ is a central player in the mediation of T cell differentiation into Th1, Th2, Th17 effector lines and a core component of the IS (Marsland and Kopf 2008). In fact, PKCθ "follows" CD28 in spatial distribution at the IS. Normally, following TCR activation and CD80 ligation upon productive APC contact, CD28 is recruited to the cSMAC. The recruitment to cSMAC is a necessary step for efficient TCR signalling as defective CD28 unable to move to the cSMAC will still recruit PKCθ, yet the downstream signalling events (NFκB activation) will be diminished (Sanchez-Lockhart et al. 2008). Within the cSMAC, PKCθ was shown to cluster with CD28 in unique compartments, which is thought to represent one core element of costimulatory signalling (Yokosuka et al. 2008).

PKCθ-mediated TCR signals also control the activity of the small GTPase Rap1, which modulates affinity and spatial organization of LFA-1 (Bos et al. 2001; Letschka et al. 2008). It is tempting to speculate that inefficient co-stimulatory activity (such as that provided by naïve B cells) fails to recruit CD28 and thus PKCθ towards the cSMAC. Failure of CD28 to induce the Rap1-inactivator RAP1GAP would lead to more active Rap1 (Rap1-GTP) which in turn would stabilize LFA-1 for enhancement of cellular adhesion and possibly enlargement of the cell–cell interface and thus the cSMAC (Reichardt et al. 2007b).

Regulation of these processes is tight and complex. Depending on ICOS surface expression and potentially other mechanisms, activatory or regulatory PI3K sub-domains are recruited to the IS (Fos et al. 2008). Thus, ICOS can participate in the control of (class 1A) PI3K signalling, a key component of T cell signalling. As for PKCθ, delayed recruitment to the IS in T cells under regulation was described earlier (Sumoza-Toledo et al. 2006). Is a regulatory synapse "simply" characterized by less costimulatory ligands being recruited to the IS? Naïve B cells are notorious for low surface expression of CD80, CD86 (and MHC-II) (Masten and Lipscomb 1999; Reichardt et al. 2007b). However, while a lack of CD28 may distract a T cell from gaining full effector function, Treg may need CTLA-4 in the IS for their functioning (Flores-Borja et al. 2008; Wing et al. 2008). In fact, CTLA-4 sounds like the perfect candidate molecule for co-stimulation-controlled immunoregulation: CTLA-4 expressed on T cells can act back on antigen-presenting DC and induce tolerogenic behaviour (Onishi et al. 2008). In addition, as stated above, Treg are shown to act via direct cell–cell contact, interfere with DC development, and require CTLA-4 for their function. CTLA-4 KO mice were found to have functional Foxp3$^+$ Tregs, however, blocking of CTLA-4 in wt mice abrogated suppression by Treg (Tang et al. 2004). In general, data from KO systems should be interpreted with special care as compensation mechanisms during development cannot be ruled out. As such, CD28 signals are potentially needed for CTLA-4 induction during thymic T cell development in the first place (Tai et al. 2005). Again, this underlines the complex interaction between these molecules. In addition, even if the overall composition of the IS may differ only slightly, the kinetics of its spatiotemporal assembly might determine the functional outcome. Thus, sophisticated imaging studies will be required to unravel differential build up of IS towards Treg cells.

8 Concluding Remarks

In the present review we have attempted to highlight several aspects of what is currently known about the IS formed by T-helper cells or precursors with surrounding, mostly antigen-presenting, cells during a life cycle of T cell generation and function. We have put together a rough overview about the current state of the art. Nevertheless, 10 years after the initial description of the structure the literature is so vast, that a full review is no longer possible. Searching 'Pubmed' for the terms "immunological synapse" or "immune synapse" yields almost 1,700 papers as of Dec. 2008. This demonstrates impressively, how the field has evolved. Table 1 represents a summary of relevant information on the subject as laid out within this review. It also serves to highlight, that despite 1,700 papers there are still many gaps in our knowledge about individual IS formation serving distinct physiological

Table 1 Key synapses involved in generation and function of helper T cells and what we know about them

Stage	Organ	T cell type	APC type	Critical synapse molecules		IS structure	References
				T cell	APC		
Bone marrow precursor	Bone marrow	HSC, different T cell precursors	Endosteal cell, stromal cell, osteoblast (?)	Notch1	Delta-like, Jagged	?	Geiger et al. (2007), Benz et al. (2008), Boehm and Bleul (2006), Visan et al. (2006b)
Thymic precursor	Thymus niche (CMJ)	Thymus seeding precursor	CMJ endothelial cell, thymic stromal cell	Notch1	Delta-like, Jagged, Lunatic-Fringe	?	Tan et al. (2005), Visan et al. (2006a, 2006b), Boehm and Bleul (2006)
Thymic positive and negative selection	Thymus cortex and medulla	DP thymocyte	Cortical and medullary EC, medullary DC	Notch1, LCK, CD3ζ, CD4, CD8	pMHC	SMAC type with LCK and CD3ζ exclusion (neg. selection), no synapse (pos. selection)	Germain (2002), Ebert et al. (2008), Ehrlich et al. (2002)
Priming of effectors	Secondary lymphatic organ (e.g. spleen, lymph node)	Naïve CD4 T cell	DC, activated B cells	αβTCR, CD28, CD3ζ, LCK, Actin, tubulin, CTLA4, PKCθ, cytokineR, LFA1	pMHCII, CD80, CD86, (secreted/membrane bound) cytokines	Multifocal (DC), cSMAC/pSMAC (B cells)	Monks et al. (1998) Krummel et al. (2000), Ehrlich et al. (2002), Penticheva-Hoang et al. (2004), Egen and Allison (2002), Grakoui et al. (1999), Brossard et al. (2005), Maldonado et al. (2004), Chang et al. (2007), Tseng et al. (2008), Reichardt et al. (2007b)
Priming of regulators	Potentially secondary lymphatic organ (e.g. spleen, lymph node)	Naïve CD4 T cell	Immature (DEC205+) DC, naïve B cells	αβTCR, Actin, tubulin, , CTLA-4, PKCθ	pMHCII, CD80, CD86	? (for DC), cSMAC/pSMAC type (for naïve B cells)	Steinman and Bancbereau (2007), Reichardt et al. (2007b)
Memory generation	Secondary lymphatic organ (e.g. spleen, lymph node)	Activated CD4 T cell	Mature DC	αβTCR, CD25, IL-7R, CD43, CD69	pMHC, CD80, CD86	IL7R is on opposite side of APC contact, otherwise ?	Chang et al. (2007), Huster et al. (2004)

Memory re-activation	Secondary lymphatic organ (e.g. spleen, lymph node), periphery	Memory CD4 T cells	DC, B cells, macrophages, other MHCII$^+$ body cells	αβTCR, IL7R (?), costimulatory receptors (?), PKCθ, LCK, LFA1, CD45	pMHC, costimulatory molecules	pSMAC/cSMAC type, CD45 in cSMAC, rapid formation	Watson and Lee (2004)
B cell helper synapse	Germinal center	T$_{FH}$	BCR-activated B cells	αβTCR, CD40-L, ICOS, SAP, OX40	pMHC, ICOSL, OX40-L, CD40, SLAM-family, SHP-1	?	Goodnow et al. (2005), Kim et al. (2003), Kato et al. (2004), Linton et al. (2003), Qi et al. (2008)

CMJ Cortico medullary junction; *HSC* Hematopoietic stem cell; *EC* Epithelial cell; *DC* Dendritic cell; *T$_{FH}$* Follicular helper T cell; *TCR* T cell receptor; *BCR* B cell receptor; *cytokineR* Any cytokine receptor; *IL7R* Interleukin 7 receptor; *PKCθ* Protein kinase C θ; *LFA-1* Leucocyte function-associated protein-1; *ICOS* Inducible costimulator; *ICOSL* ICOS-ligand; *SLAM* Signalling lymphocyte-activation molecule-associate protein; *SHP-1* Src homology phosphatase-1; *SAP* signalling lymphocyte activation molecule-associated protein

functions that warrant further study and are likely to bring about fascinating information on this key topic of immunological research.

Acknowledgments This work was supported by research grants from the German Research Community (DFG, GU769/1-3, GU769/2-1) and the European Union (EU Nest, Mamocell) to M.G.

References

Adams GB, Scadden DT (2006) The hematopoietic stem cell in its place. Nat Immunol 7:333–337

Al-Alwan MM, Rowden G, Lee TD, West KA (2001) Cutting edge: the dendritic cell cytoskeleton is critical for the formation of the immunological synapse. J Immunol 166:1452–1456

Al-Alwan MM, Liwski RS, Haeryfar SM, Baldridge WH, Hoskin DW, Rowden G, West KA (2003) Cutting edge: dendritic cell actin cytoskeletal polarization during immunological synapse formation is highly antigen-dependent. J Immunol 171:4479–4483

Banchereau J, Steinman RM (1998) Dendritic cells and the control of immunity. Nature 392:245–254

Benz C, Martins VC, Radtke F, Bleul CC (2008) The stream of precursors that colonizes the thymus proceeds selectively through the early T lineage precursor stage of T cell development. J Exp Med 205:1187–1199

Boehm T, Bleul CC (2006) Thymus-homing precursors and the thymic microenvironment. Trends Immunol 27:477–484

Bonifaz L, Bonnyay D, Mahnke K, Rivera M, Nussenzweig MC, Steinman RM (2002) Efficient targeting of protein antigen to the dendritic cell receptor DEC-205 in the steady state leads to antigen presentation on major histocompatibility complex class I products and peripheral CD8 (+) T cell tolerance. J Exp Med 196:1627–1638

Bos JL, de RJ, Reedquist KA (2001) Rap1 signalling: adhering to new models. Nat Rev Mol Cell Biol 2:369–377

Bousso P, Bhakta NR, Lewis RS, Robey E (2002) Dynamics of thymocyte-stromal cell interactions visualized by two-photon microscopy. Science 296:1876–1880

Breitfeld D, Ohl L, Kremmer E, Ellwart J, Sallusto F, Lipp M, Forster R (2000) Follicular B helper T cells express CXC chemokine receptor 5, localize to B cell follicles, and support immunoglobulin production. J Exp Med 192:1545–1552

Brocker T (1997) Survival of mature CD4 T lymphocytes is dependent on major histocompatibility complex class-II expressing dendritic cells. J Exp Med 186:1223–1232

Bromley SK, Burack WR, Johnson KG, Somersalo K, Sims TN, Sumen C, Davis MM, Shaw AS, Allen PM, Dustin ML (2001) The immunological synapse. Annu Rev Immunol 19:375–396

Brossard C, Feuillet V, Schmitt A, Randriamampita C, Romao M, Raposo G, Trautmann A (2005) Multifocal structure of the T cell – dendritic cell synapse. Eur J Immunol 35:1741–1753

Bryce PJ, Miller ML, Miyajima I, Tsai M, Galli SJ, Oettgen HC (2004) Immune sensitization in the skin is enhanced by antigen-independent effects of IgE. Immunity 20:381–392

Casamayor-Palleja M, Mondiere P, Verschelde C, Bella C, Defrance T (2002) BCR ligation reprograms B cells for migration to the T zone and B-cell follicle sequentially. Blood 99:1913–1921

Celli S, Lemaitre F, Bousso P (2007) Real-time manipulation of T cell-dendritic cell interactions in vivo reveals the importance of prolonged contacts for CD4+ T cell activation. Immunity 27:625–634

Cemerski S, Das J, Giurisato E, Markiewicz MA, Allen PM, Chakraborty AK, Shaw AS (2008) The balance between T cell receptor signaling and degradation at the center of the immunological synapse is determined by antigen quality. Immunity 29:414–422

Chang JT, Palanivel VR, Kinjyo I, Schambach F, Intlekofer AM, Banerjee A, Longworth SA, Vinup KE, Mrass P, Oliaro J, Killeen N, Orange JS, Russell SM, Weninger W, Reiner SL (2007) Asymmetric T lymphocyte division in the initiation of adaptive immune responses. Science 315:1687–1691

Delaguillaumie A, Marin-Esteban V, Setterblad N, Leh LJ, Assier E, Gelin C, Charron D, Galy A, Mooney N (2008) Contrasting cytoskeletal regulation of MHC class II peptide presentation by human B cells or dendritic cells. Eur J Immunol 38:1096–1105

Dustin ML (2008) T-cell activation through immunological synapses and kinapses. Immunol Rev 221:77–89

Ebert PJ, Ehrlich LI, Davis MM (2008) Low ligand requirement for deletion and lack of synapses in positive selection enforce the gauntlet of thymic T cell maturation. Immunity 29:734–745

Egen JG, Allison JP (2002) Cytotoxic T lymphocyte antigen-4 accumulation in the immunological synapse is regulated by TCR signal strength. Immunity 16:23–35

Egen JG, Rothfuchs AG, Feng CG, Winter N, Sher A, Germain RN (2008) Macrophage and T cell dynamics during the development and disintegration of mycobacterial granulomas. Immunity 28:271–284

Ehrlich LI, Ebert PJ, Krummel MF, Weiss A, Davis MM (2002) Dynamics of p56lck translocation to the T cell immunological synapse following agonist and antagonist stimulation. Immunity 17:809–822

Flores-Borja F, Jury EC, Mauri C, Ehrenstein MR (2008) Defects in CTLA-4 are associated with abnormal regulatory T cell function in rheumatoid arthritis. Proc Natl Acad Sci USA 105:19396–19401

Fos C, Salles A, Lang V, Carette F, Audebert S, Pastor S, Ghiotto M, Olive D, Bismuth G, Nunes JA (2008) ICOS ligation recruits the p50alpha PI3K regulatory subunit to the immunological synapse. J Immunol 181:1969–1977

Friedl P, den Boer AT, Gunzer M (2005) Tuning immune responses: diversity and adaption of the immunological synapse. Nat Rev Immunol 5:532–545

Geiger H, Koehler A, Gunzer M (2007) Stem cells, aging, niche, adhesion and Cdc42: a model for changes in cell-cell interactions and hematopoietic stem cell aging. Cell Cycle 6:884–887

Germain RN (2002) T-cell development and the CD4-CD8 lineage decision. Nat Rev Immunol 2:309–322

Gondek DC, Lu LF, Quezada SA, Sakaguchi S, Noelle RJ (2005) Cutting edge: contact-mediated suppression by CD4$^+$CD25$^+$ regulatory cells involves a granzyme B-dependent, perforin-independent mechanism. J Immunol 174:1783–1786

Goodnow CC, Cyster JG (1997) Lymphocyte homing: the scent of a follicle. Curr Biol 7: R219–R222

Goodnow CC, Sprent J, Fazekas de St GB, Vinuesa CG (2005) Cellular and genetic mechanisms of self tolerance and autoimmunity. Nature 435:590–597

Grakoui A, Bromley SK, Sumen C, Davis MM, Shaw AS, Allen PM, Dustin ML (1999) The immunological synapse: a molecular machine controlling T cell activation. Science 285:221–227

Gunsilius E, Gastl G, Petzer AL (2001) Hematopoietic stem cells. Biomed Pharmacother 55:186–194

Gunzer M (2007) Migration, cell-cell interaction and adhesion in the immune system. Earnst Schering Found Symp Proc 3:97–137

Gunzer M, Schäfer A, Borgmann S, Grabbe S, Zänker KS, Bröcker E-B, Kämpgen E, Friedl P (2000) Antigen presentation in extracellular matrix: interactions of T cells with dendritic cells are dynamic, short lived, and sequential. Immunity 13:323–332

Gunzer M, Weishaupt C, Hillmer A, Basoglu Y, Friedl P, Dittmar KE, Kolanus W, Varga G, Grabbe S (2004) A spectrum of biophysical interaction modes between T cells and different antigen presenting cells during priming in 3-D collagen and in vivo. Blood 104:2801–2809

Habicht A, Najafian N, Yagita H, Sayegh MH, Clarkson MR (2007) New insights in CD28-independent allograft rejection. Am J Transplant 7:1917–1926

Hosseini BH, Louban I, Djandji D, Wabnitz GH, Deeg J, Bulbuc N, Samstag Y, Gunzer M, Spatz JP, Hämmerling G (2009) Immune synapse formation determines interaction forces between T cells and antigen-presenting cell measured by atomic force microscopy. Proc Natl Acad Sci USA 106:17852–17857

Hsieh CS, Liang Y, Tyznik AJ, Self SG, Liggitt D, Rudensky AY (2004) Recognition of the peripheral self by naturally arising CD25$^+$ CD4$^+$ T cell receptors. Immunity 21:267–277

Huster KM, Busch V, Schiemann M, Linkemann K, Kerksiek KM, Wagner H, Busch DH (2004) Selective expression of IL-7 receptor on memory T cells identifies early CD40L-dependent generation of distinct CD8+ memory T cell subsets. Proc Natl Acad Sci USA 101:5610–5615

Itano AA, McSorley SJ, Reinhardt RL, Ehst BD, Ingulli E, Rudensky AY, Jenkins MK (2003) Distinct dendritic cell populations sequentially present antigen to CD4 T cells and stimulate different aspects of cell-mediated immunity. Immunity 19:47–57

Kamperschroer C, Roberts DM, Zhang Y, Weng NP, Swain SL (2008) SAP enables T cells to help B cells by a mechanism distinct from Th cell programming or CD40 ligand regulation. J Immunol 181:3994–4003

Kato H, Kojima H, Ishii N, Hase H, Imai Y, Fujibayashi T, Sugamura K, Kobata T (2004) Essential role of OX40L on B cells in persistent alloantibody production following repeated alloimmunizations. J Clin Immunol 24:237–248

Kim MY, Gaspal FM, Wiggett HE, McConnell FM, Gulbranson-Judge A, Raykundalia C, Walker LS, Goodall MD, Lane PJ (2003) CD4(+)CD3(−) accessory cells costimulate primed CD4 T cells through OX40 and CD30 at sites where T cells collaborate with B cells. Immunity 18:643–654

Köhler A, Schmithorst V, Filippi MD, Ryan M, Daria D, Gunzer M, Geiger H (2009) Altered cellular dynamics and endosteal location of aged early hematopoietic progenitor cells revealed by time-lapse intravital imaging in long bones. Blood 114:290–298

Kopp HG, Avecilla ST, Hooper AT, Rafii S (2005) The bone marrow vascular niche: home of HSC differentiation and mobilization. Physiology (Bethesda) 20:349–356

Krall WJ, Braun J (1992) In vivo retroviral marking of antigen-specific B lymphocytes. Semin Immunol 4:19–28

Krummel MF, Sjaastad MD, Wulfing C, Davis MM (2000) Differential clustering of CD4 and CD3 zeta during T cell recognition. Science 289:1349–1352

Lassila O, Vainio O, Matzinger P (1988) Can B cells turn on virgin T cells? Nature 334:253–255

Lee KH, Holdorf AD, Dustin ML, Chan AC, Allen PM, Shaw AS (2002) T cell receptor signaling precedes immunological synapse formation. Science 295:1539–1542

Lee KH, Dinner AR, Tu C, Campi G, Raychaudhuri S, Varma R, Sims TN, Burack WR, Wu H, Wang J, Kanagawa O, Markiewicz M, Allen PM, Dustin ML, Chakraborty AK, Shaw AS (2003) The immunological synapse balances T cell receptor signaling and degradation. Science 302:1218–1222

Letschka T, Kollmann V, Pfeifhofer-Obermair C, Lutz-Nicoladoni C, Obermair GJ, Fresser F, Leitges M, Hermann-Kleiter N, Kaminski S, Baier G (2008) PKC-theta selectively controls the adhesion-stimulating molecule Rap1. Blood 112:4617–4627

Lind EF, Prockop SE, Porritt HE, Petrie HT (2001) Mapping precursor movement through the postnatal thymus reveals specific microenvironments supporting defined stages of early lymphoid development. J Exp Med 194:127–134

Linton PJ, Bautista B, Biederman E, Bradley ES, Harbertson J, Kondrack RM, Padrick RC, Bradley LM (2003) Costimulation via OX40L expressed by B cells is sufficient to determine the extent of primary CD4 cell expansion and Th2 cytokine secretion in vivo. J Exp Med 197:875–883

Lo Celso C, Celso CL, Fleming HE, Wu JW, Zhao CX, Miake-Lye S, Fujisaki J, Cote D, Rowe DW, Lin CP, Scadden DT (2009) Live-animal tracking of individual haematopoietic stem/progenitor cells in their niche. Nature 457:92–96. doi:10.1038/nature07434

Lo CG, Xu Y, Proia RL, Cyster JG (2005) Cyclical modulation of sphingosine-1-phosphate receptor 1 surface expression during lymphocyte recirculation and relationship to lymphoid organ transit. J Exp Med 201:291–301

Maldonado RA, Irvine DJ, Schreiber R, Glimcher LH (2004) A role for the immunological synapse in lineage commitment of CD4 lymphocytes. Nature 431:527–532

Marsland BJ, Kopf M (2008) T-cell fate and function: PKC-theta and beyond. Trends Immunol 29:179–185

Masten BJ, Lipscomb MF (1999) Comparison of lung dendritic cells and B cells in stimulating naive antigen-specific T cells. J Immunol 162:1310–1317

Matzinger P (2002) The danger model: a renewed sense of self. Science 296:301–305

Mempel TR, Henrickson SE, von Andrian UH (2004) T-cell priming by dendritic cells in lymph nodes occurs in three distinct phases. Nature 427:154–159

Miller MJ, Safrina O, Parker I, Cahalan MD (2004) Imaging the single cell dynamics of CD4$^+$ T cell activation by dendritic cells in lymph nodes. J Exp Med 200:847–856

Monks CR, Kupfer H, Tamir I, Barlow A, Kupfer A (1997) Selective modulation of protein kinase C-theta during T-cell activation. Nature 385:83–86

Monks CR, Freiberg BA, Kupfer H, Sciaky N, Kupfer A (1998) Three-dimensional segregation of supramolecular activation clusters in T cells. Nature 395:82–86

M'Rini C, Cheng G, Schweitzer C, Cavanagh LL, Palframan RT, Mempel TR, Warnock RA, Lowe JB, Quackenbush EJ, von Andrian UH (2003) A novel endothelial L-selectin ligand activity in lymph node medulla that is regulated by alpha(1, 3)-fucosyltransferase-IV. J Exp Med 198:1301–1312

Muranski P, Chmielowski B, Ignatowicz L (2000) Mature CD4$^+$ T cells perceive a positively selecting class II MHC/peptide complex in the periphery. J Immunol 164:3087–3094

Nilsson SK, Johnston HM, Coverdale JA (2001) Spatial localization of transplanted hemopoietic stem cells: inferences for the localization of stem cell niches. Blood 97:2293–2299

Nurieva RI, Chung Y, Hwang D, Yang XO, Kang HS, Ma L, Wang YH, Watowich SS, Jetten AM, Tian Q, Dong C (2008) Generation of T follicular helper cells is mediated by interleukin-21 but independent of T helper 1, 2, or 17 cell lineages. Immunity 29:138–149

Okada T, Miller MJ, Parker I, Krummel MF, Neighbors M, Hartley SB, O'Garra A, Cahalan MD, Cyster JG (2005) Antigen-engaged B cells undergo chemotaxis toward the T zone and form motile conjugates with helper T cells. PLoS Biol 3:e150

Onishi Y, Fehervari Z, Yamaguchi T, Sakaguchi S (2008) Foxp3+ natural regulatory T cells preferentially form aggregates on dendritic cells in vitro and actively inhibit their maturation. Proc Natl Acad Sci USA 105:10113–10118

Osawa M, Hanada K, Hamada H, Nakauchi H (1996) Long-term lymphohematopoietic reconstitution by a single CD34-low/negative hematopoietic stem cell. Science 273:242–245

Pentcheva-Hoang T, Egen JG, Wojnoonski K, Allison JP (2004) B7-1 and b7-2 selectively recruit ctla-4 and CD28 to the immunological synapse. Immunity 21:401–413

Qi H, Cannons JL, Klauschen F, Schwartzberg PL, Germain RN (2008) SAP-controlled T-B cell interactions underlie germinal centre formation. Nature 455:764–769

Reichardt P, Dornbach B, Gunzer M (2007a) The molecular makeup and function of regulatory and effector synapses. Immunol Rev 218:165–177

Reichardt P, Dornbach B, Song R, Beissert S, Gueler F, Loser K, Gunzer M (2007b) Naive B cells generate regulatory T cells in the presence of a mature immunological synapse. Blood 110:1519–1529

Reif K, Ekland EH, Ohl L, Nakano H, Lipp M, Förster R, Cyster JG (2002) Balanced responsiveness to chemoattractants from adjacent zones determines B cell position. Nature 416:94–99

Richie LI, Ebert PJ, Wu LC, Krummel MF, Owen JJ, Davis MM (2002) Imaging synapse formation during thymocyte selection: inability of CD3zeta to form a stable central accumulation during negative selection. Immunity 16:595–606

Rudd CE, Schneider H (2003) Unifying concepts in CD28, ICOS and CTLA4 co-receptor signalling. Nat Rev Immunol 3:544–556

Sanchez-Lockhart M, Graf B, Miller J (2008) Signals and sequences that control CD28 localization to the central region of the immunological synapse. J Immunol 181:7639–7648

Sanna MG, Wang SK, Gonzalez-Cabrera PJ, Don A, Marsolais D, Matheu MP, Wei SH, Parker I, Jo E, Cheng WC, Cahalan MD, Wong CH, Rosen H (2006) Enhancement of capillary leakage and restoration of lymphocyte egress by a chiral S1P1 antagonist in vivo. Nat Chem Biol 2:434–441

Scadden DT (2006) The stem-cell niche as an entity of action. Nature 441:1075–1079

Schmitt TM, Zuniga-Pflucker JC (2002) Induction of T cell development from hematopoietic progenitor cells by delta-like-1 in vitro. Immunity 17:749–756

Scholer A, Hugues S, Boissonnas A, Fetler L, Amigorena S (2008) Intercellular adhesion molecule-1-dependent stable interactions between T cells and dendritic cells determine CD8+ T cell memory. Immunity 28:258–270

Seminario MC, Bunnell SC (2008) Signal initiation in T-cell receptor microclusters. Immunol Rev 221:90–106

Serra P, Amrani A, Yamanouchi J, Han B, Thiessen S, Utsugi T, Verdaguer J, Santamaria P (2003) CD40 ligation releases immature dendritic cells from the control of regulatory CD4$^+$CD25$^+$ T cells. Immunity 19:877–889

Shakhar G, Lindquist RL, Skokos D, Dudziak D, Huang JH, Nussenzweig MC, Dustin ML (2005) Stable T cell-dendritic cell interactions precede the development of both tolerance and immunity in vivo. Nat Immunol 6:707–714

Shevach EM, Dipaolo RA, Andersson J, Zhao DM, Stephens GL, Thornton AM (2006) The lifestyle of naturally occurring CD4$^+$ CD25$^+$ Foxp3$^+$ regulatory T cells. Immunol Rev 212:60–73

Sixt M, Kanazawa N, Selg M, Samson T, Roos G, Reinhardt DP, Pabst R, Lutz MB, Sorokin L (2005) The conduit system transports soluble antigens from the afferent lymph to resident dendritic cells in the T cell area of the lymph node. Immunity 22:19–29

Spangrude GJ, Scollay R (1990) Differentiation of hematopoietic stem cells in irradiated mouse thymic lobes. Kinetics and phenotype of progeny. J Immunol 145:3661–3668

Springer TA (1994) Traffic signals for lymphocyte recirculation and leukocyte emigration: the multistep paradigm. Cell 76:301–314

Stamper HB Jr, Woodruff JJ (1976) Lymphocyte homing into lymph nodes: in vitro demonstration of the selective affinity of recirculating lymphocytes for high-endothelial venules. J Exp Med 144:828–833

Stefanova I, Dorfman JR, Germain RN (2002) Self-recognition promotes the foreign antigen sensitivity of naive T lymphocytes. Nature 420:429–434

Steinman RM, Banchereau J (2007) Taking dendritic cells into medicine. Nature 449:419–426

Sumoza-Toledo A, Eaton AD, Sarukhan A (2006) Regulatory T cells inhibit protein kinase C theta recruitment to the immune synapse of naive T cells with the same antigen specificity. J Immunol 176:5779–5787

Tai X, Cowan M, Feigenbaum L, Singer A (2005) CD28 costimulation of developing thymocytes induces Foxp3 expression and regulatory T cell differentiation independently of interleukin 2. Nat Immunol 6:152–162

Tan JB, Visan I, Yuan JS, Guidos CJ (2005) Requirement for Notch1 signals at sequential early stages of intrathymic T cell development. Nat Immunol 6:671–679

Tang Q, Boden EK, Henriksen KJ, Bour-Jordan H, Bi M, Bluestone JA (2004) Distinct roles of CTLA-4 and TGF-beta in CD4$^+$CD25$^+$ regulatory T cell function. Eur J Immunol 34:2996–3005

Tseng SY, Waite JC, Liu M, Vardhana S, Dustin ML (2008) T cell-dendritic cell immunological synapses contain TCR-dependent CD28-CD80 clusters that recruit protein kinase Ctheta. J Immunol 181:4852–4863

Vinuesa CG, Cook MC, Angelucci C, Athanasopoulos V, Rui L, Hill KM, Yu D, Domaschenz H, Whittle B, Lambe T, Roberts IS, Copley RR, Bell JI, Cornall RJ, Goodnow CC (2005) A RING-type ubiquitin ligase family member required to repress follicular helper T cells and autoimmunity. Nature 435:452–458

Visan I, Tan JB, Yuan JS, Harper JA, Koch U, Guidos CJ (2006a) Regulation of T lymphopoiesis by Notch1 and Lunatic fringe-mediated competition for intrathymic niches. Nat Immunol 7:634–643

Visan I, Yuan JS, Tan JB, Cretegny K, Guidos CJ (2006b) Regulation of intrathymic T-cell development by Lunatic Fringe-Notch1 interactions. Immunol Rev 209:76–94

von Andrian UH, Mempel TR (2003) Homing and cellular traffic in lymph nodes. Nat Rev Immunol 3:867–878

von Boehmer H, Aifantis I, Gounari F, Azogui O, Haughn L, Apostolou I, Jaeckel E, Grassi F, Klein L (2003) Thymic selection revisited: how essential is it? Immunol Rev 191:62–78

Watson AR, Lee WT (2004) Differences in signaling molecule organization between naive and memory CD4$^+$ T lymphocytes. J Immunol 173:33–41

Wei SH, Rosen H, Matheu MP, Sanna MG, Wang SK, Jo E, Wong CH, Parker I, Cahalan MD (2005) Sphingosine 1-phosphate type 1 receptor agonism inhibits transendothelial migration of medullary T cells to lymphatic sinuses. Nat Immunol 6:1228–1235

Wilson A, Trumpp A (2006) Bone-marrow haematopoietic stem-cell niches. Nat Rev Immunol 6:93–106

Wing K, Onishi Y, Prieto-Martin P, Yamaguchi T, Miyara M, Fehervari Z, Nomura T, Sakaguchi S (2008) CTLA-4 control over Foxp3+ regulatory T cell function. Science 322:271–275

Witmer-Pack MD, Swiggard WJ, Mirza A, Inaba K, Steinman RM (1995) Tissue distribution of the DEC-205-protein is detected by the monoclonal antibody NLDC-145. II. Expression in situ in lymphoid and nonlymphoid tissues. Cell Immunol 163:157–162

Wu M, Hyog YK, Rattis F, Blum J, Zhao C, Ashkenazi R, Jackson TL, Gaiano N, Oliver T, Reya T (2007) Imaging hematopoietic precursor division in real time. Cell Stem Cell 1:541–554

Yokosuka T, Kobayashi W, Sakata-Sogawa K, Takamatsu M, Hashimoto-Tane A, Dustin ML, Tokunaga M, Saito T (2008) Spatiotemporal regulation of T cell costimulation by TCR-CD28 microclusters and protein kinase C theta translocation. Immunity 29:589–601

Index